Cardiopulmonary
Pharmacology
for Respiratory Care

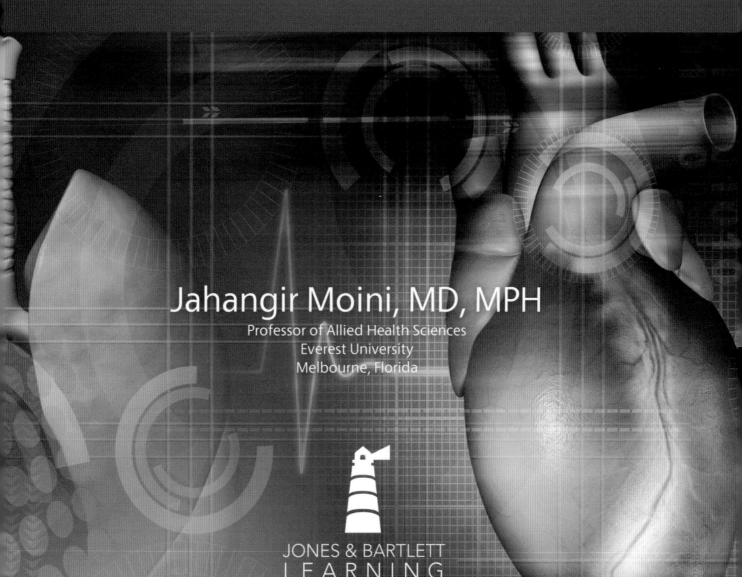

Jahangir Moini, MD, MPH

Professor of Allied Health Sciences
Everest University
Melbourne, Florida

JONES & BARTLETT
LEARNING

World Headquarters

Jones & Bartlett Learning
40 Tall Pine Drive
Sudbury, MA 01776
978-443-5000
info@jblearning.com
www.jblearning.com

Jones & Bartlett Learning Canada
6339 Ormindale Way
Mississauga, Ontario L5V 1J2
Canada

Jones & Bartlett Learning International
Barb House, Barb Mews
London W6 7PA
United Kingdom

Jones & Bartlett Learning books and products are available through most bookstores and online booksellers. To contact Jones & Bartlett Learning directly, call 800-832-0034, fax 978-443-8000, or visit our website, www.jblearning.com.

Substantial discounts on bulk quantities of Jones & Bartlett Learning publications are available to corporations, professional associations, and other qualified organizations. For details and specific discount information, contact the special sales department at Jones & Bartlett Learning via the above contact information or send an email to specialsales@jblearning.com.

The author, editor, and publisher have made every effort to provide accurate information. However, they are not responsible for errors, omissions, or for any outcomes related to the use of the contents of this book and take no responsibility for the use of the products and procedures described. Treatments and side effects described in this book may not be applicable to all people; likewise, some people may require a dose or experience a side effect that is not described herein. Drugs and medical devices are discussed that may have limited availability controlled by the Food and Drug Administration (FDA) for use only in a research study or clinical trial. Research, clinical practice, and government regulations often change the accepted standard in this field. When consideration is being given to use of any drug in the clinical setting, the health care provider or reader is responsible for determining FDA status of the drug, reading the package insert, and reviewing prescribing information for the most up-to-date recommendations on dose, precautions, and contraindications, and determining the appropriate usage for the product. This is especially important in the case of drugs that are new or seldom used.

Production Credits

Publisher: David Cella
Associate Editor: Maro Gartside
Editorial Assistant: Teresa Reilly
Associate Production Editor: Julia Waugaman
Marketing Manager: Grace Richards
Manufacturing and Inventory Control Supervisor: Amy Bacus

Composition: Shepherd Incorporated
Cover Design: Kristin E. Parker
Photo Research and Permissions Manager: Kimberly Potvin
Cover Image: © Krishnacreations/Dreamstime.com
Printing and Binding: Imago
Cover Printing: Imago

To order this product, use ISBN: 978-1-4496-1560-4

Library of Congress Cataloging-in-Publication Data
Moini, Jahangir, 1942-
  Cardiopulmonary pharmacology for respiratory care / Jahangir Moini.
      p. ; cm.
  Includes index.
  ISBN-13: 978-0-7637-8437-9 (pbk.)
  ISBN-10: 0-7637-8437-0 (pbk.)
  1. Cardiovascular agents. 2. Respiratory agents. 3. Respiratory therapists. I. Title.
  [DNLM: 1. Cardiovascular Agents--therapeutic use. 2. Cardiovascular Diseases--drug therapy. 3. Pharmacological Phenomena.
4. Respiratory System Agents--therapeutic use. 5. Respiratory Tract Diseases--drug therapy. QV 150 M712c 2011]
  RM345.M635 2011
  615'.71--dc22
                                        2010015257

6048
Printed in Singapore
14 13 12 11 10   10 9 8 7 6 5 4 3 2 1

*This book is dedicated to my wife Hengameh
and to my daughters Mahkameh and Morvarid.*

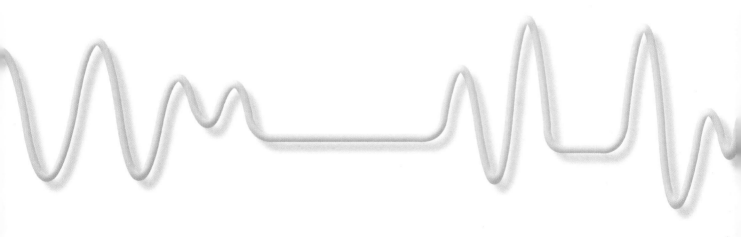

Brief Contents

Contents

Preface

Introduction

Today, respiratory care is one of the major areas of allied health. Respiratory care personnel provide evaluation, treatment, management, and monitoring of patients with many different types of respiratory-related conditions. Their job descriptions include cardiopulmonary resuscitation, oxygen administration, use of ventilators, administration of lung-specific medications, measurement of breathing capacity, and complete monitoring of the cardiopulmonary system. Cardiac and respiratory disorders are interconnected. There are some disorders of the heart that directly affect respiration, resulting in pulmonary disorders. Therefore, discussion of both of these areas is vital in understanding either of them. Drug therapy is one of the major components of respiratory care, requiring an extensive knowledge of pharmacology. The varied activities of a respiratory care technician require extensive and thorough training, as well as a complete, in-depth textbook.

Organization of Content

This book is organized into five units and contains 22 chapters, followed by appendices, an answer key, a glossary, and an index. In each chapter, drugs are discussed in relation to their mode of action, clinical implications, adverse effects, contraindications, and precautions. Each chapter contains many tables and color figures.

Features

Each chapter contains an outline of key topics, objectives that students must be able to meet upon completion of the reading, and a list of key terms (which are bolded in the chapter text). At the end of the main body of chapter text, a summary highlights important concepts, followed by learning goals, which provide answers to the objectives listed at the beginning of the chapter. Also, chapters contain critical thinking questions, related Web sites, review questions, and a case study.

Current Drug Information

The drug information in this book is current as of its printing. Remember that drug information changes often; you should always make sure you have the most up-to-date drug information before preparing or administering any medication. Consult current publications, such as *Physicians' Desk Reference, Drug Facts and Comparisons*, or drug package inserts.

Acknowledgments

would like to acknowledge David Cella, the publisher, who trusted and supported me, and all of the efforts of Maro Gartside during the creation of this book. The entire staff of Jones & Bartlett Learning has worked tirelessly on this project.

I also would like to acknowledge the hard work of Greg Vadimsky, my personal editorial assistant, as well as my daughter Morvarid, who contributed some of the figure illustrations. Additionally, I would like to sincerely thank all of the reviewers for providing their guidance in making this book thoroughly complete.

Reviewers

Lisa A. Conry, MA, RRT
Director of Clinical Education, Respiratory Care
Spartanburg Community College

Gary Jeromin, MA, RRT
Associate Professor
Ferris State University

Richelle S. Laipply, PhD
Professor, Allied Health
University of Akron

Kris Lewis, BS, RRT
Instructor
Southeast Community College

Melanie McDonough, MSHS, RRT
Cardiopulmonary Sciences Program
University of Central Florida

Pat Munzer, DHS, RRT
Chair, Allied Health Department
Washburn University

Edilberto A. Raynes, MD, PhD (candidate)
College of Health Sciences
Tennessee State University

Narciso E. Rodriguez, BS, RRT-NPS, RPFT, AE-C
Director, Respiratory Care Program-North
University of Medicine and Dentistry of New Jersey,
    School of Health Related Professions

Ray Sibberson, MS
Professor, Program Director, Respiratory Therapy
The University of Akron

Stephen G. Smith, MPA, RT, RRT
Chair, New York State Board for Respiratory Therapy
Clinical Assistant Professor
Stony Brook University
School of Health Technology and Management
Respiratory Care Program

Norman P. Tomaka, BPharm, CPh
Clinical Consultant Pharmacist

About the Author

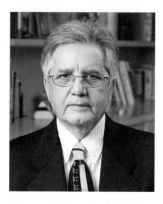

Dr. Moini was Assistant Professor at Tehran University School of Medicine for 9 years, where he taught medical and allied health students. The author is a professor and former director (for 15 years) of allied health programs at Everest University. Dr. Moini established several programs at Everest University's Melbourne campus.

As a physician and instructor for the past 35 years, he understands the importance of respiratory care therapists in the modern healthcare setting. He advocates the importance of pharmacology in the treatment of respiratory disorders because today respiratory disorders are some of the leading causes of disability and death in the United States.

Dr. Moini is actively involved in teaching and helping students to prepare for service in various health professions. He worked with the Brevard County Health Department as an epidemiologist and health educator consultant for 18 years. He has been an internationally published author of various allied health books since 1999.

Introduction to the Respiratory Care Profession

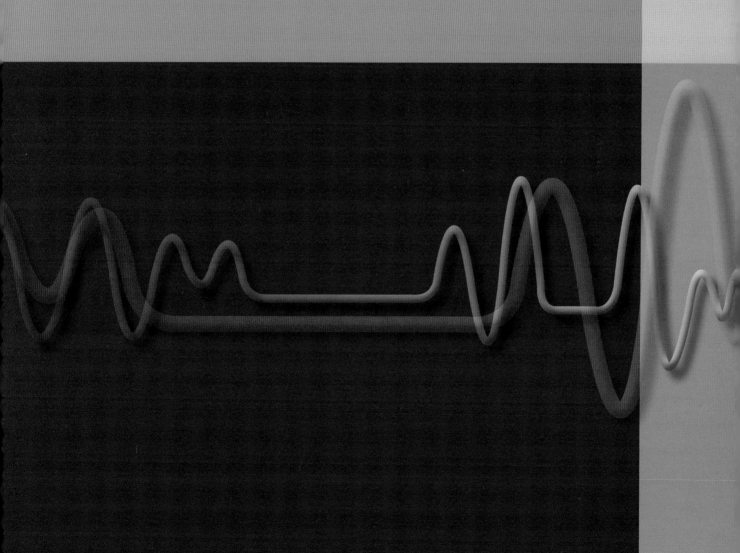

Cardiopulmonary and Central Nervous System Structures and Functions

OUTLINE

OBJECTIVES

Upon completion of this chapter, the reader should be able to do the following:

1. Name the structures that compose the cardiovascular system.
2. Distinguish among the various coverings of the heart and the layers that compose the heart wall.
3. Discuss the cardiac cycle and blood pressure.
4. Compare the structures and functions of the major types of blood vessels.
5. Identify the general functions of the respiratory system.
6. Describe the locations of the organs of the respiratory system.
7. Describe the functions of each organ of the respiratory system.
8. Explain the mechanisms of inspiration and expiration.
9. Describe the four main parts of the brain and their functions.
10. Explain the effect of the sympathetic and parasympathetic nervous systems upon the cardiopulmonary system.

KEY TERMS

Aerobic	Depolarization
Aerobic metabolism	Diaphragm
Aorta	Diastole
Aortic valve	ECG
Atria	EKG
Brainstem	Electrocardiogram
Bronchial tree	Endocardium
Carbaminohemoglobin	Epicardium
Carbonic anhydrase	Epiglottis
Cardiac cycle	Esophagus
Cardiac veins	Expiration
Coronary arteries	External respiration
Coronary sinus	Hemoglobin (Hb)
Cricoid cartilage	Inspiration

KEY TERMS (cont'd)

Internal
  respiration
Mediastinum
Medulla oblongata
Midbrain
Mitral valve
Myocardium
Nasal septum
Neurons

Parietal pleura
Pons
Pulmonary valve
Respiration
Septum
Systole
Thyroid cartilage
Tricuspid valve
Visceral pleura

INTRODUCTION

The cardiovascular system circulates blood to all parts of the body. The pumping of the heart provides oxygen to the body's cells as well as nutritive elements. It also removes waste materials and carbon dioxide. The heart is a muscular pump that is the central organ of the cardiovascular system, which also includes the arteries, veins, and capillaries.

The pulmonary system consists of the nose, pharynx, larynx, trachea, bronchi, and lungs. It furnishes oxygen for individual tissue cells and takes away their gaseous waste products. This process is accomplished through the act of respiration, which consists of external and internal processes. External respiration is the method in which the lungs are ventilated, and oxygen and carbon dioxide are exchanged between the alveoli of the lungs and the blood in the pulmonary capillaries. Internal respiration occurs when oxygen and carbon dioxide are exchanged between the blood in systemic capillaries and the body's tissues and cells (see Figures 1–1 and 1–2). The various organs, components, and functions of the cardiopulmonary system are described in this chapter.

The brain and autonomic nervous system control the operation of the cardiovascular and respiratory system. Therefore, this chapter will include a discussion of the brain's four major regions: cerebrum, diencephalon, brainstem, and cerebellum. It will also discuss the sympathetic and parasympathetic divisions of the autonomic nervous system.

Organs of the Cardiovascular System

The heart never rests; it beats approximately 100,000 times each day, pumping nearly 8000 liters of blood. The heart is a small organ that is nearly the size of an adult's closed fist.

The Heart

The heart is a hollow organ that is somewhat cone shaped. It is found within the thoracic cavity, resting upon the diaphragm. The heart contains four muscular chambers: the left and right atria, and the left and right ventricles. The heart itself weighs about 300 grams (in an

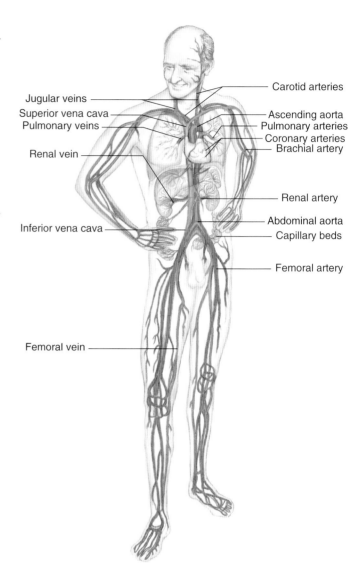

FIGURE 1–1 The cardiovascular system. Note its many similarities to a river.

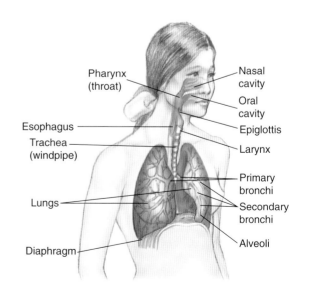

FIGURE 1–2 The respiratory system.

average adult male) and lies slightly to the left of the body's midline. It contains three layers of muscle tissue, which will be discussed later in this chapter.

The Heart Chambers

The heart consists of four hollow chambers: two on the left, and two on the right. The upper chambers are called atria and have thin walls. The lower chambers are called ventricles; they receive blood from the atria and contract to force blood out of the heart and into the arteries.

The left atrium collects blood from the pulmonary veins. It then moves this blood into the left ventricle, which pumps it into the systemic circuit (via the aorta). The right atrium collects blood from the systemic circuit (via the inferior and superior vena cava) as well as the coronary sinus and conducts it into the right ventricle. This ventricle pumps the blood into the pulmonary artery, which separates into the left and right pulmonary branches. The left and right atria, as well as the left and right ventricles, are separated from one another by wall-like structures, each of which is known as a septum. Because of the septums, blood from each side of the heart never mixes with blood from the other side (see **Figure 1–3**).

When the heart beats, the atria contract first, followed by the ventricles. The ventricles contract at the same time, ejecting equal amounts of blood into the pulmonary and systemic circuits.

The Heart Valves

An atrioventricular valve (A-V valve), including the tricuspid valve on the right and the mitral valve on the left, makes the blood flow one way between the atria and ventricles. The pulmonary valve allows blood to flow from the right ventricle while preventing backflow into the ventricle. As the left ventricle contracts, the mitral valve closes, and blood can only exit through a large artery known as the aorta. The aortic valve, located at the base of the aorta, opens to allow blood to leave the left ventricle when it contracts. Both the pulmonary and aortic valves are called semilunar valves because their cusps are shaped like half-moons. **Table 1–1** explains the locations and functions of the heart valves.

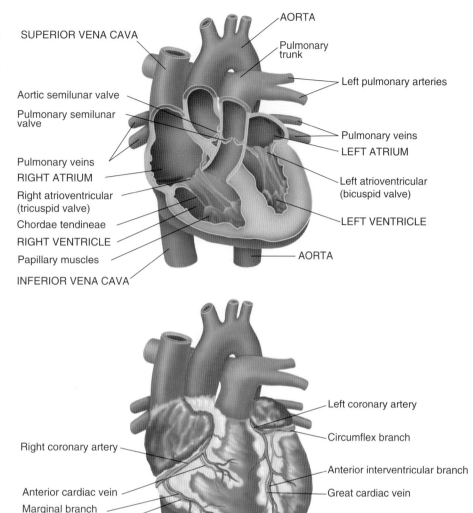

FIGURE 1–3 Anatomy of the heart.

TABLE 1-1	Heart Valves	
Valve	**Location**	**Function**
Mitral (bicuspid) valve	Opens between the left atrium and left ventricle	Prevents the blood from moving from the left ventricle into the left atrium when the ventricle contracts
Aortic valve	At the entrance to the aorta	Prevents the blood from moving from the aorta into the left ventricle when the ventricle relaxes
Tricuspid valve	Opens between the right atrium and right ventricle	Prevents the blood from moving from the right ventricle into the right atrium when the ventricle contracts
Pulmonary valve	At the entrance to the pulmonary trunk	Prevents the blood from moving from the pulmonary trunk into the right ventricle when the ventricle relaxes

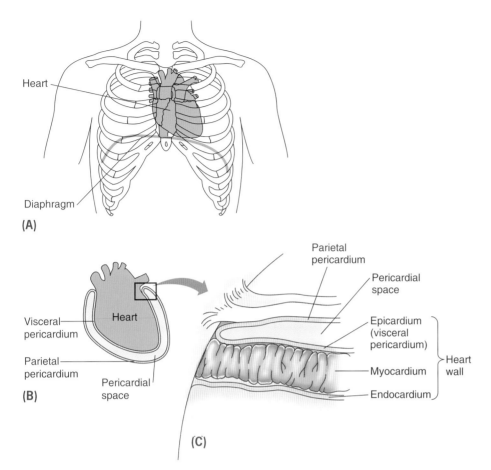

FIGURE 1–4 The heart is located in the mediastinum (**A**). It is surrounded by the pericardium, which contains the pericardial space (**B**). There are three layers to the heart wall (**C**).

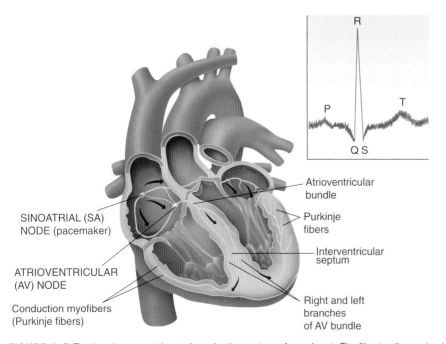

FIGURE 1–5 The impulse generation and conduction system of your heart. The fibrotendinous ring is shown in blue. Also shown is the tracking of an EKG. The p wave corresponds to atrail depolarization, the QRS complex to ventricular depolarization, and the T wave to ventricular repolarization.

The Heart Wall

The heart wall is made up of three distinct layers: the inner endocardium, the middle myocardium, and the outer epicardium. **Figure 1–4** shows these three heart layers.

The heart's inner surfaces (including the heart valves) are covered by the endocardium. The myocardium (the muscular heart wall) forms both the atria and ventricles. It contains cardiac muscle tissue, nerves, and blood vessels. The epicardium is the layer that covers the heart's outer surface.

Blood Supply to the Heart

The right and left coronary arteries are the first two branches of the aorta. They supply blood to the heart's tissues. Cardiac muscle cells require steady supplies of oxygen and nutrients because the heart works continuously. Branches of the cardiac veins drain blood from the myocardial capillaries into the coronary sinus, emptying into the right atrium.

The Conduction System of the Heart

The heart requires electrical impulses to maintain a heartbeat. A network of highly specialized muscle tissue transmits these impulses originating from the sinoatrial (SA) and atrioventricular (AV) nodes. This network includes the conducting fibers between the nodes, the bundle of His (AV bundle), the left and right bundle branches, and the Purkinje fibers (see **Figure 1–5**).

Electrocardiogram

An electrocardiogram graphically depicts, onto a moving strip of paper, a representation of the electrical impulses of the heart as it beats. The paper can be printed or the graph can be viewed on a variety of monitoring devices. An electrocardiogram is abbreviated as both ECG and EKG. Every time the heart beats, a wave of depolarization moves through the atria, reaches the AV nodes, and moves down the intraventricular septum to the apex. This wave then turns and spreads through the ventricular myocardium toward its base.

An ECG collects its electric information from electrodes at different places on the surface of the body. An ECG can reveal normal and abnormal patterns of heart conduction, such as when part of the heart has been damaged by a heart attack. The following are the components of an ECG:

- A small P wave accompanies the atrial depolarization.
- The QRS complex appears during ventricular depolarization. The ventricles begin to contract briefly after the peak of the R wave.
- A smaller T wave indicates ventricular repolarization. Note: The QRS complex helps to mask any indication of atrial repolarization, which occurs while the ventricles are depolarizing.

- The P–R interval extends from the beginning of atrial depolarization to the start of the QRS complex.
- The Q–T interval indicates the time needed for the ventricles to depolarize and repolarize one time. This is usually measured from the end of the P–R interval.

Refer back to Figure 1–5 once more to examine the appearance of the electrical phases of the heart.

Blood Vessels

The blood vessels form a closed circuit of tubes that carry blood from the heart to the cells of the body and back again. Blood leaves the heart via the pulmonary trunk (which originates at the right ventricle) and the aorta (which originates at the left ventricle). The pulmonary arteries branch from the pulmonary trunk, carrying blood to the lungs. Systemic arteries branch from the aorta, distributing blood to all other body organs (see **Figures 1–6** and **1–7**).

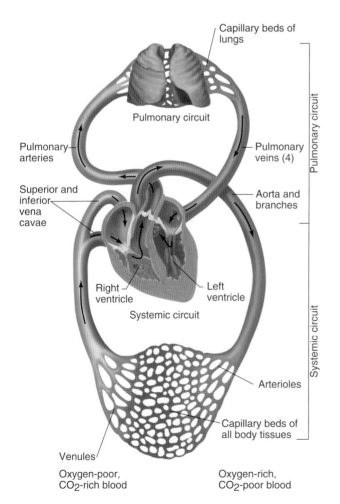

FIGURE 1–6 The blood pathway includes two circuits. The right ventricle supplies the pulmonary circuit, and the left ventricle supplies the systemic circuit.

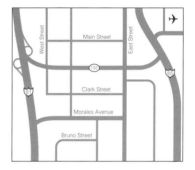

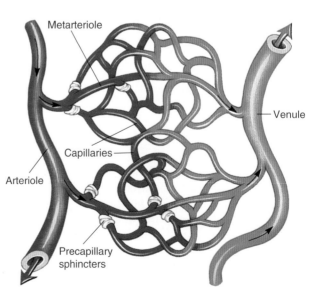

FIGURE 1–7 Just as we travel on different types of roads, our vasculature consists of several different types of vessels.

The blood vessels include arteries, arterioles, capillaries, venules, and veins. They are defined as follows:

- An artery is a blood vessel that carries blood away from the heart and toward peripheral capillaries.
- An arteriole is a smaller blood vessel that works with the arteries to carry blood to the capillaries.
- A capillary is the smallest type of blood vessel in the cardiovascular system. Capillaries allow the blood to distribute oxygen and nutrients to individual cells while picking up carbon dioxide and waste products from these cells. Blood is passed from the arterioles to the capillaries, eventually moving on to the venules.
- A venule is a small blood vessel that passes blood from the capillaries to the veins. Venules are smaller in size than veins and perform the reverse function of the arterioles.
- A vein is a blood vessel that carries blood back to the heart. Except for the pulmonary vein, all veins carry blood that is oxygen depleted and darker in color than that of oxygenated arterial blood. Veins are more numerous than arteries and hold a greater volume of blood. They contain valves that prevent blood from flowing backward. Vein walls are thinner than the walls of corresponding arteries because the blood pressure in the veins is lower than the blood pressure in the arteries. Large veins include the superior and inferior venae cavae, which carry less-oxygenated blood into the right atrium.

The Cardiac Cycle

The cardiac cycle is the period between the start of one heartbeat and the start of the next heartbeat. Atrial contraction regulates the heart chambers in an action known as atrial systole. During this action, the ventricles relax (called ventricular diastole). Next, the ventricles contract (ventricular systole) while the atria relax (atrial diastole). Finally, both the atria and ventricles relax for a brief interval.

Blood Pressure

Blood pressure is defined as the force that the blood exerts against the walls of the blood vessels. It is influenced by the amount of blood that the heart pumps, how much blood volume is in the circulatory system, and the squeezing force of the smooth muscle in the blood vessel walls. Normal blood pressure (in adults) is considered to be less than 120/80 millimeters of mercury (mm Hg).

Pulmonary and Systemic Circuits

Blood flows through the blood vessel network between the heart and peripheral tissues. This network can be subdivided into a pulmonary circuit (which carries blood between the gas exchange surfaces of the lungs) and a systemic circuit (which transports blood to and from the remainder of the body). Each circuit begins and ends at the heart. Oxygenated blood is sent from the left ventricle to the aorta and then circulated through the body (the systemic circuit). Therefore, once deoxygenated, the blood returns to the right atrium. It moves into the right ventricle and is then sent into the pulmonary trunk. Through pulmonary circulation, the exchange of oxygen and carbon dioxide occurs, and the blood returns to the left atrium. The process then begins again.

All body cells need energy for maintenance, growth, defense, and division. Energy is obtained mostly through aerobic mechanisms that require oxygen and produce carbon dioxide. Circulating blood contains oxygen, carrying it from the lungs to the peripheral tissues. This blood also transports carbon dioxide generated by the peripheral tissues to the lungs so that it can be exhaled. Deoxygenated blood is reoxygenated by the lungs.

Organs of the Respiratory System

The organs of the respiratory system can be divided into two tracts: the upper respiratory tract (nose, nasal cavity, paranasal sinuses, and pharynx) and the lower respiratory tract (larynx, trachea, bronchial tree, and lungs). The bronchial trees terminate into grapelike clusters (alveoli) in the lungs.

Nose and Nasal Cavity

The nose is the main passage that allows air to enter the respiratory system. Air moves through the two external nares (nostrils), which open into the nasal cavity. The nasal septum divides the nasal cavity into a right and a left portion, and the anterior portion of the septum consists of hyaline cartilage. The nasal cavity's lateral and superior walls are formed by the maxillary, nasal, frontal, ethmoid, and sphenoid bones of the skull (see **Figure 1–8**).

The superior, middle, and inferior nasal conchae project toward the nasal septum from the nasal cavity's lateral walls.

Pharynx

The pharynx is a hollow chamber that is also part of the respiratory and digestive systems. It is divided into the nasopharynx, oropharynx, and laryngopharynx (see **Figure 1–9**).

Larynx

The larynx (voice box) is a chamber surrounded by cartilage that

> **POINT TO REMEMBER**
>
> The most sensitive areas of the air passages are in the larynx, as well as in regions near the branches of the major bronchi.

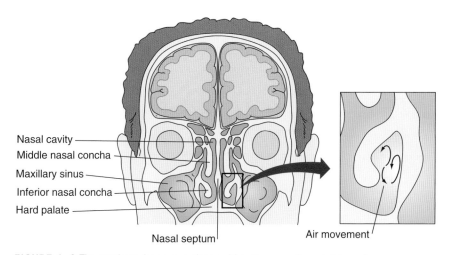

Nasal cavity
Middle nasal concha
Maxillary sinus
Inferior nasal concha
Hard palate

Nasal septum

Air movement

FIGURE 1–8 The nasal concha causes air to swirl as it passes through this cavity.

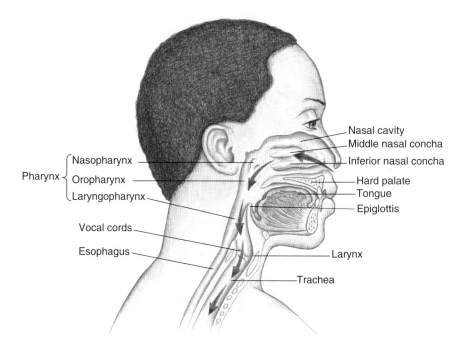

Pharynx
{ Nasopharynx
Oropharynx
Laryngopharynx }

Vocal cords

Esophagus

Nasal cavity
Middle nasal concha
Inferior nasal concha
Hard palate
Tongue
Epiglottis

Larynx

Trachea

FIGURE 1–9 The upper respiratory tract.

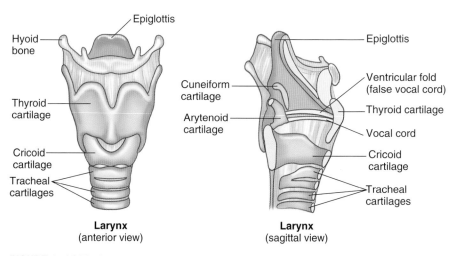

Epiglottis

Hyoid bone

Thyroid cartilage

Cricoid cartilage

Tracheal cartilages

Cuneiform cartilage

Arytenoid cartilage

Larynx (anterior view)

Epiglottis

Ventricular fold (false vocal cord)

Thyroid cartilage

Vocal cord

Cricoid cartilage

Tracheal cartilages

Larynx (sagittal view)

FIGURE 1–10 The larynx.

primarily functions to keep food and liquids out of the airway. It also contains the vocal cords (see **Figure 1–10**).

There are three types of cartilage that form the larynx:

- Thyroid cartilage: The **thyroid cartilage** is the largest of the three; it forms most of the anterior and lateral laryngeal walls.
- Cricoid cartilage: The **cricoid cartilage** is inferior to the thyroid cartilage; it also helps to protect the glottis and entrance to the trachea.
- Epiglottis: Shaped like a shoehorn, the **epiglottis** is cartilage that forms a lid over the glottis.

During swallowing, the larynx is elevated, with the epiglottis folding back over the glottis to prevent the entry of either liquids or solid food into the respiratory tract.

Trachea

The laryngeal epithelium is continuous with the trachea (windpipe), which is a tough, flexible tube about 1 inch in diameter. It contains 15 to 20 tracheal cartilages (see **Figure 1–11**). These serve to make the tracheal walls stiff, protecting the airway and preventing it from collapsing or expanding too greatly when pressures change in the respiratory system.

The tracheal cartilages are all C shaped, with the open part of the C facing posteriorly toward the **esophagus**. Because they are not continuous cartilages, the posterior wall of the trachea can distort easily when swallowing, allowing large pieces of food to pass through the esophagus.

Bronchial Tree

The primary bronchi, along with their branches, form the **bronchial tree**. The left and right primary bronchi are located outside the lungs, so they are called extrapulmonary bronchi. As the primary bronchi enter into the lungs, they divide into smaller passageways known as secondary bronchi. In each lung, one of the secondary bronchi connects to each lobe. It is important

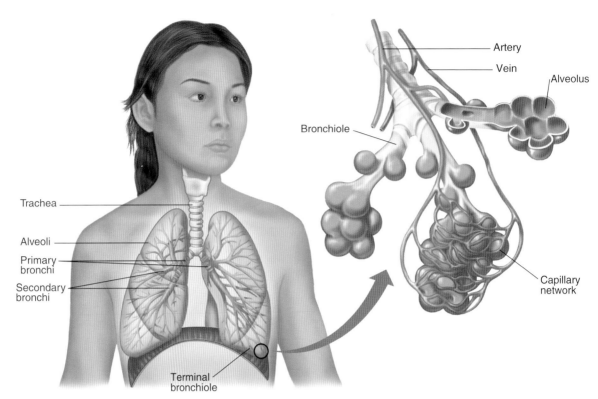

FIGURE 1–11 The trachea conveys air from the larynx to the bronchi, which distribute air throughout the lungs. The bronchioles lead to the alveoli.

to remember that the right lung has three secondary bronchi, and the left lung has only two.

Lungs

The lungs are located in the thoracic cavity and have a soft, spongy structure in a cone-shaped form. The right and left lungs are separated medially by the mediastinum, and they are enclosed by the thoracic cage and diaphragm (see **Figure 1–12**).

Each lung fills most of the thoracic space where it is located. The lungs are suspended by a bronchus and some large blood vessels, with a layer of serous membrane (the visceral pleura) attached firmly to the surface of each lung. This pleura folds back, becoming the parietal pleura, which also forms part of the mediastinum and lines the inner thoracic cavity walls.

Breathing Mechanism

The general term *respiration* refers to the processes of external and internal respiration. External respiration includes the processes involved in exchanging oxygen and carbon dioxide between the lungs and the external environment. Because the epithelium is continuous from the nares to the alveoli, the lungs are actually considered part of the external environment. External respiration occurs between the alveoli of the lungs and the pulmonary capillaries. Internal respiration is the absorption of oxygen and the release of carbon dioxide by the cells of the respiratory system. It occurs between the systemic capillaries and body tissues and cells.

Breathing (ventilation), is the physical movement of air from the outside of the body into and out of the bronchial tree and alveoli. This air movement is provided by actions collectively called inspiration (inhalation) and expiration (exhalation).

Respiratory Air Volumes and Capacities

There are four different respiratory volumes as measured by using spirometry (see **Figure 1–13**). A respiratory cycle consists of one inspiration and its subsequent

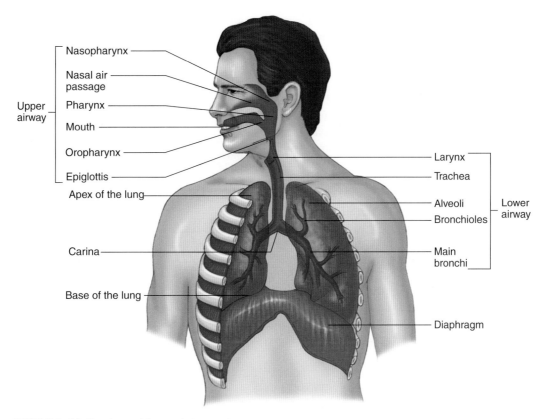

FIGURE 1–12 Structures of the respiratory system.

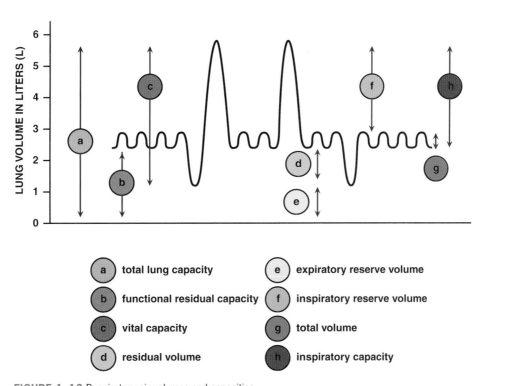

FIGURE 1–13 Respiratory air volumes and capacities.

expiration. The amount of air entering and leaving during one respiratory cycle is called the tidal volume. This consists of approximately 500 mL of air. Nearly the same amount of air leaves during a normal, resting expiration and is known as resting tidal volume.

Air that is in addition to the resting tidal volume is known as inspiratory reserve volume (complemental air) and totals about 3000 mL. The lungs can also expel about 1100 mL beyond the resting tidal volume, known as expiratory reserve volume (supplemental air). Even after forceful expiration, about 1200 mL of air remains in the lungs, known as residual volume. When fresh air is inhaled into the lungs, it mixes with the air already present and prevents wide fluctuations between oxygen and carbon dioxide concentrations.

The four respiratory capacities are as follows:

- Vital capacity (4600 mL): a combination of the inspiratory reserve volume, the tidal volume, and the expiratory reserve volume
- Inspiratory capacity (3500 mL): a combination of the tidal volume plus the inspiratory reserve volume
- Functional residual capacity (2300 mL): a combination of the expiratory reserve volume and the residual volume
- Total lung capacity (5800 mL): a combination of the vital capacity plus the residual volume (total lung capacity varies with age, body size, and gender)

Control of Breathing

The brainstem regulates the involuntary and rhythmic delivery and removal of oxygen and carbon dioxide. Control of the respiratory centers comes from the medulla oblongata and the pons (see **Figure 1–14**).

Factors That Affect Breathing

Factors that affect breathing and the depth of ventilation include certain body chemicals, level of physical activity, emotional states, and the stretchability of the lung tissues. As carbon dioxide accumulates in the blood, it stimulates breathing depth and rate. Low blood oxygen has only small direct effects on central chemoreceptors in the respiratory system. Normal breathing can be altered by emotional upset,

and fear or pain usually increases the breathing rate. Because the respiratory muscles are voluntary, conscious control of breathing is also possible.

Alveolar Gas Exchanges

Pulmonary ventilation ensures that the alveoli have adequate oxygen supply. It also removes carbon dioxide from the bloodstream, and the gas exchanges occur between the blood and alveolar air across the respiratory membranes (see **Figure 1–15**).

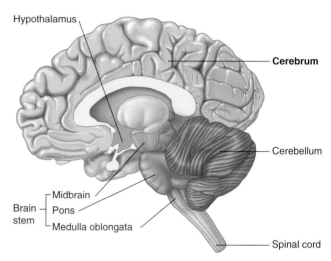

FIGURE 1–14 Cross-section of the brain.

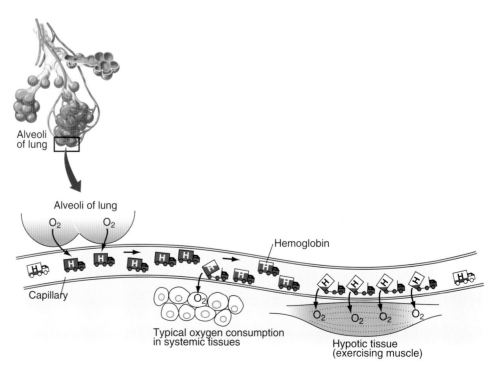

FIGURE 1–15 The relationship between the partial pressure of oxygen and hemoglobin.

Gas Transport

Oxygen (O_2) and carbon dioxide (CO_2) are not readily soluble in blood plasma. This situation of limited solubility is a problem because peripheral tissues need more oxygen than plasma can absorb and transport. The peripheral tissues also generate more carbon dioxide than the plasma can absorb and transport. Gases that are dissolved are bound to **hemoglobin (Hb)** molecules. This action forms oxyhemoglobin (HbO_2). This reversible reaction is summarized as follows:

$$Hb + O_2 \longleftrightarrow HbO_2$$

Aerobic metabolism generates carbon dioxide in body tissues. When a CO_2 molecule enters the bloodstream, it is either converted to a carbonic acid molecule, bound to the protein in hemoglobin molecules inside red blood cells, or dissolved in the blood plasma. These three reactions can be completed in reverse order.

Most of the carbon dioxide that is absorbed in the blood, which is almost 70% of the total amount, is transported as carbonic acid molecules. Carbon dioxide is converted to carbonic acid through **carbonic anhydrase** enzyme activity in the red blood cells. Carbonic acid molecules dissociate immediately into hydrogen and bicarbonate ions. This reaction can be summarized as follows:

$$CO_2 + H_2O \longleftrightarrow H^+ + HCO_3^-$$

Approximately 23% of the carbon dioxide in the blood is bound to the protein of the Hb molecules inside the red blood cells. This compound is then called **carbaminohemoglobin**.

Plasma becomes saturated with carbon dioxide. This process is rapid. Approximately 7% of the carbon dioxide is absorbed by the peripheral capillaries and transported as dissolved molecules of gas. The remainder is absorbed by the red blood cells, where it is converted (via carbonic anhydrase) or stored as carbaminohemoglobin.

> **POINT TO REMEMBER**
>
> Exposure to high oxygen concentration for a prolonged time may damage lung tissue, particularly capillary walls.

Overview of the Nervous System

The nervous system is made up of the central nervous system, which contains the brain and the spinal cord. The peripheral nervous system is composed of the peripheral nerves, which connect the central nervous system to the rest of the body. It also contains the autonomic nervous system, which utilizes autonomic neurotransmitters to function. See **Figure 1–16** for a depiction of the central and peripheral nervous systems, and also see **Figure 1–17** for the major subdivisions of the nervous system.

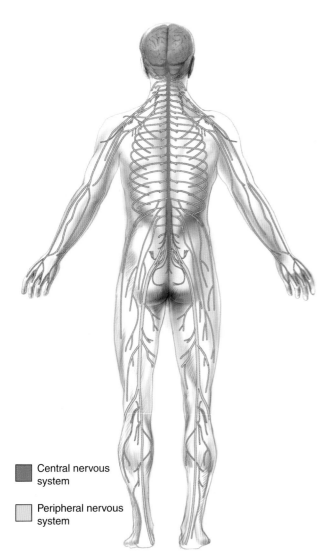

Central nervous system

Peripheral nervous system

FIGURE 1–16 The nervous system can be divided into the central nervous system and peripheral nervous system.

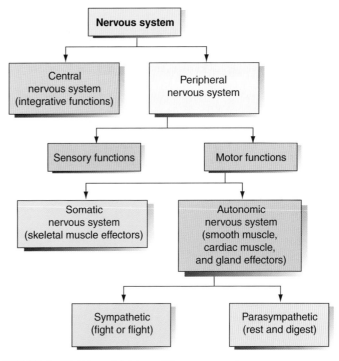

FIGURE 1–17 Major subdivisions of the nervous system.

Central Nervous System

The central nervous system (CNS) is made up of the brain and the spinal cord. It functions by utilizing sensory receptors that detect changes both inside and outside the body. These receptors transmit impulses over peripheral nerves to the CNS. Nervous tissue consists of masses of nerve cells (neurons), which are the structural and functional units of the nervous system. They transmit information as nerve impulses to other neurons and also to cells that are outside of the nervous system.

Nerves are bundles of axons. An axon is an extension from a neuron's cell body that sends out nerve impulses. Another type of extension, the dendrite, receives electrochemical messages. The junction between any two neurons is called a synapse. Synaptic transmission is accomplished by biochemicals known as neurotransmitters, which may be either excitatory (increasing the chance that a nerve impulse will occur) or inhibitory (decreasing the chance that a nerve impulse will occur). Nerves that conduct impulses to the brain or spinal cord are called sensory nerves, and those that carry impulses to muscles or glands are called motor nerves. Most nerves have both types of fibers and are called mixed nerves.

Brain

The brain receives and processes large amounts of information. The 100 billion **neurons** of the brain control many activities simultaneously. The brain is divided into four major portions: cerebrum, diencephalon, brainstem, and cerebellum (see **Figure 1–18**). The brain can respond to various stimuli in many diverse ways.

Cerebrum

The cerebrum is made up of the two large hemispheres of the brain. It is the center of conscious thought, sensory perception, memory, and motor activities. Its outer layer is known as gray matter (the cerebral cortex), and its inner layer is known as white matter. Its surface is

covered with elevated ridges (gyri) separated by grooves called sulci and fissures. The cerebrum contains many neurons required for analytical functions. Each cerebral hemisphere is divided into five lobes.

The cerebrum is categorized into three functional areas: motor, sensory, and association. The motor areas are located within the frontal lobes. The sensory areas are located within the parietal, temporal, and occipital lobes. The association areas are located throughout various lobes.

Diencephalon

The diencephalon is located between the inferior regions of the two cerebral hemispheres. It contains the epithalamus, thalamus, and hypothalamus. The epithalamus contains the pineal gland, which is important for the regulation of the body's day and night cycles. The thalamus is the main point of processing sensory information. The hypothalamus is attached to the pituitary gland by a thin funnel-like stalk called the infundibulum. The hypothalamus controls the autonomic nervous system, endocrine system, body temperature, emotions, eating, drinking, and sleeping.

Brainstem

The brainstem helps to connect the cerebellum to the spinal cord and is divided into three regions: mes-

> **POINT TO REMEMBER**
>
> Injuries to the respiratory center or to spinal nerve tracts that transmit motor impulses may paralyze the breathing muscles.

encephalon, pons, and medulla oblongata. The brainstem houses the nuclei of many of the cranial nerves and contains many critical autonomic and reflex centers. The mesencephalon is also known as the **midbrain**. It contains cranial nerves, motor tracts, axons, sensory nuclei, and other important structures.

The pons bulges out on the anterior brainstem and houses sensory and motor tracts connecting the brain and spinal cord. The medulla oblongata is continuous with the spinal cord and even resembles it. All communication between the brain and spinal cord flows through the medulla oblongata. The most important autonomic centers of the medulla oblongata regulate the heart, blood pressure, and breathing.

Cerebellum

The cerebellum is the second largest section of the brain. Similar to the cerebrum, it also consists of two hemispheres primarily composed of white matter, with a thin gray matter layer on its surface. The cerebellum controls skeletal muscle movements and contractions to control equilibrium and posture. It is important in keeping the skeletal muscle activity fine-tuned so that the body has correct and adequate muscle tone and strength.

The cerebellum interacts with the CNS via three paired nerve tracts called the cerebellar peduncles. It is basically a reflex center concerned with body position.

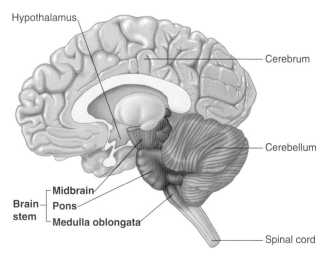

FIGURE 1–18 Major portions of the brain.

Hypothalamus

Cerebrum

Cerebellum

Brain stem —⎰ Midbrain, Pons, Medulla oblongata

Spinal cord

When damaged, the results often include tremors, impaired muscle control, imbalance, and reduced muscle tone.

Spinal Cord

The spinal cord occupies the vertebral canal inside the vertebral column. Between the bony coverings and soft tissues of the CNS, layered membranes called meninges are found. Meninges have three layers: dura mater, arachnoid mater, and pia mater. The dura mater is attached to the cranial cavity and continues into the vertebral canal. The arachnoid mater is a weblike membrane between the dura and pia maters. The pia mater contains nerves and blood vessels that are important for nourishing brain and spinal cells. Between the arachnoid and pia maters is the subarachnoid space, which contains the clear and watery cerebrospinal fluid (CSF).

The spinal cord itself is a slender column of nerves that passes from the brain into the vertebral canal. It begins where nervous tissue exits the cranial cavity, and it ends near the intervertebral disc that separates the first and second lumbar vertebrae. The spinal cord has 31 segments that each have a pair of spinal nerves attached. It is divided by two grooves that separate the cord into right and left halves. Gray matter divides the spinal cord's white matter into anterior, lateral, and posterior funiculi regions, which contain bundled nerve fibers.

The spinal cord functions primarily to conduct nerve impulses and control spinal reflexes. The axons inside the spinal cord allow two-way communication between the brain and body parts. The ascending tracts of the spinal cord carry sensory information to the brain, and the descending tracts conduct motor impulses from the brain to the muscles and glands.

Peripheral Nervous System

The peripheral nervous system (PNS) contains the cranial and spinal nerves, which branch out from the CNS. These nerves connect to the rest of the body. The PNS is divided into the somatic and autonomic nervous systems. The somatic nervous system oversees conscious activities and actions of the skin and skeletal muscles. The autonomic nervous system oversees the actions of the heart, stomach, intestines, and other viscera. It controls unconscious activities.

Cranial Nerves

There are 12 pairs of cranial nerves that extend from the underside of the brain, all of which (except for the first pair) originate in the brainstem. These nerves lead to various areas of the head, neck, and trunk. **Table 1-2** lists the 12 pairs of cranial nerves.

Spinal Nerves

The 31 pairs of spinal nerves are grouped by the level of the spinal cord from which they arise. In general, they are associated with their respective spinal vertebrae.

TABLE 1-2 Cranial Nerves

Number	Nerve	Type
I	Olfactory	Sensory (smell)
II	Optic	Sensory (vision)
III	Oculomotor	Primarily motor (eye muscles)
IV	Trochlear	Primarily motor (eye muscles)
V	Trigeminal (ophthalmic, maxillary, mandibular)	Mixed (eyes, tear glands, scalp, forehead, upper eyelids, teeth, gums, lips, palate, face, jaw)
VI	Abducens	Primarily motor (eye muscles)
VII	Facial	Mixed (taste and tongue, expression, tear glands, salivary glands)
VIII	Vestibulocochlear	Sensory (equilibrium, hearing)
IX	Glossopharyngeal	Mixed (pharynx, tonsils, tongue, carotid arteries, swallowing, salivary glands)
X	Vagus	Mixed (speech, swallowing, transmission of impulses to heart, smooth muscles, thoracic glands, abdominal glands; also impulses from pharynx, larynx, esophagus, and viscera)
XI	Accessory (cranial and spinal)	Primarily motor (soft palate, pharynx, larynx, neck, back)
XII	Hypoglossal	Primarily motor (muscles that move the tongue)

There are 8 pairs of cervical nerves, 12 pairs of thoracic nerves, 5 pairs of lumbar nerves, 5 pairs of sacral nerves, and 1 pair of coccygeal nerves. Except for the thoracic region, the main portions of spinal nerves form complex networks (plexuses), wherein nerve fibers are sorted and recombined. This allows them to innervate certain peripheral body parts even though they originate from different spinal nerves.

Autonomic Nervous System

The autonomic nervous system (ANS) governs involuntary actions and works with the somatic nervous system to regulate body organs and functions. Both are part of the central as well as the peripheral nervous systems. The ANS functions mostly unconsciously, such as the stomach's process of digestion or the blood vessels' processes of coordinating blood pressure. It is activated by visceral sensory neurons. The ANS is subdivided into the parasympathetic and sympathetic divisions, which focus on the control of the body's internal environment.

Parasympathetic Division

The parasympathetic division arises from the brainstem and the sacral region of the spinal cord (see **Figure 1–19**). It conserves energy and replaces nutrients, so it is called the rest-and-digest division. It helps to maintain homeostasis in the body. Its preganglionic axons are longer, and the relatively short postganglionic fibers continue from the ganglia to specific muscles or glands within the viscera. Only one or a few structures become innervated by this system at the same time.

Sympathetic Division

The sympathetic division prepares the body for emergencies, hence its fight-or-flight name. The preganglionic fibers originate from the neurons of the spinal cord (see Figure 1–19). Increased sympathetic activity causes increased alertness and metabolism. When this system causes innervation, all of its components become stimulated.

Autonomic Neurotransmitters

The sympathetic and parasympathetic divisions secrete the neurotransmitter known as acetylcholine from their preganglionic fibers (cholinergic fibers). Most sympathetic postganglionic neurons secrete norepinephrine (noradrenaline), so they are also called adrenergic fibers. Most body organs are innervated by the actions of these various autonomic neurotransmitters. The sympathetic and parasympathetic nervous systems use these neurotransmitters to achieve opposing actions.

Other neurotransmitters released from the brain include dopamine, serotonin, and gamma-aminobutyric acid (GABA). However, their actions may not be directly opposed to one another (antagonistic). **Table 1–3** explains the opposing actions of the sympathetic and parasympathetic nervous system neurotransmitters.

Patient Education

Respiratory therapists should be familiar with the structures and functions of the cardiovascular system. They should advise patients who are suffering

TABLE 1–3 Opposing Neurotransmitter Actions

Body structure or function	Sympathetic	Parasympathetic
Eye pupils	Dilation	Constriction
Tear glands	No action	Secretion
Salivary glands	Decreased secretion	Increased secretion
Lung bronchioles	Dilation	Constriction
Heart rate	Increased	Decreased
Blood distribution	Increased to skeletal muscles, decreased to digestive organs	Decreased to skeletal muscles, increased to digestive organs
Blood glucose	Increased	Decreased
Intestinal wall muscles	Peristalsis decreased	Peristalsis increased
Intestinal glands	Secretion decreased	Secretion increased
Gallbladder muscles	Relaxed	Contracted
Urinary bladder muscles	Relaxed	Contracted

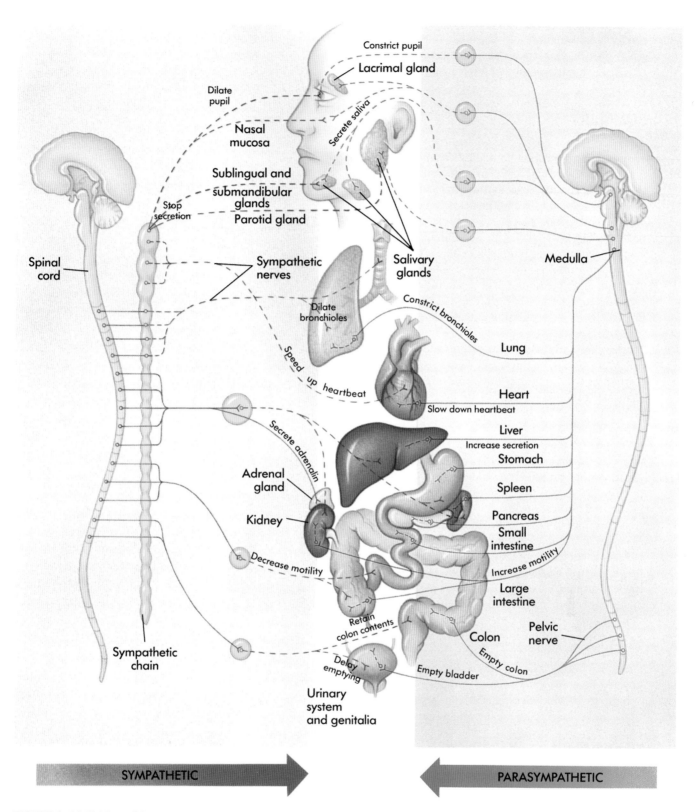

FIGURE 1–19 Divisions of the autonomic nervous system.

from congestive heart failure to restrict their intake of sodium, lose weight, avoid smoking, and see their physician on a regular basis. Respiratory therapists should also instruct patients to take their medications exactly as prescribed.

SUMMARY

The heart pumps nearly 8000 liters of blood per day, yet is only about the size of an adult's clenched fist. It consists of two hollow atria and two hollow ventricles. When the heart beats, the atria contract first, followed by the ventricles. Special valves in the heart control blood flow and keep it from flowing back into areas where it should not flow. The heart valves include the mitral (bicuspid), aortic, tricuspid, and pulmonary valves. The heart wall is made up of three distinct layers: endocardium, myocardium, and epicardium. The heart requires electrical impulses to maintain a heartbeat. These impulses may be charted on a graph known as an electrocardiogram (ECG or EKG).

The cardiopulmonary vessels include arteries, arterioles, capillaries, venules, and veins. Blood pressure is defined as the force that the blood exerts against the walls of the blood vessels. The organs of the respiratory system include the upper respiratory tract (nose, nasal cavity, paranasal sinuses, and pharynx) and the lower respiratory tract (larynx, trachea, bronchial tree, and lungs). The pharynx is also part of the digestive system because food and liquids pass through it. The lungs are the primary organs of respiration, and the processes of inspiration and exhalation are controlled by the brainstem, primarily the medulla oblongata and pons. However, because the respiratory muscles are voluntary, conscious control of breathing is also possible.

The central nervous system (CNS) is made up of the brain and spinal cord. The four major parts of the brain are the cerebrum, diencephalon, brainstem, and cerebellum. The spinal cord is a slender column of nerves that passes from the brain through the vertebral canal. The peripheral nervous system (PNS) contains the cranial and spinal nerves. The autonomic nervous system (ANS) governs involuntary actions to stimulate or inhibit the activity of the visceral organs. It consists of the sympathetic and parasympathetic nervous systems.

LEARNING GOALS

These learning goals correspond to the objectives at the beginning of the chapter, providing a clear summary of the chapter's most important points.

1. The structures of the cardiovascular system include the heart (including its chambers, valves, and wall) and the blood vessels.

2. The heart's inner surfaces (including the heart valves) are covered by the endocardium. The myocardium (the muscular heart wall) forms both the atria and ventricles. It contains cardiac muscle tissue, nerves, and blood vessels. The epicardium is the layer that covers the heart's outer surface.

3. The cardiac cycle is the period between the start of one heartbeat and the start of the next heartbeat. Atrial contraction regulates the heart chambers in an action known as atrial systole. During this action, the ventricles relax (called ventricular diastole). Next, the ventricles contract (ventricular systole) while the atria relax (atrial diastole). Finally, both the atria and ventricles relax for a brief interval.

   Blood pressure is defined as the force that the blood exerts against the walls of the blood vessels. It is influenced by the amount of blood that the heart pumps, how much blood volume is in the circulatory system, and the squeezing force of the smooth muscle in the blood vessel walls. Normal blood pressure (in adults) is considered to be 120/80 millimeters of mercury (mm Hg).

4. The blood vessels include arteries, arterioles, capillaries, venules, and veins. They are defined as follows:

   - An artery is a blood vessel that carries blood away from the heart and toward peripheral capillaries.

   - An arteriole is a smaller blood vessel that works with the arteries to carry blood to the capillaries.

   - A capillary is the smallest type of blood vessel in the cardiovascular system. Capillaries allow the blood to distribute oxygen and nutrients to individual cells while picking up carbon dioxide and waste products from these cells. Blood is passed from the arterioles to the capillaries, eventually moving on to the venules.

   - A venule is a small blood vessel that passes blood from the capillaries to the veins. Venules are smaller than veins and perform the reverse function of the arterioles.

   - A vein is a blood vessel that carries blood back to the heart. Except for the pulmonary vein, all veins carry blood that is oxygen depleted and darker in color than that of oxygenated arterial blood. Veins are more numerous than arteries and hold a greater volume of blood. They contain valves that prevent blood from flowing backward. Vein walls are thinner than the walls of corresponding arteries because the blood pressure in the veins is lower than the blood pressure in the arteries. Large veins include the superior and inferior venae cavae, which carry less-oxygenated blood into the right atrium.

5. The respiratory system furnishes oxygen for individual tissue cells and takes away their gaseous waste products. Through the act of respiration, consisting of external and internal processes, this process is accomplished. External respiration is the method in which the lungs are ventilated, and oxygen and carbon dioxide are exchanged between the air in the alveoli of the lungs and the blood in the pulmonary capillaries. Internal respiration occurs when oxygen and carbon dioxide are exchanged between the blood in systemic capillaries and the body's tissues and cells.

6. The locations of the respiratory system organs are in the upper respiratory tract (nose, nasal cavity, and paranasal sinuses in the skull; and pharynx in the neck) and the lower respiratory tract (larynx and trachea in the neck; and bronchial tree and lungs in the thoracic cavity).

7. The nose is the main passage that allows air to enter the respiratory system. Air moves through the two external nares (nostrils), which open into the nasal cavity. The pharynx is a hollow chamber that is also part of the respiratory and digestive systems. It is divided into the nasopharynx, oropharynx, and laryngopharynx. The larynx (voice box) is a chamber surrounded by cartilage that primarily functions to keep food and liquids out of the airway. It also contains the vocal cords. During swallowing, the larynx is elevated, with the epiglottis folding back over the glottis to prevent the entry of either liquids or solid food into the respiratory tract. The laryngeal epithelium is continuous with the trachea (windpipe), which is a tough, flexible tube about 1 inch in diameter. It contains 15 to 20 tracheal cartilages. These serve to make the tracheal walls stiff and protect the airway, as well as preventing it from collapsing or expanding too greatly when pressures change in the respiratory system. The primary bronchi, along with their branches, form the bronchial tree. The right lung has three secondary bronchi, and the left lung has only two. The lungs are located in the thoracic cavity, with a soft, spongy structure in a cone-shaped form. The right and left lungs are separated medially by the mediastinum and are enclosed by the thoracic cage and diaphragm.

8. The general term *respiration* refers to the processes of external and internal respiration. External respiration includes the processes involved in exchanging oxygen and carbon dioxide between the lungs and the external environment. Internal respiration is the absorption of oxygen and the release of carbon dioxide by the cells of the respiratory system. Breathing (ventilation) is the physical movement of air from the outside of the body into and out of the bronchial tree and alveoli. This air movement is provided by actions collectively called inspiration (inhalation) and expiration (exhalation).

9. The four main parts of the brain and their functions are as follows:
   - Cerebrum: The cerebrum is the center of conscious thought, sensory perception, memory, and motor activities; it contains many neurons required for analytical functions. There are three functional areas: motor, sensory, and association.
   - Diencephalon: The diencephalon contains the pineal gland, which is important for the regulation of the body's day and night cycles. Another structure, the thalamus, is the main point of processing sensory information. The part of the thalamus known as the hypothalamus controls the autonomic nervous system, endocrine system, body temperature, emotions, eating, drinking, and sleeping.
   - Brainstem: The brainstem is divided into three regions: mesencephalon (midbrain), pons, and medulla oblongata. It contains many critical autonomic and reflex centers. All communication between the brain and spinal cord flows through the medulla oblongata, and its most important autonomic centers regulate the heart, blood pressure, and breathing.
   - Cerebellum: The cerebellum controls skeletal muscle movements and contractions to control equilibrium and posture, and it is important in keeping the skeletal muscle activity fine-tuned so the body has correct and adequate muscle tone and strength.

10. The cardiopulmonary system is affected by the parasympathetic and sympathetic nervous systems as follows:
   - Parasympathetic: The parasympathetic nervous system conserves energy and replaces nutrients; therefore it is called the rest-and-digest division. It helps to main homeostasis in the body.
   - Sympathetic: The sympathetic nervous system prepares the body for emergencies, hence its fight-or-flight name. Increased sympathetic activity causes increased alertness and metabolism.

CRITICAL THINKING QUESTIONS

1. Cigarette smoke contains thousands of chemicals, including nicotine and carbon monoxide. Nicotine constricts blood vessels. Carbon monoxide prevents

oxygen from binding to hemoglobin. How do these two components of smoke affect the cardiovascular system?

2. If a tracheostomy bypasses the upper respiratory passages, how might the air entering the trachea differ from air normally passing through this tube? What problems might this cause for the patient?

WEB SITES

http://hes.ucfsd.org/gclaypo/repiratorysys.html

http://science.nationalgeographic.com/science/health-and-human-body/human-body/lungs-article.html

http://users.rcn.com/jkimball.ma.ultranet/BiologyPages/C/CNS.html

http://www.americanheart.org/presenter.jhtml?identifier=4463

http://www.cardiovascularcs.org/

http://www.cvphysiology.com/Heart%20Disease/HD002.htm

http://www.daviddarling.info/encyclopedia/B/bronchial_tree.html

http://www.fi.edu/learn/heart/structure/structure.html

http://www.tutorvista.com/content/biology/biology-ii/respiration/breathing-mechanism.php

REVIEW QUESTIONS

Multiple Choice

Select the best response to each question.

1. Breathing is regulated by the
   A. thalamus
   B. cerebellum
   C. hypothalamus
   D. pons

2. The artery that carries deoxygenated blood from the heart to the lungs is the
   A. coronary artery
   B. renal artery
   C. pulmonary artery
   D. aorta

3. Which part of the heart receives oxygenated blood from the pulmonary veins?
   A. right atrium
   B. left atrium
   C. right ventricle
   D. left ventricle

4. Where in the lung does the exchange of gases take place?
   A. trachea
   B. alveoli
   C. bronchioles
   D. larynx

5. Which of the following is *not* a function of the sympathetic division of the autonomic nervous system?
   A. It increases the heart rate and breathing rate.
   B. It prepares the body for an emergency.
   C. It increases digestive system motility and activity.
   D. It dilates the pupils.

6. Which of the following is *not* part of the respiratory system?
   A. larynx
   B. pharynx
   C. thoracic duct
   D. bronchi

7. Which of the following is *not* a function of the hypothalamus?
   A. It regulates the sleep–wake cycle.
   B. It controls the autonomic nervous system.
   C. It initiates voluntary skeletal muscle movement.
   D. It controls the endocrine system.

8. Which valve is located between the left atrium and left ventricle?
   A. bicuspid valve
   B. tricuspid valve
   C. aortic valve
   D. pulmonary valve

9. The heart's pacemaker is located in the
   A. right ventricle
   B. right atrium
   C. left ventricle
   D. left atrium

10. Which structure contains some autonomic centers involved in regulating respiration?
    A. pons
    B. cerebellum
    C. thalamus
    D. cerebrum

11. Which part of the pleura is attached to the lung surface?
    A. parietal
    B. apical
    C. visceral
    D. mediastinum

12. Which of the following keeps the airways of the trachea open?
    A. ciliated epithelium
    B. surfactant
    C. smooth muscle
    D. cartilage

13. Which of the following large vessels drains low-oxygen blood from the majority of the lower body into the right atrium?
    A. hepatic vein
    B. inferior vena cava
    C. superior vena cava
    D. azygos vein

14. Which of the following is a part of both the respiratory and digestive systems and allows the passage of food, drink, and air?
    A. nasopharynx
    B. trachea
    C. oropharynx
    D. glottis

15. In the respiratory system, which of the following is the last and smallest conducting portion?
    A. terminal bronchiole
    B. respiratory bronchiole
    C. nasopharynx
    D. alveolus

CASE STUDY

In 1799, a 67-year-old man had flulike symptoms for a few days during the winter. He began having trouble breathing and swallowing, and his voice became muffled. His doctors tried a variety of therapies that were popular, including bleeding and using beetles to bite his legs to produce blisters. One of the doctors suggested a tracheostomy so the patient could breathe, but the other doctors said it would not help. The man later died with no improvement in his condition. If a tracheostomy had been performed, would it likely have saved his life?

Overview of Cardiopulmonary Disorders and Conditions

OBJECTIVES

Upon completion of this chapter, the reader should be able to do the following:

1. Compare emphysema and chronic bronchitis.
2. Define atelectasis and discuss possible causes.
3. Contrast the pathologic course of acute bronchitis with that of chronic bronchitis.
4. Describe the condition known as angina pectoris.
5. List the leading causes of lung cancer.
6. Distinguish among endocarditis, myocarditis, and pericarditis.
7. Compare left-sided heart failure with right-sided heart failure.
8. Name the causes of cardiac arrhythmias.
9. Describe the causes of pulmonary edema and explain how it affects oxygen levels.
10. Explain the possible consequences of emboli.

KEY TERMS

Angina pectoris	Gag reflex
Anoxia	Granuloma
Anthracosis	Hemagglutinin
Arrhythmia	Hemoptysis
Asbestosis	Histoplasmosis
Asthma	Hypercapnia
Atelectasis	Hypoxemia
Atherosclerosis	Ischemia
Bronchiectasis	Myocardial infarction
Bronchiolectasis	Nasal flaring
Bronchiolitis	Neuraminidase
Bronchitis	Pathogen
Bronchogenic carcinoma	Pleural effusion
Carcinogens	Pleurisy
Consolidation	Pneumoconiosis
Dyspnea	Pneumonia
Dysrhythmia	Pneumothorax
Emphysema	Pulmonary edema
Epithelial	Pulmonary embolism

Pulmonary fibrosis   Stridor
Pulmonary hypertension   Surfactant
Respiratory acidosis   Thrombus
Respiratory failure   Tuberculosis
Sepsis   Ventricular asystole
Silicosis   Ventricular fibrillation

INTRODUCTION

Cardiovascular disease is the number one cause of death in the United States. Coronary heart disease, as of 2000, is responsible for more than one out of every five deaths in the country annually. Common heart diseases include hypertensive heart disease, angina and heart attacks, cardiac arrhythmias, and congestive heart failure. Risk factors for heart diseases include obesity, smoking, alcoholism, and lack of exercise. Pulmonary diseases result from circulatory disorders, immune diseases, congenital defects, central nervous system damage or diseases, environmental conditions, and infection.

This chapter focuses on major cardiopulmonary disorders.

Cardiovascular Disorders

Cardiovascular disease is described as any abnormal condition characterized by heart or blood vessel dysfunction. Cardiovascular disease is the leading cause of death in the United States.

Coronary Artery Disease

Coronary artery disease is an abnormal condition that may affect the arteries of the heart and produce varying pathologic effects, primarily reduced flow of oxygen and nutrients to the myocardium. Atherosclerosis is the most common type of coronary artery disease, and it is now the leading cause of death in North America. Angina pectoris is the classic symptom of coronary artery disease; it results from myocardial ischemia.

Angina Pectoris

Angina pectoris is a sudden outburst of chest pain frequently caused by myocardial anoxia as a result of atherosclerosis or coronary artery spasm. Atherosclerosis is a deposition of fat-containing substances collectively known as plaque in the lumen (opening) of the coronary arteries that causes them to narrow (see **Figure 2–1**). Anginal pain usually radiates along the neck, jaw, shoulder, and down the left arm. It is often accompanied by feelings of suffocation that may seem to indicate impending death.

Angina pectoris attacks are often related to emotional stress, eating, exertion, and exposure to intense cold. There are four types of angina:

- Stable angina: The pain is predictable in frequency and duration and is relieved by rest and nitroglycerin.
- Unstable angina: The pain increases in frequency and duration and is more easily induced. It indicates a worsening of coronary artery disease, which may progress to myocardial infarction.
- Variant angina: The pain is caused by coronary artery spasm and may occur spontaneously. It may not be related to physical exercise or emotional stress. It is also known as Prinzmetal angina.
- Microvascular angina: Impairment of the vasodilator reserve causes angina-like chest pain even though the patient's coronary arteries are normal.

The pain of angina may be relieved by rest and vasodilation of the coronary arteries with medication. Angina pectoris is also referred to as cardiac pain.

Myocardial Infarction

When coronary blood flow is interrupted for extended periods, necrosis (tissue death) of part of the cardiac muscle occurs. Necrosis results in **myocardial infarction**. When the coronary arteries are obstructed, this may result in either atherosclerosis, a spasm, or a **thrombus**. Myocardial infarction (MI) is also called heart attack.

Of the various types of cardiovascular disorders, heart attack is the leading cause of death in the United States. When treatment is delayed, mortality is high. Nearly one-half of sudden myocardial infarction deaths occur before the patient can be hospitalized, usually within

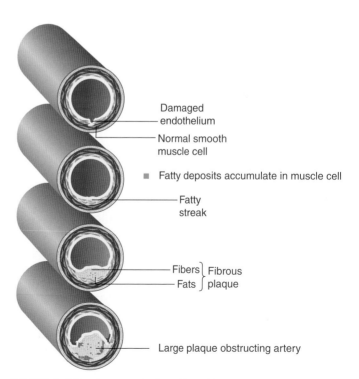

Damaged endothelium

Normal smooth muscle cell

- Fatty deposits accumulate in muscle cell

Fatty streak

Fibers ⎫ Fibrous
Fats ⎭ plaque

Large plaque obstructing artery

FIGURE 2–1 Development of a deposition of fat-containing substances which form plaque and lead to arterial occlusion.

1 hour of the onset of symptoms. Risk factors for myocardial infarction include the following:

- family history of MI
- aging
- gender
- hypertension
- elevated total cholesterol
- obesity
- lifestyle
- smoking
- stress or type A personality
- drug use (especially cocaine and amphetamines)

The occlusion of a coronary artery may result in ischemia and infarct (death) of the myocardium, causing sudden and severe left-sided chest pain (see **Figure 2–2**).

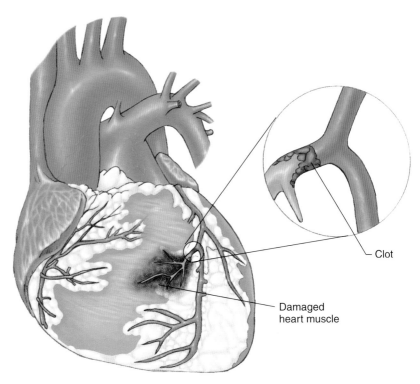

Clot

Damaged heart muscle

FIGURE 2–2 Damage caused by myocardial infarction.

Dysrhythmias

A **dysrhythmia** (**arrhythmia**) is a disturbance of heart rhythm. The sinoatrial (SA) node generates normal heart rhythms that travel through the heart's conduction system. This causes the atrial and ventricular myocardium to contract and relax at a regular rate. This rate maintains circulation during various levels of physical activity. Dysrhythmias range from mild to catastrophic ventricular fibrillation.

Arrhythmias are usually classified according to their origin (either ventricular or supraventricular). Their effect on blood pressure as well as cardiac output (which may be influenced from where they originate) determines how clinically significant they are. Common causes of arrhythmias include the following:

- congenital defects
- drug toxicity
- electrolyte imbalances
- myocardial infarction or **ischemia**

Hypertension

Hypertension is an elevation in either systolic or diastolic blood pressure. It occurs as either essential (primary) hypertension or secondary hypertension. Primary hypertension is the most common type. Secondary hypertension results from renal disease or other identifiable causes. Malignant hypertension is a severe form of hypertension that may be either primary or secondary. Hypertension is a major cause of cardiac disease, renal failure, and stroke.

Hypertension affects nearly 20% of adults in the United States. Risks for hypertension increase with age. Hypertension is more prevalent in the black population than in the white population. It is also more prevalent in people with less education and lower income. During young and middle adulthood, men have a higher incidence of hypertension, but thereafter, women have a higher incidence.

Risk factors for essential hypertension include the following:

- the aging process
- family history
- obesity
- high intake of sodium
- high intake of saturated fat
- sleep apnea
- stress
- excessive alcohol consumption
- sedentary lifestyle
- diabetes mellitus
- tobacco use

Cardiomyopathy

Cardiomyopathy is a term that generally applies to a disease of the heart muscle fibers. It is the second most common direct cause of sudden death (after coronary artery disease). The most common type of cardiomyopathy is the dilated form. Men and blacks are at greatest risk for dilated cardiomyopathy. Other risk factors include coronary artery disease, hypertension, pregnancy, viral infections, and use of alcohol or illegal drugs. Hypertrophic cardiomyopathy is different in that it is caused by a genetic abnormality.

Carditis

Carditis is defined as inflammation of the heart and its surrounding structures. The several types of carditis include pericarditis, myocarditis, and endocarditis, each of which describes the portion of the heart that is inflamed in the specific condition. Common causes of the various forms of carditis include viral infections, bacterial infections, fungal infections, immune conditions, myocardial infarction, trauma, uremia, cancers, certain medications, radiation, and other causes.

Heart Failure

Heart failure is the inability of the heart muscle to contract with enough force to properly circulate the blood throughout the body. Dysfunction of the left ventricle is the most common cause of heart failure. However, the right ventricle may also be dysfunctional, especially in pulmonary disease (right ventricular failure).

The most common form of heart failure is congestive heart failure. It is called this because of the collection of fluid (congestion) in the lungs and extremities. Heart failure may be classified as left- or right-sided heart failure according to the side of the heart that is affected. It may also be classified as systolic or diastolic dysfunction based on the cardiac cycle involved.

Left-sided heart failure is caused by ineffective left ventricular contraction. As the left ventricle's pumping ability fails, cardiac output falls. Because blood is no longer effectively pumped out, it backs up into the left atrium and then into the lungs. This causes activity intolerance and dyspnea. If the condition persists, pulmonary edema and right-sided heart failure can result. Common causes of left-sided heart failure include hypertension, aortic and mitral valve stenosis, and left ventricular infarction.

Right-sided heart failure is caused by ineffective right ventricular contraction. As a result, blood is not pumped with enough force through the right ventricle to the lungs. This causes blood to back up into the right atrium as well as the peripheral circulation. The patient gains weight, develops peripheral edema, and the kidneys (and other organs) become engorged. Right-sided heart failure may be caused by pulmonary hypertension, pulmonary embolus, or acute right ventricular infarction.

Cardiac Arrest

Cardiac arrest is a sudden cessation of cardiac output and effective circulation. It is usually precipitated by ventricular fibrillation or ventricular asystole. When cardiac arrest occurs, delivery of oxygen and removal of carbon dioxide ceases. Tissue cell metabolism becomes anaerobic, and metabolic and respiratory acidosis occurs. Immediate initiation of cardiopulmonary resuscitation (CPR) is required to prevent heart, lung, kidney, and brain damage and death. Cardiac arrest is also called cardiopulmonary arrest.

Respiratory Disorders

A respiratory disorder is any abnormal condition of the respiratory system. Respiratory disorders are characterized by coughing, chest pain, dyspnea, hemoptysis, production of sputum, and stridor. Less common symptoms include anxiety, arm and shoulder pain, headache, hoarseness, and drowsiness. There are several varieties of respiratory diseases and disorders.

Newborn and Adult Respiratory Distress Syndrome

Respiratory distress syndrome is an acute lung disease of newborns characterized by airless alveoli, inelastic lungs, a respiration rate greater than 60 breaths per minute, nasal flaring, intercostal and subcostal retractions, grunting on expiration, and peripheral edema. The condition occurs most often in premature babies. It is caused by a deficiency of pulmonary surfactant, resulting in alveolar collapse. Sometimes other symptoms include hyaline membrane formation, alveolar hemorrhage, decreased cardiac output, and severe hypoxemia. The disease is self-limited; infants either die in 3 to 5 days or recover completely with no aftereffects.

In adults, this condition causes severe pulmonary congestion characterized by diffuse injury to alveolar-capillary membranes. Fulminating sepsis, especially when gram-negative bacteria are involved, is the most common cause. Adult respiratory distress syndrome may occur after trauma, near drowning, aspiration of gastric acid, ingestion of certain herbicidal chemicals, and inhalation of corrosive chemicals (such as chlorine and ammonia) or certain drugs including barbiturates, chlordiazepoxide, heroin, methadone, propoxyphene, and salicylates.

> **POINT TO REMEMBER**
>
> Adults with sleep apnea may cease breathing for 10 to 20 seconds hundreds of times a night. The greatest danger of adult sleep apnea is the fatigue, headache, drowsiness, and depression that follows during waking hours.

Influenza

Influenza is caused by a virus and manifests itself as the most common, yet serious, acute upper respiratory tract infection in humans. Prior to acquired immunodeficiency syndrome (AIDS), influenza was the most recent uncontrolled pandemic infection in human beings. Each year in the United States, nearly 36,000 people die because of influenza-related illness during nonpandemic years. Although children are infected more than any age group, influenza causes serious illness and even death, most commonly in people aged 65 years or older.

Two types of influenza virus exist in humans: type A and type B. Type A is the most common form, causing the most severe disease symptoms. It is further divided into subtypes that are based on two surface antigens: **hemagglutinin** (H) and **neuraminidase** (N). Influenza type B does not have any subtypes. Influenza is more contagious than respiratory tract infections that arise from a bacterial source. The disease is transmitted by aerosol droplets or by direct contact with an infected person.

A person may inhale as few as three infected particles and then contract influenza. Most people who become infected will develop symptoms of influenza, which increases the likelihood of contagion. Because young children are most likely to become infected with influenza, they are also most likely to spread the infection.

Swine Flu (H1N1)

Swine flu was the original name used to describe novel H1N1, a new influenza virus that causes illness in humans. It was detected in the United States in April 2009, and also has been reported in Mexico, Canada, and other countries. This virus spreads from person to person, similar to the way that regular seasonal influenza viruses spread.

The term *swine flu* was originally used because laboratory testing showed that many genes in this new virus were very similar to influenza viruses that normally occur in pigs in North America. The virus has spread throughout the country as well as other parts of the world, and is very contagious.

The symptoms of the novel H1N1 flu virus in people are similar to the symptoms of seasonal flu and include fever, cough, sore throat, runny or stuffy nose, body aches, headache, chills, and fatigue. A significant number of people who have been infected with this virus also have reported diarrhea and vomiting. Also, like seasonal flu, severe illnesses and deaths have occurred as a result of illness associated with this virus. Vaccines that are currently available may be given either by injection or by nasal instillation.

There are everyday actions that can help prevent the spread of germs that cause respiratory illnesses like influenza. The CDC recommends the use of oseltamivir (Tamiflu) or zanamivir (Relenza) for the treatment or prevention of infection with novel H1N1 flu virus. Complications of H1N1 may include worsening of chronic conditions, such as heart disease, diabetes, asthma, pneumonia, and respiratory failure.

Asthma

Asthma is a disease that is characterized by increasing irritability of the tracheobronchial tree. It involves acute, episodic paroxysmal (sudden, intense) narrowing of the

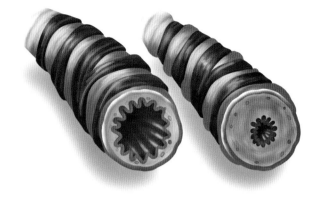

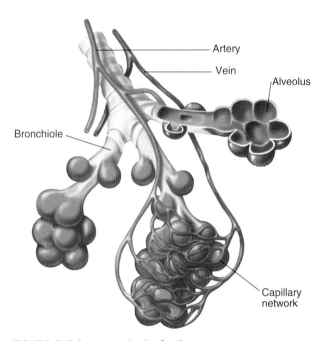

FIGURE 2–3 An acute episode of asthma.

airways. This narrowing may reverse spontaneously or as a result of pharmacologic therapy (see **Figure 2–3**). Asthma may result from either allergic or nonallergic stimuli.

Hyperreactivity in asthma may lead to airway obstruction because of acute muscle spasms in the smooth tracheobronchial tree muscles. In addition to muscle spasms, the mucosa swells, which leads to edema. The mucous glands then increase their production of thick mucous.

Bronchitis

Bronchitis is defined as inflammation of the mucous membranes of the bronchi. Bronchitis is a type of chronic obstructive pulmonary disease of the larger airways. When the airway mucosa becomes inflamed, it leads to edema and submucosal gland enlargement. Damage occurs to the epithelial cells and cilia in the respiratory tract. The most obvious symptom is the production of sputum.

Acute bronchitis has a short, severe course of duration, which subsides without any long-term effects. Chronic bronchitis leads to excessive mucous production and coughing. It can be reversed after the removal of the irritant and is complicated by respiratory tract infections. Chronic bronchitis can lead to right-sided heart failure, acute respiratory failure, and pulmonary hypertension.

Acute bronchitis is often caused by viruses, and the primary cause of chronic bronchitis is smoking or exposure to certain respiratory irritants. Risk factors include the following:

- history of smoking
- air pollution
- occupational exposure
- heredity
- reduced lung function

Children of parents who smoke are at higher risk for pulmonary infections, which may cause bronchitis.

Bronchiolitis

Bronchiolitis (respiratory syncytial viral infection) commonly affects the lower respiratory tract and is usually caused by the respiratory syncytial virus (RSV). It causes inflammation that obstructs the small respiratory airways. Bronchiolitis can range from a minor infection lasting only a few days to a severe infection causing dangerous respiratory distress. In older children and adults, usually a mild upper respiratory infection occurs because these patients have larger airways and can tolerate the swelling of the airways with fewer symptoms than when it affects infants.

Bronchiectasis

Bronchiectasis is characterized by permanent bronchi and bronchiole dilation. This occurs because of the destruction of muscle and elastic supporting tissue caused by inflammation and infection. Bronchiectasis is a secondary disease to either obstruction or a persistent infection. In past decades, necrotizing bacterial pneumonia conditions that were complications of measles, influenza, pertussis, or tuberculosis often caused

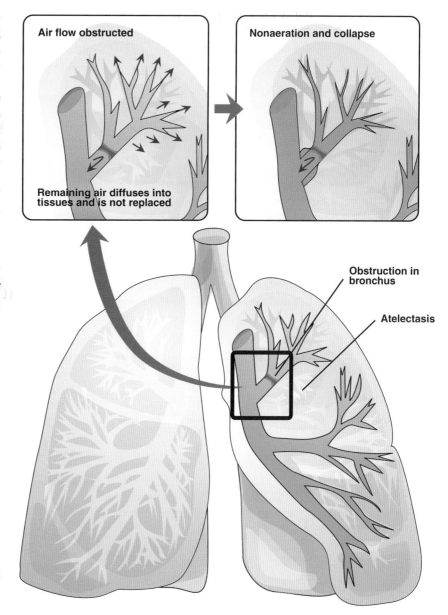

FIGURE 2–4 Obstructive atelectasis.

bronchiectasis. Today, more effective antibiotics exist to treat the conditions that previously led to bronchiectasis, so its occurrence is rarer.

Atelectasis LUNG COLLAPSE

Atelectasis is defined as imperfect expansion, which refers to incomplete expansion of a lung or part of a lung (see **Figure 2–4**). This condition can occur due to airway obstruction, increased lung recoiling (due to loss of pulmonary surfactant), or lung compression (which may occur in **pleural effusion** or **pneumothorax**). Atelectasis may be present at birth, develop in the neonatal period, or develop later in life.

Emphysema GAS EXCHANGE IS POOR

Emphysema causes the destruction of alveolar ducts, alveoli, and respiratory bronchioles, which creates enlarged air spaces. The loss of many of the alveoli reduces air exchange with the blood. As emphysema progresses, the patient experiences increased shortness of breath following only minimal exertion. The most common cause of emphysema is the inhaling of smoke from tobacco products. Stopping smoking usually stops, or at least slows, the progression of the disease. However, lung damage from emphysema is usually irreversible. Chronic obstructive pulmonary disease has, as its most common components, both emphysema and chronic bronchitis.

Cystic Fibrosis

Cystic fibrosis is a chronic dysfunction of the exocrine glands that affects multiple organ systems. The disease affects both males and females, and it is the most common fatal genetic disease in white children. Cystic fibrosis is accompanied by many complications and now carries an average life expectancy of 32 years. The disorder is characterized by chronic airway infection leading to bronchiectasis, **bronchiolectasis**, exocrine pancreatic insufficiency, intestinal dysfunction, abnormal sweat gland function, and reproductive dysfunction. Cystic fibrosis is inherited, and the gene on chromosome 7 is responsible for the disease.

Signs and symptoms may become apparent soon after birth, or they may develop in childhood. Cystic fibrosis primarily attacks the lungs and digestive system, producing copious thick, sticky mucus that accumulates to block glandular ducts. Pancreatic changes occur, with fat and fiber replacing normal tissue. Sweat gland dysfunction results in increased concentrations of salt in the sweat, and normal growth and health are reduced.

Cystic fibrosis is considered a fatal disease. However, early diagnosis and treatment have greatly increased life expectancy during the past few decades. Treatment involves supportive measures that help the child to lead as normal a life as possible, along with the prevention of pulmonary infections. lung transplant doesn't rid of CF

CO_2 floods lungs @ end of life

Pneumonia

Pneumonia is defined as lung inflammation with fluid that fills the alveoli and bronchioles. It may develop either as a primary acute lung infection or secondary to another condition that reduces lung tissue resistance (either a respiratory or systemic condition). Pneumonia is a risk after any aspiration or lung inflammation, when fluids may collect, or when defense mechanisms (such as the cilia in the trachea) are reduced.

Primary pneumonia may be caused by the inhalation or aspiration of a bacterium or virus. Bacterial pneumonia is caused by a bacterium such as staphylococcus, klebsiella, or streptococcus. Viral pneumonia is caused by a virus that attacks bronchiolar **epithelial** cells, eventually spreading to the lung alveoli. Secondary pneumonia ensues from lung damage caused by bacteria spreading from another infection (anywhere in the body) or a noxious chemical. Aspiration pneumonia occurs from the inhalation of foreign matter (such as food or vomitus) into the bronchi. An impaired **gag reflex**, old age, debilitating diseases, decreased levels of consciousness, and surgical procedures are all potential causes of aspiration pneumonia.

Legionnaires' Disease

Legionnaires' disease is a type of bronchopneumonia. It is caused by a gram-negative, rod-shaped microorganism known as *Legionella pneumophila*. It is one of the three or four most common causes of community-acquired pneumonia. The microorganism is often found in warm standing water. BACTERIA IN LUNGS

It was recognized for the first time as an epidemic of severe (and even fatal) pneumonia that developed among delegates to the 1976 American Legion convention, hence its name. The convention was held in a Philadelphia hotel, with the infection traced to the hotel's water-cooled air conditioning system. Healthy people can contract legionnaires' disease, but the risk is highest among those who smoke tobacco products and persons with chronic diseases and impaired cell-mediated immunity.

Pulmonary Vascular Disease

Vascular lung disorders include pulmonary edema, pulmonary hypertension, and pulmonary embolus, all of which are discussed in the following sections.

Pulmonary Edema Right HF

Pulmonary edema is a condition wherein fluid collects in the lung alveoli and interstitial tissues. This accumulation of fluid reduces diffused oxygen levels in the blood and interferes with the lungs' ability to expand. Pulmonary edema may result from predisposing factors, such as acute respiratory distress syndrome, heart disease, and inhalation of toxic gases. Of these factors, heart disease is the most common cause of pulmonary edema.

Pulmonary Hypertension

Pulmonary hypertension is the elevation of pressure in the pulmonary vessels. This condition is common in preexisting cardiac or pulmonary diseases, but it may also result from the condition known as **pulmonary fibrosis**. The actual cause of pulmonary hypertension is unknown, but it tends to occur in members of the same family. Conditions that produce **hypoxemia**, such as alveolar hypoventilation, chronic obstructive pulmonary disease, high altitudes, and smoke inhalation, often cause secondary pulmonary hypertension.

Pulmonary Embolism

Pulmonary embolism is a condition resulting from a blood clot or fat (lipid) deposit that has formed in a peripheral blood vessel and then broken free to lodge in a blood vessel in one of the lungs (see **Figure 2–5**). Pulmonary embolism is a potentially life-threatening condition. Its major risk factors include any conditions that produce *[not moving]* venous stasis, increased coagulation ability, or changes in the walls of blood vessels.

Pathological changes that can cause pulmonary embolism include dehydration, immobility, decreased venous return, or injury. Conditions that are related to the previously mentioned risk factors include pregnancy, **sepsis**, congestive heart failure, and tumors. *[VIRUSES]*

Tuberculosis *[MAYBE DORMANT]*

Tuberculosis is the main cause of death from a single infectious agent throughout the world. More than 8 million new cases of tuberculosis occur every year worldwide, with approximately 3 million people dying from the disease. It is caused by *Mycobacterium tuberculosis*, a bacterium resistant to destruction that can survive in calcified, necrotic lesions for long periods of time.

Tuberculosis mostly affects the lungs, but the **pathogen** can also invade other body organs, such as the bones, gastrointestinal tract, and kidneys. Tuberculosis lesions cause the death of affected tissue, which is sloughed off, and the formation of cavities.

Resistance to secondary tuberculosis depends on the patient's environment and health status. Reinfection occurs more often when a patient is malnourished, in poor health, living in crowded or unsanitary conditions, or has various other illnesses. An increase of tuberculosis has been seen in the United States due to the prevalence of human immunodeficiency virus (HIV) infection and acquired immunodeficiency syndrome (AIDS).

Histoplasmosis *[MAY BE DORMANT]*

Histoplasmosis is a fungal disease that originates in the lungs from the inhalation of dust containing *Histoplasma capsulatum*. It is common in the midwestern United States and occurs as an opportunistic infection, commonly in AIDS patients. In these cases, the fungus disseminates or spreads quickly throughout the entire body. Histoplasmosis is similar to tuberculosis in that its first stage usually involves an asymptomatic, limited infection followed by a second active infection. This second infection involves the formation of **granuloma** and necrosis and **consolidation** in the lungs, sometimes spreading to other organs.

Pneumoconiosis

Pneumoconiosis involves any change in the lungs due to inhaling inorganic dust particles (usually in the workplace). Environmentally acquired lung diseases such as

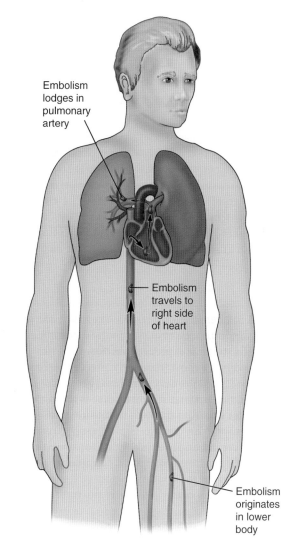

FIGURE 2–5 The development of pulmonary embolism.

pneumoconiosis relate to the patient's history of exposure, and this factor is important in correctly diagnosing the patient's individual lung condition. Pneumoconiosis often occurs after years of inhaling inorganic dust particles, resulting in progressive fibrosis of lung tissue. The most common causes of pneumoconiosis are the dusts of coal, asbestos, and silica. Other potential causes are beryllium, cadmium, cement, clays, fiberglass, cobalt, aluminum, iron, and talc. The most common types of pneumoconiosis are discussed in the following sections.

Silicosis

Silicosis affects workers who have continually inhaled the inorganic dust compound known as silicon dioxide, which is found in sand, flint, quartz, and many other stones. Silicosis is characterized by the development of nodular fibrosis in the lungs. The incidence is highest among industrial workers exposed to silica powder during manufacturing, in those who work with ceramics, sand, or stone, and in those who mine silica. Silicosis is also known as grinder's disease or quartz silicosis.

Anthracosis

Anthracosis is a chronic lung disease characterized by the deposit of coal dust in the lungs. It is also characterized by the formation of black nodules on the bronchioles that result in focal emphysema. The condition occurs in coal miners and is aggravated by cigarette smoking. There is no specific treatment for anthracosis, which is also known as black lung disease or coal worker's pneumoconiosis.

Asbestosis

Asbestosis is a chronic lung disease caused by the inhalation of asbestos fibers, resulting in the development of alveolar, interstitial, and pleural fibrosis. Asbestos miners and workers are most frequently affected. Asbestosis sometimes occurs in others who have been exposed to asbestos building materials. The disease is characterized by small linear opacities throughout the lungs, as shown on chest X-rays. The disease is progressive, results in shortness of breath, and eventually develops into respiratory failure. Cigarette smoking and continuous asbestos exposure aggravate the condition, and fatal mesothelial tumors sometimes occur. There is no treatment for asbestosis.

Berylliosis

> **POINT TO REMEMBER**
>
> Severe altitude sickness includes a condition called high-altitude pulmonary edema. This condition causes nausea and vomiting, rapid heart rate and breathing, and a cyanotic (blue) cast to the skin.

Beryllium is an element used in fluorescent powders, metal alloys, and in the nuclear power industry. A small percentage of workers exposed to beryllium dust or vapor develop an immune response, which damages the lungs. Symptoms include fever, fatigue, cough, shortness of breath, night sweats, loss of appetite, and weight loss. Radiographs show granuloma scars in the lungs, and pulmonary function tests show impaired breathing.

Respiratory Failure

Respiratory failure is the inability of the cardiovascular and pulmonary systems to maintain an adequate exchange of oxygen and carbon dioxide in the lungs. It may be caused by a failure in either oxygenation or ventilation. Oxygenation failure is characterized by hypoxemia, which can initially lead to hyperventilation.

However, oxygenation failure is not caused by hyperventilation. Oxygenation failure occurs in diseases that affect the alveoli or interstitial lung tissues. These diseases include the following:

- alveolar edema
- emphysema
- fungal infections
- leukemia
- lobar pneumonia
- lung carcinoma
- tuberculosis
- various pneumoconioses

Ventilatory failure is characterized by increased arterial carbon dioxide. Ventilation may also be reduced by the following:

- depression of the respiratory center by barbiturates or opiates
- hypercapnia
- hypoxia
- intracranial diseases
- lesion of the neuromuscular system or thoracic cage
- trauma

Respiratory failure in preexisting chronic lung diseases may be precipitated by added stress, such as with cardiac failure, anesthesia, surgery, or upper respiratory tract infections.

Pleural Disorders

The pleura is a double-layered membrane that encases the lungs. The mediastinum separates the right and left pleural cavities. Pleural disorders include pleurisy, pleural effusion, pneumothorax, hemothorax, and flail chest.

Pleurisy

Pleurisy is an inflammation of the pleura, also called pleuritis. It causes intense pain during breathing and is usually secondary to other diseases or infections. Pleurisy also may result from injury or the presence of a tumor.

Pleural Effusion

Pleural effusion is defined as the presence of excessive fluid in the pleural cavity. Normally, small amounts of fluid are present, providing lubrication for the pleural membranes. Usually only one lung is affected by pleural effusion, but sometimes both lungs are affected. This is because each lung is enclosed in a separate pleural membrane. The effects of pleural effusion depend on the amount, rate of accumulation, and type of fluid.

Pneumothorax

Pneumothorax is a collection of air or gas in the pleural cavity. This results in a collapsed or partially collapsed lung (see **Figure 2–6**). When pneumothorax is caused by

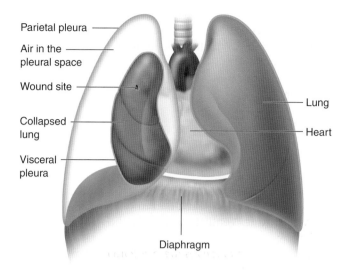

FIGURE 2–6 Pneumothorax.

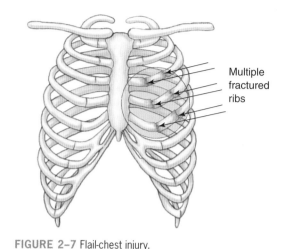

FIGURE 2–7 Flail-chest injury.

trauma or a malignant tumor, blood or fluid may also be present in the cavity. Tension pneumothorax describes a life-threatening condition of excessive pleural cavity pressure.

> **POINT TO REMEMBER**
>
> Pneumothorax may be treated by covering the chest wound with an impermeable bandage, passing a chest tube through the thoracic wall into the pleural cavity, and applying suction to the tube.

Pneumothorax can be either spontaneous or traumatic. Spontaneous pneumothorax occurs when an opening is present on a lung's surface. It can be caused by erosion of the alveoli (due to disease or tumors), increased respiratory pressure, or a spontaneous tear in tissue. Traumatic pneumothorax occurs when the pleural cavity's integrity is breached due to trauma (including stabbing, gunshots, or crushing of the chest).

Hemothorax

Hemothorax is the accumulation of blood and fluid in the pleural cavity. The patient experiences symptoms that are similar to those of pneumothorax. Hemothorax is life threatening and requires emergency medical care. Trauma or the erosion of a pulmonary vessel may cause blood to enter the pleural space. *aspirations*

Flail Chest *OPPOSITE DIRECTION*

Flail chest is a condition of instability in the chest wall due to multiple rib fractures. If it is not corrected, hypoxia will occur. The most common chest injuries occur from automobile accidents and falls (see **Figure 2–7**). This condition is characterized by sharp pain, shallow and rapid respiration, decreased breath sounds, and uneven chest expansion. Flail chest is a medical emergency and may be life threatening. *one of the hardest to treat and repair*

Lung Cancer

The lungs are common sites of both primary and secondary types of cancer. Lung cancer is the leading cause of cancer deaths in both men and women in the United States. Increases in lung cancer incidence and deaths during the past 60 years are closely related to increased smoking of tobacco products. Nearly 95% of primary lung tumors are of the type known as **bronchogenic carcinoma**. The remaining 5% includes bronchial gland tumors, fibrosarcomas, and lymphomas. The lung is also a common site of metastasis from cancers in other parts of the body. There are four major categories of bronchogenic carcinomas:

- adenocarcinoma
- large cell carcinoma
- small cell carcinoma
- squamous cell lung carcinoma

Secondhand smoke in the environment has resulted in a significant number of cases of bronchogenic carcinoma. The risk of developing cancer is higher in persons who begin smoking early in life, continue for many years, and smoke more than one pack of cigarettes per day (considered to be heavy smokers).

Not all smokers develop lung cancer; therefore, there is probably a genetic factor involved. Occupational exposure to **carcinogens** such as silica, asbestos, or vinyl chloride is another major cause of lung cancer. The risk is greatly increased if a second factor (such as cigarette smoking) is also present in an occupationally exposed individual.

Patient Education

Respiratory therapists must be up to date on the latest information concerning H1N1 flu (commonly referred to as swine flu). They should advise patients who are at highest risk of contracting H1N1 flu to be especially careful. These include pregnant women, children younger than age 5 years, adults older than age 65 years, and those with chronic medical conditions, such as diabetes, heart disease, asthma, and kidney disease. Respiratory therapists must educate patients about proper hand washing, wearing protective masks, avoiding using utensils that other family members might use, and avoiding going to work if they show signs of infection.

SUMMARY

Cardiovascular diseases include carditis, coronary artery disease, hypertension, heart failure, and myocardial infarction. Angina pectoris is a condition of chest pain often caused by anoxia, atherosclerosis, or coronary artery spasm. Hypertension is a major cause of cardiac disease, renal failure, and stroke. A common form of heart disease is called congestive heart failure, which may be related to pulmonary conditions. Common respiratory conditions include asthma, bronchitis, and emphysema—all of which are aggravated by smoking. Common forms of pulmonary vascular disease include edema, hypertension, and embolism, as well as other potentially deadly pulmonary conditions, including pneumonia, tuberculosis, histoplasmosis, and pneumoconiosis. When the lungs cannot adequately exchange oxygen and carbon dioxide, respiratory failure may occur. Lung cancer is the deadliest type of cancer in the United States.

LEARNING GOALS

These learning goals correspond to the objectives at the beginning of the chapter, providing a clear summary of the chapter's most important points.

1. Emphysema causes the destruction of alveolar ducts, alveoli, and respiratory bronchioles, causing enlarged air spaces. As emphysema progresses, the patient experiences increased shortness of breath following only minimal exertion. The most common cause of emphysema is the inhaling of smoke from tobacco products. Lung damage from emphysema is usually irreversible. Chronic obstructive pulmonary disease has, as its most common components, both emphysema and chronic bronchitis. Bronchitis is defined as inflammation of the mucous membranes of the bronchi. Bronchitis is a type of chronic obstructive pulmonary disease of the larger airways. The most obvious symptom is the production of sputum. Chronic bronchitis leads to excessive mucous production and coughing. Chronic bronchitis can lead to right-sided heart failure, acute respiratory failure, and pulmonary hypertension.

2. Atelectasis is defined as imperfect expansion, referring to incomplete expansion of a lung or part of a lung. This condition can occur due to airway obstruction, increased lung recoiling (due to loss of pulmonary surfactant), or lung compression (which may occur in pleural effusion or pneumothorax). Atelectasis may be present at birth, develop in the neonatal period, or develop later in life.

3. Acute bronchitis has a short, severe duration, which subsides without any long-term effects. Chronic bronchitis leads to excessive mucous production and coughing. It can be reversed after the removal of the irritant and is complicated by respiratory tract infections. Chronic bronchitis can lead to right-sided heart failure, acute respiratory failure, and pulmonary hypertension. Acute bronchitis is often caused by viruses, and the primary cause of chronic bronchitis is smoking or exposure to certain respiratory irritants. Risk factors include history of smoking, air pollution, occupational exposure, heredity, and reduced lung function.

4. Angina pectoris is a sudden outburst of chest pain frequently caused by myocardial anoxia, atherosclerosis, or coronary artery spasm. Anginal pain usually radiates along the neck, jaw, shoulder, and down the left arm. It is often accompanied by feelings of suffocation that may seem to indicate impending death. Angina pectoris attacks are often related to emotional stress, eating, exertion, and exposure to intense cold. Angina pectoris is also referred to as cardiac pain.

5. Increases in lung cancer incidence and deaths during the past 60 years are closely related to increased smoking of tobacco products. Secondhand smoke in the environment has resulted in a significant number of cases of bronchogenic carcinoma. The risk of developing cancer is higher in persons who begin smoking early in life, continue for many years, and smoke more than one pack of cigarettes per day (considered to be heavy smokers). Not all smokers develop lung cancer; therefore, there is probably a genetic factor involved. Occupational exposure to carcinogens, such as silica, asbestos, or vinyl chloride, is another major cause of lung cancer. The risk is greatly increased if a second factor (such as cigarette smoking) is also present in an occupationally exposed individual.

6. Endocarditis is inflammation of the inner layer of the heart, known as the endocardium. Myocarditis is inflammation of the middle layer of the heart, known as the myocardium. Myocarditis is the type of carditis that is most likely to

cause sudden death. Pericarditis is inflammation of the outer layer of the heart, known as the pericardium.

7. Left-sided heart failure is caused by ineffective left ventricular contraction. As the left ventricle's pumping ability fails, cardiac output falls. Because blood is no longer effectively pumped out, it backs up into the left atrium and then into the lungs. This causes activity intolerance and dyspnea. If the condition persists, pulmonary edema and right-sided heart failure can result. Common causes of left-sided heart failure include hypertension, aortic and mitral valve stenosis, and left ventricular infarction.

   Right-sided heart failure is caused by ineffective right ventricular contraction. As a result, blood is not pumped with enough force through the right ventricle to the lungs. This causes blood to back up into the right atrium as well as the peripheral circulation. The patient gains weight, develops peripheral edema, and the kidneys (and other organs) become engorged. Right-sided heart failure may be caused by pulmonary hypertension, pulmonary embolus, or acute right ventricular infarction.

8. A dysrhythmia (arrhythmia) is a disturbance of heart rhythm. Common causes of arrhythmias include congenital defects, drug toxicity, electrolyte imbalances, and myocardial infarction or ischemia.

9. Pulmonary edema is a condition wherein fluid collects in the lung alveoli and interstitial tissues. This accumulation of fluid reduces diffused oxygen levels in the blood and interferes with the lungs' ability to expand. Pulmonary edema may result from predisposing factors, such as acute respiratory distress syndrome, heart disease, and inhalation of toxic gases. Of these factors, heart disease is the most common cause of pulmonary edema.

10. An emboli may cause eventual death if untreated. When an embolism occurs in the pulmonary system, it may be caused by any conditions that produce venous stasis, increased coagulation ability, or changes in the walls of blood vessels. Pathological changes that can cause pulmonary embolism include dehydration, immobility, decreased venous return, or injury. Conditions that are related to the previously mentioned risk factors include pregnancy, sepsis, congestive heart failure, and tumors.

CRITICAL THINKING QUESTIONS

1. Explain why there is an extensive network of capillaries in skeletal muscles and in the liver.
2. Explain why an embolus may cause a larger infarction than an atheroma with a thrombus.
3. Describe how cystic fibrosis affects the lungs and the sweat glands.
4. List the factors that interfere with oxygenation of the blood in patients with emphysema.

WEB SITES

http://hypertensionweb.info/result.php?Keywords=Hypertension

http://www.cancer.org/docroot/PED/content/PED_10_2X_Cigarette_Smoking.asp

http://www.cdc.gov/niosh/topics/pneumoconioses/

http://www.emedicinehealth.com/angina_pectoris/article_em.htm

http://www.healthnewsflash.com/conditions/respiratory_failure.php

http://www.lungcancer.org/

http://www.medicinenet.com/high_blood_pressure/article.htm

http://www.nei.nih.gov/health/histoplasmosis/index.asp

http://www.webmd.com/asthma/

http://www.webmd.com/a-to-z-guides/pneumonia-topic-overview

REVIEW QUESTIONS

Multiple Choice

Select the best response to each question.

1. Cancer in which of the following sites is the leading cause of cancer death in males?
   A. prostate
   B. pancreas
   C. lung
   D. colon

2. Chronic dilation and distention of the bronchial walls is called
   A. hemoptysis
   B. pneumoconiosis
   C. bronchiectasis
   D. atelectasis

3. An area of dead cells due to lack of oxygen is called
   A. ischemia
   B. infarction
   C. atresia
   D. gangrene

4. A collection of air or gas in the pleural cavity that results in a collapsed lung is referred to as
   A. emphysema
   B. pneumoconiosis
   C. bronchiectasis
   D. pneumothorax

5. When the heart is pumping inadequately to meet the needs of the body, the condition is called
   A. cor pulmonal
   B. congestive heart failure
   C. arrhythmia
   D. myocardial infarction

6. An abnormally slow heart rate is known as
   A. bradycardia
   B. tachycardia
   C. heart block
   D. ventricular fibrillation

7. Stasis of blood flow from immobility, injury to a vessel, or predisposition to clot formation increases the risk of
   A. pulmonary embolism
   B. emphysema
   C. pneumothorax
   D. chronic obstructive pulmonary disease

8. Which of the following is an occupational disease that causes progressive, chronic inflammation and infection in the lungs due to inhalation of inorganic dust?
   A. emphysema
   B. pneumothorax
   C. pneumoconiosis
   D. bronchiectasis

9. Fluid shift into the extravascular spaces of the lungs with accompanying dyspnea and coughing is indicative of
   A. myocardial infarction
   B. pulmonary edema
   C. angina pectoris
   D. pneumothorax

10. Which of the following is a common disease of the lower respiratory tract that frequently is caused by the respiratory syncytial viral infection?
    A. bronchiolitis
    B. atelectasis
    C. bronchiectasis
    D. pulmonary edema

11. Which of the following is a major cause of cardiac disease, renal failure, and stroke?
    A. emphysema
    B. heart failure
    C. hypertension
    D. asthma

12. Which of the following is the most common cause of emphysema?
    A. bronchogenic cancer
    B. pneumothorax
    C. pulmonary edema
    D. smoking cigarettes

13. Which of the following cardiovascular disorders is the leading cause of death in the United States?
    A. myocardial infarction
    B. hypertension
    C. stroke
    D. angina pectoris

14. Which of the following is the cause of primary pulmonary hypertension?
    A. hypoxemia
    B. pulmonary embolism
    C. pneumonia
    D. unknown

15. Tuberculosis primarily affects the
    A. brain
    B. liver
    C. kidneys
    D. lungs

CASE STUDY

A 52-year-old man who worked for 15 years in the nuclear power industry began to have symptoms of lung problems, including coughing, shortness of breath, fatigue, loss of appetite, fever, night sweats, and weight loss. Chest X-rays showed granuloma scars in his lungs. His pulmonary function tests revealed impaired breathing.

1. What is the probable diagnosis of his condition?
2. What medication should this patient receive to relieve his symptoms?

Principles of Pharmacology

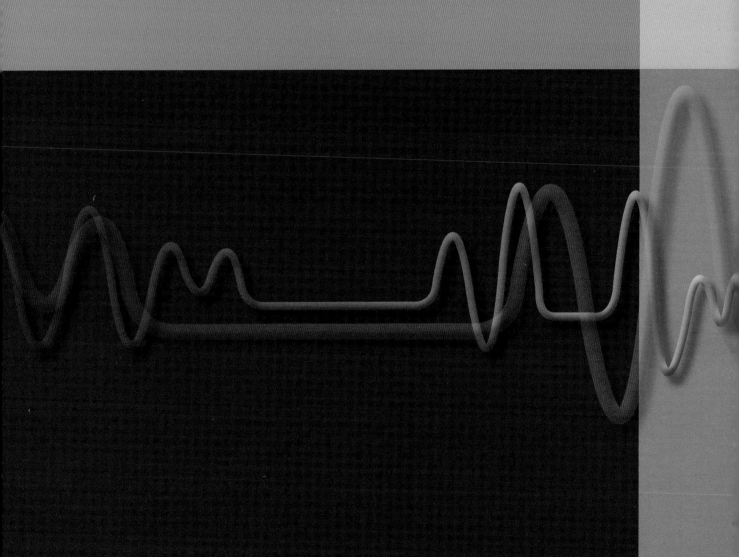

Fundamentals of Pharmacology

OUTLINE

OBJECTIVES

Upon completion of this chapter, the reader should be able to do the following:

1. Describe drug names and classifications.
2. Define prefixes and suffixes.
3. Explain abbreviations used in pharmacology.
4. Explain the Orphan Drug Act.
5. Explain how, under the Combat Methamphetamine Epidemic Act, ephedrine and pseudoephedrine must be stored and sold.
6. Describe the items contained in a prescription.
7. List the generic names for the top 10 most commonly used brand name drugs in the United States.
8. For each of the following controlled substances, list the drug schedule in which it appears: anabolic steroids, cough medicines with codeine, diazepam, marijuana, and methamphetamine.
9. Define controlled substances and drug schedules.
10. Explain a medication administration record.

KEY TERMS

Abbreviations	Heredity
Biopharmaceutical	Prototype
Genes	Standing orders

INTRODUCTION

Pharmacology may be defined as the study of medicinal substances. It involves the actions of these substances upon humans and animals. Drug therapy is used to diagnose, cure, treat, or reduce the symptoms of disease. Pharmacology utilizes knowledge of drug properties, anatomy, physiology, pathology, and the mechanisms of drug actions. Pulmonary care practitioners must be familiar with the fundamentals of pharmacology, a brief history of pharmacology, terminology, abbreviations, the content of prescriptions, and drug classifications. They also must be knowledgeable about drug names and controlled substances.

History of Pharmacology

For centuries, humans have used plants to treat various illnesses. As far back as 3000 BC, people in various countries, such as Egypt, India, China, and Mesopotamia, documented their knowledge of pharmaceutical properties. The *Papyrus Ebers* (pronounced pah-PY-rus EE-bers) of 1550 BC was an Egyptian document that listed more than 700 medical compounds and more than 800 prescriptions. In China, the *Pen T'sao Ching* (pronounced PEN SOW CHING) of 2750 BC lists more than 1000 medicinal compounds and more than 11,000 prescriptions. Likewise in India, the *Dravyaguna* (pronounced drahv-yah-GOO-nah) of 2500 BC lists hundreds of medicinal materials and their sources, uses, and properties.

The father of pharmacology was a Greek physician known as Theophrastus (pronounced thee-oh-FRAS-tus) who lived circa 300 BC. He is credited as such because of his study of plants and their uses in medicine. Another Greek physician, Dioscorides (pronounced dee-os-coh-REE-des) complied the *De Materia Medica*, which lists more than 600 medicinal plants including some still in use today (such as belladonna and opium).

In the 20th century, many new medicinal substances were discovered, including insulin, antiretrovirals, and anti-infectives. Study began to focus on **genes** and **heredity** in determining how they affect the progression of specific diseases. Bioengineering has been developed to produce **biopharmaceutical** agents, such as human insulin and erythropoietin. A brief time line of the history of pharmacology is shown in **Table 3–1.**

Terminology

Pulmonary care practitioners must understand the language of medicine. This is based on medical terminology that was originated by mostly Greek and Latin sources. Word parts used in medicine include prefixes, roots, and suffixes. Pulmonary care practitioners must learn general pharmacological terms and concepts and understand common medical terms, abbreviations, and word building.

Prefixes

A prefix is a structure at the beginning of a word that modifies the word's root. **Table 3–2** shows common general prefixes.

Word Roots

A word root is the main part of a word. The root gives the word its central meaning. It is the basic foundation, which can be modified by adding prefixes or suffixes. Examples of word roots that are used in Table 3–2 are partum, biotic, lateral, scopic, dermic, etc.

Suffixes

A suffix is a word ending that modifies the meaning of a root. **Table 3–3** shows common general suffixes.

Combining Vowels

Medical terms are formed by utilizing many different word parts. Often these parts are joined by combining vowels. The most common combining vowel is the letter

> **POINT TO REMEMBER**
>
> If a vowel comes before the letter *x*, such as *ax* or *ix*, change the *x* to the letter *c*. Thus, the word *thorax* (chest) can be enlarged into the word *thoracotomy* (incision into the chest). Also, the word *cervix* (neck) can be enlarged into the word *cervical* (pertaining to the neck).

TABLE 3–1 Time Line of the History of Pharmacology		
2750 BC	Shen Nung	Chinese emperor who wrote the *Pen T'sao Ching*
2500 BC	*Dravyaguna*	Indian manuscript of medicinal herbs
1550 BC	*Papyrus Ebers*	Egyptian manuscript that lists hundreds of medical compounds and prescriptions; may be as old as circa 3000 BC
400 BC	Hippocrates	The father of medicine
300 BC	Theophrastus	The Greek father of pharmacology
120 to 200 AD	Galen	The father of pharmacotherapy
Circa 1500 AD	Paracelsus	The father of the pharmaceutical revolution
1700s	Discoveries of medicines	The following were discovered during this period: digitalis, iodine, quinine, nicotine, etc.
1800s	Louis Pasteur	Proved that microorganisms cause disease, and they can be killed by heat
1900s	Modern discoveries	Insulin for the treatment of diabetes; sulfonamide becomes the first anti-infective; penicillin is produced from a fungus; and the Bayer company develops diuretics, anti-infectives, and other drugs

o, and occasionally the letter *i* is a combining vowel. For example, *o* serves as the combining vowel in the term *chemotherapy*:

chem / o / therapy

Vocabulary

Common vocabulary terms used for respiratory system disorders are shown in **Table 3–4**.

Common vocabulary terms for pharmacology are shown in **Table 3–5**.

TABLE 3–2 Common General Prefixes

Prefix	Meaning	Example
Ante-	Before	Antepartum
Anti-	Against	Antibiotic
Bi-	Two, both	Bilateral
Endo-	Into, within	Endoscopic
Epi-	Upon, above	Epidermic
Hemi-	Half, one side	Hemisphere
Multi-	Many	Multigravida
Poly-	Many, much	Polymorphous
Quadri-	Four	Quadriplegia
Semi-	Half	Semiconscious
Tetra-	Four parts	Tetralogy
Ultra-	Beyond, excessive	Ultrasound

TABLE 3–3 Common General Suffixes

Suffix	Meaning	Example
-ectomy	Excision, removal	Splenectomy
-emesis	Vomiting	Hyperemesis
-ic	Neurotic	Pertaining to a neurosis
-ism	Condition	Cryptorchidism
-itis	Inflammation	Pericarditis
-logy	Study of	Physiology
-oma	Tumor	Sarcoma
-pathy	Disease	Myopathy
-phobia	Abnormal fear	Hydrophobia
-scope	Instrument used to view	Ophthalmoscope
-stasis	Stopping or controlling	Hemostasis
-tomy	Incision into	Phlebotomy

Abbreviations

Abbreviations are shortened forms of words or phrases. Respiratory care practitioners must memorize many different abbreviations that relate to their practice.

> **POINT TO REMEMBER**
>
> An acronym is an abbreviation. The use of an acronym may save time; however, an acronym can also cause confusion if it is not universally understood.

Common Medical Abbreviations

Table 3–6 lists the abbreviations commonly used in the field of respiratory care.

Common Abbreviations Used in Prescriptions

Abbreviations that are commonly used in prescriptions are listed in **Table 3–7**.

Common Abbreviations for Measurements

Abbreviations that are commonly used for measurements are listed in **Table 3–8**.

Abbreviations to Be Avoided

In 2004, The Joint Commission issued a list of abbreviations that should be avoided for the safety of patients. This includes abbreviations, acronyms, and symbols that may be confused, easily misinterpreted, or that may have more than one meaning. **Table 3–9** shows The Joint Commission's abbreviation recommendations.

Another organization, the Institute for Safe Medication Practices (ISMP), has established its own list of other potentially dangerous abbreviations, acronyms, and symbols. The most commonly used terms are shown in **Table 3–10**.

Prescription Ingredients

Prescriptions are most effective when they are clearly written and contain specific, required information. Their ingredients relate to five of the seven rights of drug administration (right patient, right drug, right dose, right route, and right time). A prescription's ingredients include the following:

- the patient's name and address
- the prescriber's office address
- the date of the prescription
- the medication that is being prescribed (the inscription)
- the Rx symbol (the superscription)
- the directions concerning dispensing for the pharmacist (the subscription)

TABLE 3-4 Common Vocabulary Terms for Respiratory Disorders

Term	Definition
Acute pulmonary disease	A medical condition characterized by an abrupt onset and short duration
Acute rhinitis	Severe inflammation of the nasal mucosa
Aspiration	Accidental inhalation of food or foreign materials into the lungs
Asthma	Respiratory disease caused by spasm of the bronchial tubes or by swelling of bronchial tube mucous membranes
Atelectasis	Incomplete expansion of a lung or part of a lung
Bronchiectasis	Chronic dilation of one or more bronchi
Bronchitis	Inflammation of a bronchus
Chronic obstructive pulmonary disease (COPD)	A group of respiratory diseases that are chronic and progressive, including asthma, bronchiectasis, bronchitis, and emphysema
Cyanosis	Bluish skin discoloration due to lack of blood oxygen
Cystic fibrosis	An inherited disease characterized by mucus accumulating in the bronchi
Diphtheria	Acute upper respiratory disease with formation of a surface pseudomembrane of cells and coagulates
Dyspnea	Difficult or labored breathing
Emphysema	A COPD with enlargement and destruction of alveoli
Hemothorax	Blood in the pleural space
Hydrothorax	Fluid in the pleural space
Hyperventilation	Increased breathing rate and depth
Hypoventilation	Decreased breathing rate and depth
Influenza	Acute, contagious respiratory infection; also known as the flu
Pertussis	Whooping cough; an acute, infectious condition
Pleural effusion	Fluid that may contain blood or pus in the pleural space
Pleurisy	Pleuritis; inflammation of the pleura around the lungs
Pneumoconiosis	Respiratory tract disease caused by inhalation of various types of dust particles
Pneumonia	Inflammation of the lungs caused by an infection
Pneumonitis	Inflammation of the lungs because of allergies, asthma, infections, or inhalation of irritants
Pneumothorax	Air or gas in the pleural space
Pyothorax	Pus in the pleural space
Respiratory distress syndrome	A condition affecting infants who were born with insufficient amounts of surfactant in the lungs
Sudden infant death syndrome	Crib death; the sudden, unexplained death of an otherwise healthy infant
Tuberculosis	A bacterial infection that usually involves the lungs but may also affect other organs and become life threatening

TABLE 3–5 Common Vocabulary Terms for Pharmacology

Term	Definition
Analgesic	An agent that relieves pain
Anesthetic	An agent that prevents sensation of pain
Antacid	An agent that neutralizes stomach acid
Antiarrhythmic	An agent that normalizes heartbeat rhythm
Antibiotic (or anti-infective)	An agent that slows or stops the growth of microorganisms
Anticholinergic	An agent that blocks parasympathetic nerve impulses
Anticoagulant	An agent that prevents blood clotting
Anticonvulsant	An agent that relieves or controls convulsion (seizures)
Antidepressant	An agent that relieves depression
Antidiabetic	An agent that reduces glucose
Antidiarrheal	An agent that relieves diarrhea
Antidote	An agent that counteracts another drug
Antiemetic	An agent that relieves or prevents nausea and vomiting
Antifungal	An agent that slows or stops the growth of fungi
Antihelmintic (or anthelmintic)	An agent that slows or stops the growth of parasitic worms
Antihistamine	An agent that relieves symptoms of allergies
Antihypertensive	An agent that reduces blood pressure
Anti-inflammatory	An agent that reduces inflammation
Antilipidemic	An agent that lowers blood lipids
Antineoplastic	An agent that poisons cancer cells
Antipsychotic	An agent that controls symptoms of psychosis
Antipyretic	An agent that reduces fever
Antiseptic	An agent that inhibits growth of microorganisms
Antitussive	An agent that inhibits coughing
Bronchodilator	An agent that dilates bronchial airways in the lungs
Cathartic (laxative)	An agent that induces defecation to alleviate constipation
Contraceptive	An agent that reduces the risk of pregnancy
Decongestant	An agent that relieves nasal swelling and congestion
Diuretic	An agent that increases urine output, which reduces blood pressure and cardiac output
Expectorant	An agent that thins bronchial mucus, allowing expectoration of mucus as well as phlegm and sputum
Hemostatic	An agent that controls or stops bleeding by promoting coagulation
Hormone replacement	An agent that replaces hormones to resolve deficiency
Hypnotic (sedative)	An agent that induces sleep or relaxation based on the dosage
Muscle relaxant	An agent that relaxes skeletal muscles
Mydriatic	An agent that constricts blood vessels (such as in the eye or nasal passage) to raise blood pressure; also dilates the pupils when included in ophthalmic preparations
Stimulant	An agent that affects the central nervous system to increase activity of the brain and other organs; also decreases appetite
Vasoconstrictor	An agent that constricts blood vessels to increase blood pressure
Vasodilator	An agent that dilates blood vessels to decrease blood pressure

TABLE 3-6 Common Medical Abbreviations

Abbreviation	Meaning	Abbreviation	Meaning
A&P	Auscultation and percussion	GSW	Gunshot wound
Abd	Abdomen	HIV	Human immunodeficiency virus
ABE	Acute bacterial endocarditis	HTN	Hypertension
ABGs	Arterial blood gases	Hx	History
ACS	Acute cardiac syndrome	ICU	Intensive care unit
Adm	Admission	IHD	Ischemic heart disease
A-Fib	Atrial fibrillation	Lat	Lateral
AHD	Arteriosclerotic heart disease	LLL	Left lower lobe
AI	Aortic insufficiency	LOC	Loss of consciousness
AIDS	Acquired immunodeficiency syndrome	LUL	Left upper lobe
Amb	Ambulatory	MI	Myocardial infarction
AMI	Acute myocardial infarction	MVP	Mitral valve prolapse
ARDS	Adult respiratory distress syndrome	N&V	Nausea and vomiting
ASCVD	Arteriosclerotic cardiovascular disease	O_2	Oxygen
ASD	Atrial septal defect	OP	Outpatient
ASHD	Arteriosclerotic heart disease	OR	Operating room
BA	Bronchial asthma	OSA	Obstructive sleep apnea
BBB	Bundle branch block	PE	Pulmonary embolism
BP	Blood pressure	Peds	Pediatrics
BR	Bed rest	PEEP	Positive end expiratory pressure
Bx	Biopsy	PFTs	Pulmonary function tests
CA	Cancer; carcinoma	PICU	Pediatric intensive care unit
CABG	Coronary artery bypass graft	PRBC	Packed red blood cells
CAD	Coronary artery disease	Pt	Patient
CBC	Complete blood count	Px	Prognosis
CCU	Coronary care unit	RBC	Red blood cell
CF	Cystic fibrosis	resp	Respirations
CHD	Coronary heart disease	RLL	Right lower lobe
CHF	Congestive heart failure	RR	Recovery room
CO	Carbon monoxide	RT	Respiratory therapy
CO_2	Carbon dioxide	RUL	Right upper lobe
COLD	Chronic obstructive lung disease	RXT	Radiation therapy
COPD	Chronic obstructive pulmonary disease	SARS	Severe acute respiratory syndrome
CPR	Cardiopulmonary resuscitation	SICU	Surgical intensive care unit
CRD	Chronic respiratory disease	SIDS	Sudden infant death syndrome
CVA	Cerebrovascular accident	SVN	Small-volume nebulizer
DVT	Deep vein thrombosis	TB	Tuberculosis
Dx	Diagnosis	trach	Tracheostomy
ECG or EKG	Electrocardiogram	Tx	Treatment
Echo	Echocardiogram	URI	Upper respiratory infection
Flu	Influenza	VS	Vital signs
Fx	Fracture	WBC	White blood cell

TABLE 3-7 Common Abbreviations Used in Prescriptions

Abbreviation	Meaning
®	Right; registered trademark
a	Before
a.c.	Before meals
ad lib.	As desired
AM, a.m.	Morning
amt	Amount
aq	Water
b.i.d., BID	Twice a day
buc	Buccal
c̄	With
cap	Capsule
d	Day
Fl.	Fluid
h, hr	Hour
h.s.	At bedtime; at the hour of sleep
ID	Intradermal
IM	Intramuscular
IV	Intravenous
noc., n.	Night
NPO	Nothing by mouth
oint., ung.	Ointment
p̄	After
p.c.	After meals
per	By; through
PM, p.m.	After noon
p.o., P.O.	By mouth
PR	Through the rectum
p.r.n., PRN	As needed
PV, vag.	Through the vagina
q	Every
q2h	Every two hours
qh	Every hour
q.i.d., QID (Note: The Joint Commission now recommends that these abbreviations be avoided)	Four times a day
Rx	Prescription; take
s̄	Without
SC, sub-Q, SQ, subcu	Subcutaneous
Sig:	Instruction to patient
soln.	Solution
sp.	Spirits
s̄s̄	One-half
stat	Immediately
supp., suppos.	Suppository
syr.	Syrup
T	Topical
tab	Tablet
t.i.d., TID	Three times a day
x	Times; for

TABLE 3-8 Common Abbreviations for Measurements

Abbreviation	Meaning
C	Celsius
cc	Cubic centimeter
dr	Dram
F	Fahrenheit
fl dr	Fluidram
fl oz	Fluidounce
g or gm	Gram
gal	Gallon
gr	Grain
gtt	Drop
kg	Kilogram
L	Liter
lb	Pound
mcg	Microgram
mg	Milligram
min	Minim
mL or ml	Milliliter
oz	Ounce
pt	Pint
qt	Quart

- the directions for the patient (the signa)
- refill information (repetatur) and special labeling
- the prescriber's signature and license or Drug Enforcement Administration (DEA) number

A sample prescription is shown in **Figure 3-1**.

In Figure 3-1, the blue colored letters to the left signify the following ingredients of the prescription: (a) the prescriber's office name, address, phone number, and DEA number; (b) the patient's name, address, and date of the prescription; (c) the superscription (the Rx symbol); (d) the inscription (the main part of a prescription); (e) the subscription (instructions to the pharmacist by the physician about which drugs and quantities are to be used); (f) the signa (sig.), which the pharmacist will translate into instructions for the patient, such as "Take one tablet by mouth three times per day"; (g) the signature area (where the prescriber signs the prescription); (h) the repetatur (which tells how many refills; note that none of the choices are marked or circled, which indicates that no refills are allowed); and (i) the label instructions area (which tells the pharmacist how to

TABLE 3-9 The Joint Commission's Abbreviations to Be Avoided

Abbreviation	Meaning	Reason	Suggestion
A.S., A.D., A.U.	Left ear, right ear, both ears	Can be mistaken for O.S., O.D., O.U.	Write out *left ear*, *right ear*, or *both ears*
c.c. or cc	Cubic centimeter	Can be mistaken for U (units)	Use *mL* for milliliter instead because it is the equivalent unit
D/C	Discharge	Can be interpreted as discontinue whatever medications follow	Write out *discharge*
H.S.	Half-strength or hour of sleep (bedtime)	Meanings can be mistaken for each other; also, if q.H.S. is used, it can be mistaken for every hour	Write out *half-strength* or *at bedtime*
IU	International unit	Can be mistaken as IV or the number 10	Write out *international unit*
μg	Microgram	Can be mistaken for milligrams, resulting in a massive overdose	Write out *mcg*
MS, MSO$_4$, MgSO$_4$	Morphine sulfate or magnesium sulfate	Meanings can be confused for one another	Write out *morphine sulfate* or *magnesium sulfate*
O.S., O.D., O.U.	Left eye, right eye, both eyes	Can be mistaken for A.S., A.D., A.U.	Write out *left eye*, *right eye*, or *both eyes*
Q.D., Q.O.D., QD, QOD, qd, qod, q.d., q.o.d.	Once daily; once every other day	Meanings can be mistaken for one another; the period after the letter Q may be mistaken for the letter I, and the letter O may be mistaken for the letter I	Write out *daily* and *every other day*
QID, Q.I.D., qid, q.i.d.	Four times a day	Can be mistaken for QOD, qod, Q.O.D., q.o.d.	Write out *four times a day*
S.C. or S.Q.	Subcutaneous	Can be mistaken for SL (sublingual) or 5 every	Write out *Sub-Q*, *subQ*, or *subcutaneously*
T.I.W.	Three times a week	Can be mistaken for three times a day or twice weekly	Write out *3 times weekly* or *three times weekly*
U	Unit	Can be mistaken for zero, four, or cc	Write out *unit*
x.0 mg or .x mg	Trailing zero or lack of a leading zero	The decimal point may not be seen, causing incorrect dosing	Never write a zero by itself after a decimal point; always use a zero before a decimal point

TABLE 3-10 ISMP's Abbreviations to Be Avoided

Abbreviation	Meaning	Reason	Suggestion
ʒ	Dram	Can be misread as the number 3	Use the metric system instead
> or <	Greater than or less than	Meanings can easily be confused with each other	Use the terms *greater than* and *less than*
/	Slash mark; separates two doses or indicates the term *per*	Can be misread as the number 1	Do not use; instead, use the term *per*
AZT	Zidovudine (Retrovir)	Can be misread as azathioprine	Write out the drug name
BT	Bedtime	Can be mistaken as BID (twice daily)	Use *hs* instead
CPZ	Prochlorperazine (Compazine)	Can be misread as chlorpromazine	Write out the drug name
o.d.	Once daily	Can be misread as right eye	Use the word *daily* instead
per os	Orally	The os can be misread as left eye	Use *PO*, *by mouth*, or *orally* instead
qhs	Nightly at bedtime	Can be misread as every hour	Use *nightly* instead
qn	Nightly or at bedtime	Can be misread as qh (every hour)	Use *nightly* instead
ss	Sliding scale (when using insulin) or ½ (in the apothecary system)	Can be mistaken for the number 55	Spell out *sliding scale*, *one-half*, or use the fraction ½
x3d	For three days	Can be mistaken for three doses	Use the phrase *for three days*

label the medication; note that there are no specific labeling instructions listed).

Sometimes a physician must prescribe a medication for a patient who will take it at another time besides when the patient can be present. This is true when a physician phones in a prescription to a pharmacist to be filled or even to a nurse who will then administer the medication to the patient. When this occurs, the physician must, as soon as possible, write out the drug order on a prescription pad, sign it, and make sure that the pharmacist or nurse receives it. The physician's actual signature must be on these follow-up written prescriptions. In certain care settings, standing orders are used. These are written orders left by physicians as ongoing prescriptions. They are still required to be properly written, dated, and signed, as with all other types of prescriptions.

A			**Dr. Greg Roberts and Associates** 1111 First Ave., Melbourne FL 32901 (321) 555-0000 CR1424326
B	Name	John Jones	
	Address	99 Smith St.	Melbourne, FL 32935
	Date	7/11/2010	
C	℞		
D		Lopid 600 mg Tabs	
E		60	
F		Sig 600 mg PO tid	
G	Generic Substitution Allowed Dispense As Written		Greg Roberts, M.D. _____, M.D.
H	REPETATUR 0 1 2 3 PRN		
I	LABEL		

FIGURE 3–1 Sample prescription.

Medication Administration Records

POINT TO REMEMBER

An order written in the chart of a hospital patient is considered a legal prescription when it is signed by the physician.

Medication administration records (also known as individually as a MAR) are the forms upon which prescriptions are transcribed in hospitals. In the hospital, a prescription is usually first written on a drug chart or physician order sheet and then transcribed onto the MAR. These documents may be many pages in length to cover the different medications administered to each patient. These forms require the following:

- Approved drug names must be used.
- Existing orders should not be altered.
- When drugs were administered or not administered, this information must be recorded with the reasons for the actions.
- IV fluid orders must be recorded on a separate IV order chart.
- Nurse-initiated therapies must be countersigned by a physician (these include administration of antacids, mild analgesics, laxatives, etc.).

A sample MAR is shown in **Figure 3–2**.

Drug Classifications

Drugs are commonly classified according to either their therapeutic classification or their pharmacological classification. The therapeutic classification refers to exactly what conditions the drug is used to treat. Examples of therapeutic classifications include antianginals, anticoagulants, antidysrhythmics, antihyperlipidemics, and antihypertensives. The pharmacological classification refers to how the drug works in the body's systems, tissues, and molecules. Examples of pharmacological classifications include adrenergic antagonists, angiotensin-converting enzyme inhibitors, calcium channel blockers, diuretics, and vasodilators.

A drug's mechanism of action is how it produces its effects in the body. Pharmacological classifications are more specific than therapeutic classifications because they define the actual effects of the drug being used. A prototype drug is one that other drugs in the same pharmacological class are compared to. For example, penicillin V is the prototype to which all other types of penicillins are compared. It is important that pulmonary care practitioners become familiar with the various prototype drugs in each class that they use in their daily work.

Drug Names

Drugs have three basic types of names: chemical, generic, and trade names. A drug's chemical name is unique and one of a kind, but it is often complicated and lengthy. Rather than using many drugs' entire chemical names, they are often classified by a chemical group name that uses part of their chemical structure, such as cephalosporins, fluoroquinolones, benzodiazepines, and thiazides.

In the United States, a drug's generic name is assigned by the U.S. Adopted Name Council. Generic names are less complicated than chemical names. There is only one generic name for each drug. Generic names are also known as nonproprietary names. Examples of generic names include diphenhydramine, ibuprofen, acetaminophen, diazepam, and alprazolam. Generic names are usually expressed in only lowercase letters.

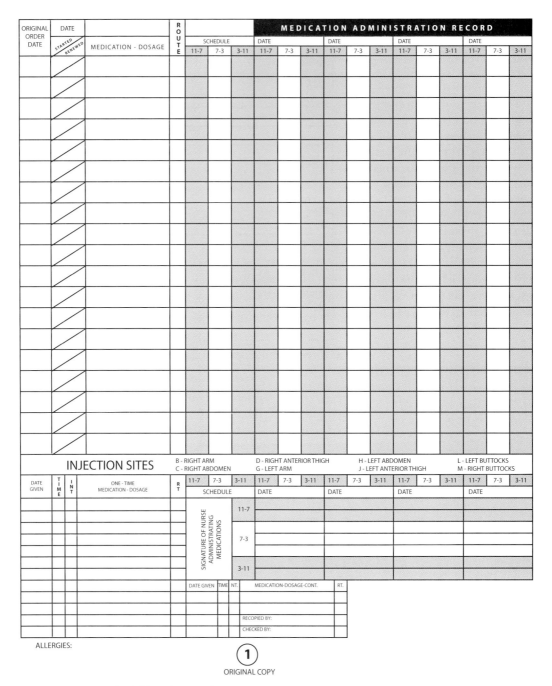

FIGURE 3–2 Medical administration record.

A drug's trade name is created by a manufacturer to establish a product name that belongs to them. Trade names are also known as brand names, product names, and proprietary names. Drug manufacturers in the United States have exclusive rights to name and market a drug for 17 years after they submit their new drug application to the Food and Drug Administration (FDA).

There may be many different trade names for the same generic drug after this period has passed. Trade names of drugs are usually capitalized. The following list shows examples of generic names (shown first) and their related trade names (shown second):

- diphenhydramine: Benadryl, Aler-Tab, Dytuss, etc.
- ibuprofen: Advil, Motrin, Nurofen, etc.
- acetaminophen: Tylenol, Actamin, Tactanol, etc.
- diazepam: Valium
- alprazolam: Xanax, Niravam, etc.

It is also important to understand combination drugs, which are those that may contain more than one active, generic ingredient. It is vital to check the active ingredients in drugs to ascertain whether they contain more than one of these ingredients. Medication errors may be prevented more effectively if possible interactions, contraindications, and adverse effects for each active ingredient are understood before a drug is prescribed or purchased over the counter (OTC). **Table 3–11** shows generic and brand names of the 100 most commonly used drugs in the United States.

Drug Legislation

The Pure Food and Drugs Act (1906) paved the way for many different laws that regulated drug manufacture and distribution. The Food, Drug, and Cosmetic Act (1938) required manufacturers to ensure the purity, strength, safety, and packaging of foods, drugs, and cosmetics. It also gave the FDA the power to approve or deny new drug applications and ensure compliance via inspections. The Durham-Humphrey Amendment (1951) separated legend drugs (those requiring a prescription bearing the Rx symbol) from over-the-counter (OTC) drugs (those that can safely be used without a prescription or supervision by a healthcare practitioner). The Kefauver-Harris Amendment (1962) requires drugs to be safe and effective, meaning that investigational new drugs cannot be sold to the general public until their clinical studies have proven them safe and effective.

The Comprehensive Drug Abuse Prevention and Control Act (1970) required the maintenance of physical security and strict record keeping for many drugs. It divided controlled substances into five schedules based upon the abuse and addiction potential of various drugs. Controlled substances are those with restricted use in the United States, as defined by the Controlled Substances Act of 1970. Those who prescribe controlled substances must be registered with the DEA to obtain them legally. The drug schedules are shown in **Table 3–12**.

The Poison Prevention Packaging Act (1970) created standards for child-resistant packaging, which affected nearly all legend drugs and a few OTC drugs. The Occupational Safety and Health Act (OSHA) (1970) was designed to help prevent workplace disease and injuries and requires all employers to ensure protective standards. The Drug Listing Act (1972) assigned a unique, permanent National Drug Code (NDC) number to identify manufacturers, distributors, drug formulations, and packaging.

The Orphan Drug Act (1983) offered federal financial incentives to manufacturers to develop new drugs that affect less than 200,000 patients in the United States. Such orphan drugs have included those used to treat AIDS, blepharospasm, cystic fibrosis, and snakebites. The Drug Price Competition and Patent Term Restoration Act (1984) streamlined the drug approval process for drugs that are no longer patented. Normally, a manufacturer has 20 years of exclusivity to produce a proprietary drug until the patent protection expires. The Prescription Drug Marketing Act (1987) ensures that prescription drug products are safe, effective, untainted, not counterfeited, and not misbranded.

The Omnibus Budget Reconciliation Act (1990) reduced Medicaid costs and created a tax limit cap on taxable income for Medicare patients. The Anabolic Steroids Control Act (1990) regulated these substances that are used to promote muscle growth and curbed their illegal use by athletes. The Health Insurance Portability and Accountability Act (HIPAA) (1996) was designed to improve continuity and portability of health insurance and to improve healthcare insurance and records administration.

More recently, the Medicare Prescription Drug, Improvement, and Modernization Act (2003) overhauled Medicare and introduced tax breaks and subsidies for prescription drugs. The Combat Methamphetamine Epidemic Act (2005) was designed to stop the illegal manufacture and use of crystal meth and the drug products that are combined to create this illegal drug. Drugs that are regulated by this act must be kept secure, behind a counter or in a locked case. Customers who buy ephedrine or pseudoephedrine (which may be used to illegally manufacture crystal meth) must provide their identification and sign a logbook that tracks the sale of these substances.

Patient Education

Respiratory therapists should educate patients about their prescriptions, instruct them to keep prescriptions out of the reach of children, and store them in an appropriate location. For example, if a medication must be kept in a refrigerator, it should not be stored at room temperature except when being administered. The use of medical terminology that the patient may not be familiar with should be avoided. Common medical abbreviations should also be avoided when educating patients.

SUMMARY

As far back as 3000 BC, humans have used plants to treat various illnesses. The Greek physician Theophrastus is considered the father of pharmacology because of his study of plants and their uses in medicine. In more recent times, many new sources of medicines have been developed, including the use of bioengineering to develop biopharmaceutical agents. Pharmacological terms include word parts such as prefixes, roots, suffixes, and combining vowels. Pharmacologic agents are commonly classified according to either their therapeutic classification or their pharmacological classification. Drugs have three basic types of names: chemical, generic, and trade names. There is only one chemical name and one

TABLE 3–11 Commonly Used Drugs (Generic and Brand Names)

Number	Generic Name	Brand Name	Number	Generic Name	Brand Name
1	atorvastatin	Lipitor	41	alprazolam	Xanax
2	hydrocodone / acetaminophen	Vicodin	42	ezetimibe	Zetia
3	hydrocodone / acetaminophen	Lortab 2.5/500	43	fluoxetine	Sarafem
4	levothyroxine sodium	Levothroid	44	fenofibrate	Tricor
5	amoxicillin	Amoxil	45	trazodone	Desyrel
6	lisinopril	Prinivil	46	ztenolol	Tenormin
7	esomeprazole magnesium	Nexium	47	celecoxib	Celebrex
8	levothyroxine sodium	Synthroid	48	insulin glargine	Lantus
9	escitalopram oxalate	Lexapro	49	amlodipine besylate / atorvastatin	Caduet
10	montelukast sodium	Singulair	50	zolpidem	Ambien
11	clopidogrel	Plavix	51	metoprolol succinate	Toprol XL
12	simvastatin	Zocor	52	lisinopril / hydrochlorothiazide	Pinzide
13	hydrochlorothiazide / triamterene	Dyazide	53	mometasone	Nasonex
14	amlodipine	Norvasc	54	prednisone	Dectasone
15	azithromycin	Zithromax	55	propoxyphene napsylate / acetaminophen	Darvocet-N
16	warfarin	Coumadin	56	clonazepam	Klonopin
17	furosemide	Lasix	57	albuterol	AccuNeb
18	azithromycin	Zmax	58	sertraline hydrochloride	Sertraline
19	levothyroxine sodium	Levoxyl	59	ibuprofen	Motrin
20	fluticasone	Advair Diskus	60	hydrochlorothiazide	Microzide
21	metoprolol tartrate	Lopressor	61	alprazolam	Niravam
22	valsartan	Diovan	62	pregabalin	Lyrica
23	venlafaxine (extended-release)	Effexor XR	63	donepezil	Aricept
24	rosuvastatin	Crestor	64	drospirenone / ethinyl estradiol	Yaz-28
25	oxycodone / acetaminophen	Percocet	65	metoprolol	Dutoprol
26	cephalexin	Keflex	66	gabapentin	Neurotin
27	hydrochlorothiazide	Lopressor HCT	67	alprazolam	Xanax XR
28	albuterol	ProAir HFA	68	sildenafil	Viagra
29	metformin	Fortamet	69	oxycodone / acetaminophen	Roxicet
30	ezetimibe / simvastatin	Vytorin	70	acetaminophen / codeine	Tylenol-Codeine
31	lansoprazole	Prevacid	71	amoxicillin / clavulanate potassium	Augmentin
32	quetiapine	Seroquel	72	omeprazole	Prilosec
33	simvastatin /niacin (extended-release)	Simcor	73	alendronate sodium	Fosamax
34	duloxetine	Cymbalta	74	losartan	Cozaar
35	sertraline	Zoloft	75	conjugated estrogens	Premarin
36	valsartan / hydrochlorothiazide	Diovan HCT	76	risedronate	Actonel
37	levofloxacin	Levaquin	77	valacyclovir	Valtrex
38	lisinopril	Zestril	78	hydrocodone / acetaminophen	Norco
39	tamsulosin	Flomax	79	atenolol	Tenormin I.V.
40	pioglitazone	Actos	80	tramadol hydrochloride	Tramadol Hydrochloride

TABLE 3-11 (Continued)

Number	Generic Name	Brand Name	Number	Generic Name	Brand Name
81	amlodipine besylate/benazepril	Lotrel	90	fexofenadine	Allegra
82	linisopril/hydrochlorothiazide	Zestoretic	91	zolpidem	Ambien CR
83	amphetamine/dexgtroamphetamine mixed salts	Adderall XR	92	fluticasone propionate	Flovent
			93	pantoprazole sodium	Protonix I.V.
84	metoprolol tartrate/hydrochlorothiazide	Lopressor HCT	94	tiotropium bromide	Spiriva HandiHaler
			95	triamterene	Dyrenium
85	paroxetine	Paxil	96	methylphenidate extended-release	Concerta
86	omeprazole/sodium bicarbonate	Zegerid	97	clonidine	Catapres
87	topiramate	Topamax	98	atenolol	Tenormin
88	amoxicillin	Augmentin Chewable Tablets	99	olmesartan	Benicar
89	metformin	Glumetza	100	lantanoprost	Xalatan

TABLE 3-12 Drug Schedules

Schedule	Abuse Level	Dependence Level	Examples	Prescription Requirement
I	Highest	High	Heroin, LSD, marijuana, methaqualone, etc.	No prescription permitted
II	High	High	Morphine, PCP, cocaine, methadone, methamphetamine, etc.	Prescription required; no refills permitted without a new written prescription
III	Medium	Medium to high	Anabolic steroids, codeine, hydrocodone, certain barbiturates, etc.	Prescription required; five refills permitted in 6 months
IV	Low	Low	Diazepam, alprazolam, pentazocine, meprobamate, etc.	Prescription required; five refills permitted in 6 months
V	Lowest	Lowest	OTC cough medicines that contain codeine	No prescription required, with a few exceptions

generic name for each drug, but the same drug may have many different trade names. Controlled substances are those with restricted use in the United States, and they are listed in five drug schedules based primarily on their potential for addiction and abuse.

Until 1906, there was no drug legislation in the United States. Congress passed the Pure Food and Drugs Act in that year to regulate drug manufacture and distribution. The Durham-Humphrey Amendment of 1951 separated legend drugs from OTC drugs. The Comprehensive Drug Abuse Prevention and Control Act of 1970 divided controlled substances into five schedules based on abuse and addiction potentials. The Poison Prevention Packaging Act of 1970 created standards for child-resistant packaging. The Drug Listing Act of 1972 assigned National Drug Code (NDC) numbers to drugs that identify manufacturers, distributors, formulations, and packaging. The Combat Methamphetamine Epidemic Act of 2005 was designed to stop the illegal manufacture of crystal meth by regulating the legal drug products used to make it.

LEARNING GOALS

These learning goals correspond to the objectives at the beginning of the chapter, providing a clear summary of the chapter's most important points.

1. Drugs have three basic types of names: chemical, generic, and trade names. A drug's chemical

name is unique and one of a kind, but it is often complicated and lengthy. In the United States, a drug's generic name is assigned by the U.S. Adopted Names Council. There is only one generic name for each drug. Generic names are also known as nonproprietary names. Generic names are usually expressed only in lowercase letters. A drug's trade name is created by a manufacturer to establish a product name that belongs to them. Trade names are also known as brand names, product names, and proprietary names. There may be many different trade names for the same generic drug after this period has passed. The trade names of drugs are usually capitalized.

2. A prefix is a structure at the beginning of a word that modifies the word's root. A suffix is a word ending that modifies the meaning of a root.

3. Abbreviations are shortened forms of words or phrases. Respiratory care practitioners must memorize many different abbreviations that relate to their practice. Most abbreviations used in pharmacology consist of between two and five characters, with three characters most often being used for each abbreviation.

4. The Orphan Drug Act (1983) offered federal financial incentives to manufacturers to develop new drugs that affect less than 200,000 patients in the United States. Such orphan drugs have included those used to treat AIDS, blepharospasm, cystic fibrosis, and snakebites.

5. Because ephedrine and pseudoephedrine are commonly used to illegally manufacture crystal meth, these drugs must be kept secure, behind a counter or in a locked case. Customers who buy ephedrine or pseudoephedrine must provide their identification and sign a logbook that tracks the sale of these substances.

6. A prescription's ingredients include the following: patient's name and address, prescriber's office address, date of the prescription, medication that is being prescribed (the inscription), Rx symbol (the superscription), directions concerning dispensing for the pharmacist (the subscription), directions for the patient (the signa), refill information (repetatur) and special labeling, the prescriber's signature, and the prescriber's license or Drug Enforcement Administration (DEA) number.

7. The top 10 generic and brand name drugs in the United States are as follows (in order of rank): atorvastatin (Lipitor), hydrocodone/acetaminophen (Vicodin), hydrocodone/acetaminophen (Lortab 2.5/500), levothyroxine sodium (Levothroid), amoxicillin (Amoxil), lisinopril (Prinivil), esomeprazole magnesium (Nexium),

levothyroxine sodium (Synthroid), escitalopram oxalate (Lexapro), and montelukast sodium (Singulair).

8. Each of the following controlled substances are included in the indicated schedule: anabolic steroids (Schedule III), cough medicines with codeine (Schedule V), diazepam (Schedule IV), marijuana (Schedule I), and methamphetamine (Schedule II).

9. Controlled substances are those with restricted use in the United States, as controlled by the Controlled Substances Act of 1970. Those who prescribe controlled substances must be registered with the Drug Enforcement Administration (DEA) to obtain them legally. Because many drugs have a high potential for abuse and addiction, drug schedules have been adopted that list these substances and classify them accordingly.

10. Medication administration records (also known individually as a MAR) are the forms upon which prescriptions are transcribed in hospitals. In the hospital, a prescription is usually first written on a drug chart or physician order sheet and then transcribed onto the MAR. These documents may be many pages in length to cover the different medications administered to each patient.

CRITICAL THINKING QUESTIONS

1. Why are certain drugs classified in schedules? What extra precautions must be taken by practitioners when prescribing scheduled drugs?

2. If a pharmacist decides to switch from a trade name drug that was ordered by the physician to a generic equivalent drug, what advantages does this substitution have for the patient? What disadvantages might be caused by the switch?

WEB SITES

http://media.wiley.com/product_data/excerpt/95/04712335/0471233595.pdf

http://pubs.acs.org/subscribe/journals/mdd/v04/i05/html/05timeline.html

http://www.biologie.uni-hamburg.de/b-online/e01/01a.htm

http://www.biopharma.com/biopharmacopeia/

http://www.bostonreed.com/students/coursematerials/cma/medterm1–2.pdf

http://www.ciesin.org/docs/002–256c/002–256c.html

http://www.deadiversion.usdoj.gov/schedules/

http://www.macroevolution.net/medical-suffixes.html

http://www.medilexicon.com/medicalabbreviations.php

http://www.medword.com/prefixes.html

http://www.nicd.us/nicddrugclassifications.html

http://www.rxlist.com/script/main/hp.asp

REVIEW QUESTIONS

Multiple Choice

Select the best response to each question.

1. A prefix is
   A. the first part of a word
   B. a word structure at the end of a term that modifies the root
   C. a word structure at the beginning of a term that modifies the root
   D. the last part of a word that gives the word its root meaning

2. An agent that relieves symptoms of allergies is called an
   A. antiemetic
   B. antihistamine
   C. anti-inflammatory
   D. anticholinergic

3. Drugs with high abuse potential and no accepted medical use are classified in Schedule
   A. I
   B. II
   C. III
   D. IV

4. The abbreviation for the word *treatment* is
   A. Dx
   B. Tx
   C. Px
   D. Bx

5. Which of the following acts classified legend and OTC drugs?
   A. Kefauver-Harris Amendment
   B. Drug Listing Act
   C. Comprehensive Drug Abuse Prevention and Control Act
   D. Durham-Humphrey Amendment

6. Which of the following agents relieves nasal swelling and blockage?
   A. decongestant
   B. diuretic
   C. bronchodilator
   D. anticoagulant

7. Heroin is an example of a drug from which schedule?
   A. Schedule II
   B. Schedule I
   C. Schedule V
   D. Schedule III

8. Which of the following suffixes means inflammation?
   A. -iasis
   B. -trophy
   C. -itis
   D. -desis

9. The five controlled substance schedules were established by which of the following acts?
   A. Harrison Narcotics Tax Act
   B. Drug Regulation Reform Act
   C. Drug Listing Act
   D. Comprehensive Drug Abuse Prevention and Control Act

10. The prefix hemi- means
    A. two, both
    B. half, one side
    C. into, within
    D. beyond, excessive

11. Which of the following abbreviations used in prescriptions means as needed?
    A. PRN
    B. NPO
    C. Stat
    D. BID

12. The part of a prescription that includes directions for the pharmacist is referred to as the
    A. inscription
    B. superscription
    C. signature
    D. subscription

13. The brand name of albuterol is
    A. Toprol
    B. Proventil
    C. Zithromax
    D. Tenormin

14. An inherited disease characterized by mucus accumulating in the bronchi is known as
    A. bronchiectasis
    B. atelectasis
    C. emphysema
    D. cystic fibrosis

15. A condition affecting infants who were born with insufficient amounts of surfactant in the lungs is known as
    A. sudden infant death syndrome
    B. respiratory distress syndrome
    C. pneumoconiosis
    D. cystic fibrosis

CASE STUDY

A pharmacist decides to switch a patient's prescription from a trade name drug (that was ordered by the physician) to a generic-equivalent drug.

1. What advantages may this substitution have for the patient?
2. What disadvantages might be caused by this substitution?

Biopharmaceutics

OBJECTIVES

Upon completion of this chapter, the reader should be able to do the following:

1. Explain the mechanisms of drug actions.
2. Discuss the factors that influence a patient's response to drug therapy.
3. Describe the metabolism of drugs.
4. Discuss anaphylactic reactions.
5. Define and differentiate the terms *adverse effects* and *side effects* of drugs.
6. Identify the four components of pharmacokinetics.
7. Explain drug allergies.
8. Discuss how drugs are distributed throughout the body.
9. Define the term *idiosyncratic reaction*.
10. Explain the excretion of drugs through the kidneys.

KEY TERMS

Absorption	Efficacy
Adverse effects	Excretion
Affinity	First-pass effect
Agonist	Half-life
Albumin	Lipophilic
Antagonist	Metabolism
Bioavailability	Metabolites
Biotransformation	Potency
Blood–brain barrier	Receptor
Clearance	Side effects
Distribution	Therapeutic effects
Dose–effect relationship	Therapeutic index

INTRODUCTION

Medications are given to achieve desirable effects within the body. For this to occur, the drug must reach its target cells. This is an easy task for certain medications, such as topical agents used for superficial skin conditions. Other medications have more difficulty in reaching target cells in sufficient quantities to cause a physiological change. Some medications affect the body more rapidly than other medications. A medication may affect one patient dramatically but have no affect or a different affect on another patient. Sometimes the difference between drug effects in different patients can be predicted based on pharmacokinetic principles.

Pharmacodynamics

Pharmacodynamics is the study of how drugs interact with their sites of action. It examines how drugs bind with their receptors, the concentration that is needed to obtain a response, and the amount of time required for each of these events to occur. To determine a drug's pharmacologic actions, the blood is the most commonly tested bodily fluid. Drugs are absorbed into the bloodstream and metabolized before they reach their site of action. A drug's therapeutic effects and its adverse effects are influenced by the processes of absorption, metabolism, reabsorption, and excretion. Pharmacodynamics, along with pharmacokinetics (discussed later in this chapter) help determine the dose–effect relationship of a drug. There are variable factors that influence the dose of a drug, including potency and efficacy, the effective dose, lethal dose, and therapeutic index.

- Potency and efficacy: Potency describes the amount of a drug that must be given to produce a particular response. A highly potent drug can produce its effect with only a small amount. A drug's affinity is related to its potency. Drugs bind to a receptor for which they have a high affinity in small amounts. They are therefore highly potent. Efficacy describes how well a drug produces its desired effect.
- Effective dose: Each patient responds to a specific drug dose differently. To determine what constitutes a usual dose, the doses needed to cause a response in a large number of people from different populations is statistically calculated. The dose required to produce the therapeutic response in 50% of the population is called the effective dose 50% (ED_{50}). This dose is considered the standard or typical dose, and it is usually chosen as the starting dose.

> **POINT TO REMEMBER**
>
> The effect of a drug in the body's fluids may be determined by the relationship between the amount of the drug in the body and the drug concentration.

- Lethal dose: The lethal dose of a drug is computed in a laboratory setting and analyzed statistically. The point at which a drug's dose would be fatal in 50% of the population is called lethal dose 50% (LD_{50}).
- Therapeutic index: To determine drug safety, the ED_{50} is compared to the LD_{50}. The relationship of these two doses is called a drug's therapeutic index (TI). It can be explained by the following equation:

$$TI = \frac{ED_{50}}{LD_{50}}$$

If the amount required for the ED_{50} is similar to the amount required for the LD_{50}, the mathematical ratio of these two values will be a number close to 1. For example, if the ED_{50} is 99 mg and the LD_{50} is 100 mg, the therapeutic index would be computed as follows:

$$TI = \frac{99}{100}$$

Therefore, the TI = 0.99, which can be rounded to 1.00.

When the ED_{50} and the LD_{50} do not differ greatly, the drug is considered to have a narrow therapeutic index. These drugs are not considered to be very safe. Accurate doses are difficult to determine because the dose needed to be effective in half of the population can also potentially kill half of the population.

Drug Action

Drugs alter how cells, tissues, and even microorganisms function in the body. Every drug has a unique affinity for a target receptor (cell recipient). These receptors are usually specific proteins. Receptors may be located in cell membranes or within the cell's cytoplasm, or they may be intracellular. When the drug binds to its receptor, either an agonist or antagonist reaction is produced.

An agonist is a drug that binds to a specific receptor, producing a stimulatory response. This is similar to how hormones and other endogenous substances actually work. Adrenaline is an example of an agonist at beta adrenoceptors (β-adrenoceptors); it stimulates the heart rate, thus causing it to increase.

An antagonist is a drug that prevents an agonist from binding to its specific receptor. This action blocks the effects of the agonist. Antagonists themselves have no pharmacologic actions that are controlled by receptors. Propranolol is an example of an antagonist at β-adrenoceptors, which causes the opposite effect of adrenaline and prevents the heart rate from increasing. There are two main subtypes of β-adrenoceptors called $β_1$ and $β_2$. It is important to understand that some antagonists target both types, and some only target one of them.

Factors Affecting Drug Action

Various factors determine how a drug will affect the human body. These factors, listed in the following sections, should be taken into consideration when determining the correct drugs for each patient.

Age

Age often affects the body's metabolism. This means that drug effects vary according to each patient's metabolic rate. Drug dosages, therefore, may require adjustment for children and the elderly. For safety, remember the following rule of thumb: start low and go slow.

Gender

Females and males have different responses to drugs due to a variety of factors. Men absorb intramuscular drugs more quickly than women, but these same drugs stay in a female's tissues longer than in men's tissues because women have a higher body fat content.

Body Weight
The weight of a patient influences how dosages of medication affect the body. Correct drug dosages must be calculated accurately so that the patient is not over- or undermedicated. This is especially true for children because they have much lower body weight than adults. The most accurate method of determining a child's correct drug dosage is by considering his or her body surface area, which is done by using a chart called a nomogram.

Drug Half-Life
The half-life of a drug is the major determining factor of the length of its action in the body. The longer the half-life, the longer the drug stays in the body. Each drug's half-life is different. The half-life of a drug is expressed in equations as "t ½" and refers to how long the blood or plasma concentration of the drug takes to decrease from full concentration to one-half (50%) concentration.

Diurnal Body Rhythms
Diurnal body rhythms, also called circadian rhythms, influence how a drug affects each patient. These rhythms adjust the body for periods of wakefulness and sleep. When the body starts to adjust itself for sleep at nighttime, the effects of sedatives are increased as a result. Drugs with the reverse effect are better administered during the day.

Diseases
Certain diseases may greatly affect drug action. This is true because in the body, the liver is the main site of detoxification, and the kidneys are responsible for most of the elimination of chemicals. Thus, any patient with a disease affecting the liver or kidneys may have altered responses to certain drugs as compared to healthy individuals.

Adverse Effects and Side Effects of Drugs

Harmful, unexpected effects caused by a drug are referred to as adverse effects. This term differs from the term side effects, which refers to effects that were not necessarily intended (and may be either beneficial or harmful). Adverse drug reactions (which include nausea, vomiting, or diarrhea) are responses to a drug that may be noxious, unintended, and may occur at normal dose levels. These reactions may be responded to by discontinuing the drug, hospitalizing the patient, modifying the dose, or providing supportive treatment. Among the elderly, adverse drug reactions commonly cause morbidity and mortality. In children, they exist partially due to the lack of new drug studies in this population.

Drug Interactions

Drug interactions occur when a drug's effects are altered by another drug's effects. This may result in either an increased or decreased effect of the drug in question. Sometimes, both drugs' effects are altered, and sometimes the drug interaction may actually be beneficial. Examples of drug interactions include the following:

- Amiodarone: can reduce metabolism of warfarin to increase anticoagulant effects
- Carbamazepine: can reduce anticoagulant effects of warfarin
- Phenytoin: when used with phenobarbital, results in both drugs' effects being altered
- Diuretics: when used with ACE inhibitors, become more beneficial when treating hypertension

Drug Allergies

Drug allergies are abnormal responses to drugs that occur in a small number of individuals. Allergic reactions may be characterized by previous exposure to the same or a chemically-related drug, with rapid development of an allergic reaction after reexposure. The term *hypersensitivity* is often used synonymously with the term *allergy*. A drug allergy may be difficult to diagnose because no reliable laboratory tests exist to identify the causative drug, and symptoms of a drug allergy may resemble symptoms of infectious diseases. Drug intolerance must be ruled out when determining whether a patient has a specific drug allergy. Drug allergies may cause the following classifications of reactions:

- Class I: immediate hypersensitivity (e.g., penicillins, streptomycin)
- Class II: antibody dependent, cytotoxic (e.g., quinine, quinidine)
- Class III: complex mediated (e.g., anticonvulsants, antibiotics)
- Class IV: cell mediated or delayed hypersensitivity (e.g., local anesthetic creams, antihistamine creams)

Anaphylactic Reactions

The term *anaphylactic shock* is defined as an idiosyncratic, severe, sudden allergic reaction that may be life threatening. Anaphylactic reactions commonly cause a sharp loss of blood pressure, urticaria (skin rash), diaphragm paralysis, and oropharynx swelling. The end result of an anaphylactic reaction can be cardiac collapse. Therefore, these reactions signify a true medical emergency. They can occur very rapidly. As a result, a thorough history of previous allergic reactions to drugs, serum, blood transfusions, or vaccines must be obtained from every patient before use of a medication. The drug frequently used to combat anaphylactic shock, which must be administered quickly after shock begins, is epinephrine (adrenaline).

Idiosyncratic Reactions

Idiosyncratic reactions are strange, unique, unpredicted drug reactions. They may be caused by enzyme deficiencies due to genetics and hormone imbalances. An example is the drug carisoprodol, which may cause transient quadriplegia, dizziness, and temporary vision loss.

Synergism

Synergism occurs when two drugs combine to produce an effect greater than that which would have been expected from the two drugs acting separately. This may be harmful or beneficial. Examples of synergism include the following:

- Trimethoprim: With sulfamethoxazole, these drugs become more effective against infections than either drug alone.
- Aspirin: With warfarin, this combination can reduce blood clotting to result in hemorrhaging if their doses are not controlled carefully.

Tolerance

Drug tolerance is the development of resistance to a drug's effects to the degree that doses must be raised continually to achieve the desired response. Drug tolerance often occurs with abused drugs, such as nitrates, barbiturates, alcohol, opiates, and tobacco. Cross-tolerance occurs when a patient develops a resistance to chemically similar drugs. Dependence is often confused with tolerance. However, dependence refers to the drug's ability to stimulate the brain and cause the patient to desire more or continued use of the drug.

Potentiation

Potentiation is an interaction between two drugs that causes a greater effect than the effect that would occur from the additive properties of the two drugs. An example is alcohol, which potentiates the sedative effects of diazepam when ingested at the same time.

Cumulative Effect

A cumulative effect occurs when the body cannot completely metabolize and excrete one dose of a drug before the next dose is given. As the doses are repeated, the drug collects in the blood and tissues, resulting in cumulative toxicity. This may occur rapidly or slowly over time. Ethyl alcohol accumulates rapidly in the body, and lead poisoning occurs slowly.

Toxicity and Overdose

Toxicity is the state of being noxious. It refers to a drug's ability to poison the body. A drug that has the opposite effect and can reverse the toxic symptoms is known as an antidote. A drug overdose is a toxic dose of a drug that harms the patient. Overdoses may occur through medication errors, poor judgment, or as the result of attempted suicide. Any drug can act like a poison if taken in too large a dose.

Pharmacokinetics

Pharmacokinetics is the movement of a drug's particles inside the body and the processes that occur during this movement. In general, pharmacokinetics describes the affect of the body on a specific drug. Pharmacokinetics is made up of four phases: absorption, distribution, metabolism, and excretion. The science of pharmacokinetics explains, in many cases, why different people have different reactions to the same drug.

> **POINT TO REMEMBER**
>
> Pharmacokinetics can be thought of as what the body does to a drug.

Drug Absorption

Absorption is the movement of a drug from the site of administration into the bloodstream. Drug absorption depends on a drug's ability to cross the cellular membranes and resist stomach, liver, or intestinal breakdown. Presystemic metabolism affects the amount of a drug that can reach the systemic metabolism intact and how fast this happens. This concept is the definition of the term **bioavailability**, which is dependant upon pharmaceutical factors (such as rate of dissolution) and variable factors in the gastrointestinal tract (such as the presence or lack of food). The small intestine absorbs most drugs because it has a very large surface area that drugs can diffuse across.

> **POINT TO REMEMBER**
>
> Drug metabolism refers to the body's process of transforming drugs.

Factors Affecting Absorption

Several variables affect the completeness and rate of a drug's absorption. The completeness of absorption describes the portion of the drug that is absorbed. Drugs given orally may not be completely absorbed because of other drugs in the body or because of food that is ingested before or after taking the drug.

Routes of Administration

The rate of absorption of a drug depends on the route of administration. This rate is also affected by the speed at which the drug dissolves, which is known as the rate of dissolution. The routes of administration and their absorptions rates are as follows:

- Drugs administered orally generally take the longest to be absorbed because they must be broken down into small particles before they can move into the bloodstream. The presence of other drugs or food may impair the rate of oral drug absorption. Orally administered medications are usually absorbed in the upper gastrointestinal tract, immediately exposing them to metabolism by liver enzymes prior to reaching systemic circulation. This process is called the **first-pass effect**. Medications that are metabolized too quickly in the liver should not be given orally; they should be administered parenterally instead. Drugs administered parenterally bypass the liver and directly enter the systemic circulation. The advantages of oral administration include convenience and fewer abrupt changes of serum drug concentrations than with parenteral administration. Disadvantages include first-pass metabolism by the liver and systemic exposure to the drug.

- Drugs given parenterally are already dissolved and are in a liquid form. Therefore, these drugs are absorbed more rapidly than drugs given orally.
- Drugs administered subcutaneously or intramuscularly are absorbed into the body's small capillaries fairly rapidly. Intramuscular absorption is somewhat more rapid than subcutaneous absorption.
- Drugs administered intravenously are placed directly into the bloodstream and are not technically absorbed. However, some sources describe IV drugs as being instantly absorbed.

The rate of absorption is increased by large surface areas; therefore, most orally-administered drugs are absorbed in the small intestine because it has a larger surface area than the stomach. The greater the volume of blood flow, the faster absorption occurs. Increased blood flow carries more absorbed particles of a drug into the general circulation. High concentrations of a drug move into areas of the blood system where there are low concentrations of the drug. Patients with impaired circulation absorb drugs less rapidly than those with normal circulation. Lipid solubility also affects how a drug is absorbed. Drugs with higher lipid solubility are absorbed more rapidly than drugs with lower lipid solubility. When the pH at the site of administration and in the blood plasma are different, the drug molecules may or may not be ionized in the plasma more quickly. Absorption is more rapid when ionization occurs in the plasma than when it does not occur. A patient's physiologic condition affects drug absorption because of the following factors:

- Health condition: Diseases, trauma, exercise, and drug therapy all have varying effects.
- Contact time and absorptive surface: Absorptive surfaces may be affected by radiation, disease, or surgery.
- Gastrointestinal factors: Absorption may be affected by the presence of food, constipation, or diarrhea.
- Age and gender: Many drugs are metabolized very slowly in both young children and the elderly. Also, women's stomachs empty solids more slowly than liquids, and they have lower gastric acidity and lower gastric levels of alcohol dehydrogenase than men.
- Diet and lifestyle habits: High acidity, application of heat or massage, shock, and vasoconstriction all affect absorption.

Different administration sites affect how biologic fluids absorb different drugs. This is because each drug's solubility and thermodynamics are unique. These physiochemical properties should be taken into account when considering the drug's absorption rates.

Presence of Food

Food in the stomach or intestine is an important consideration concerning drug absorption. Many medications are absorbed more slowly if food is present than if the stomach or intestine is relatively empty. Because food acts as a buffer against irritation, medications that cause irritation should be taken with food.

Stomach Acidity

The difference between the stomach and intestine when it comes to absorption of drugs is easy to remember. The stomach is acidic, and the intestine is alkaline (basic). Drugs that are acidic, such as aspirin, are more readily absorbed in the stomach. Drugs that are alkaline are more readily absorbed in the intestine. It is also important to remember that the stomach's pH is influenced by consuming milk products and antacids. Thus, certain drugs should not be taken with these products. Infants who drink milk or formula may need to be given certain drugs when their stomach is empty.

Drug Distribution

Distribution is the movement of a drug through the bloodstream into the tissues and eventually into the cells. Drug distribution throughout the body depends on blood flow to the kidneys, the drug's ability to leave the blood, and the drug's ability to enter the cells.

After the drug has moved through the blood to the tissues, it leaves the bloodstream and enters the tissues themselves. This transition is necessary because most drugs do not produce their effects while in the blood. The drug moves from the vascular space in the capillary bed. Because the capillary wall cells have fairly wide spaces between them, drug molecules easily move between the cells to leave the capillaries and enter the tissues.

Many drugs bind to circulating proteins, specifically albumin. Because albumin is a large molecule, it cannot pass through capillary walls. Therefore, when the drug particle is attached to the albumin, the drug is prevented from passing through the capillary walls. Changes in protein binding can affect rates of drug distribution. Drugs that are lipid soluble enter the central nervous system (CNS) quickly. However, some drugs are more poorly distributed to the CNS because they must pass through the blood–brain barrier.

The purpose of the blood–brain barrier is to keep toxins and poisons from reaching the brain. This mechanism promotes health in normal situations, but sometimes it prevents the treatment of certain conditions. For example, many antibiotics cannot cross the blood–brain barrier. This

> **POINT TO REMEMBER**
>
> Some drugs are actively or passively transported by carrier proteins, but the movement of drugs across cell membranes is conducted by diffusion.

makes treatment of life-threatening brain infections (such as bacterial meningitis) difficult.

The placental membrane (which separates the maternal circulation from the fetal circulation) is not as strong as the blood–brain barrier. Any drug that can pass through a membrane can pass through the placenta. To do this, however, the drug must be lipophilic, not ionized, and not protein bound.

Drug Metabolism

Metabolism is the conversion of a drug into another substance or substances. Drug metabolism occurs primarily in the liver. Some metabolism also occurs in other tissues, most notably the gastrointestinal tract, lungs, kidneys, and skin. When drugs are metabolized, they are changed from their original form to a new form. The process of conversion of drugs is known as biotransformation.

Microsomal enzymes convert most drugs into metabolites during metabolism, primarily in the liver. Cytochrome P-450 describes specific liver enzymes essential for metabolism of drugs, which results in end products known as metabolites. Active metabolites may affect either pharmacologic action or a drug's adverse effects. Toxic drugs can be influenced by drug metabolism, which includes the duration of drug effects, drug interactions, drug activation, drug toxicity, and adverse effects.

POINT TO REMEMBER
In response to the chronic administration of certain drugs, the liver will increase its enzyme production.

Drug Excretion

POINT TO REMEMBER
The majority of drugs are eliminated through the kidneys. Therefore, good renal function is essential.

Excretion is the removal of a drug, or what the drug became after metabolism, from the body. The most common route of drug excretion is through the urine. Other routes include bile in the gastrointestinal (GI) tract, air exhaled from the lungs, breast milk, sweat from the skin, tears, feces, and saliva. Sweat and saliva are not therapeutically important routes of excretion. Diseases of the kidneys, such as renal failure, decrease the effectiveness of the kidneys in drug excretion.

Drug Clearance

Several pharmacokinetic factors work together to affect the rate in which drug molecules disappear from the circulation. This rate is called the clearance rate of a drug. The major modes of drug clearance are renal excretion and hepatic metabolism. Some drugs are cleared mostly by one mechanism, and certain drugs are cleared by both mechanisms actively.

A patient's gender can also affect the clearance of some drugs. In women, some drugs are cleared more rapidly (such as erythromycin, theophylline, and clozapine). Other drugs are cleared more rapidly in men (such as acetaminophen, lorazepam, and digoxin). Slower drug clearance means that drug particles stay in the circulation for a longer period of time, increasing the half-life and potential for increased therapeutic effects, as well as adverse effects, of the drug.

Patient Education
The patient must understand the concept of the effects of drugs on the body because some factors change the effects of drugs. Scheduled drugs should be administered by patients precisely as prescribed and on time. If a medication is ordered to be administered on an empty stomach, the patient must take it prior to eating. Patients should understand the importance of drug allergies and anaphylactic reactions. If there are any serious adverse effects, patients should notify their physician.

SUMMARY
For medications to be effective within the body, it is important that respiratory therapists understand how drugs interact with the site of action. The time required for each drug to be absorbed into the bloodstream and then metabolized before reaching the site of action is unique. Practitioners must also be aware of a drug's therapeutic effects and its adverse effects, as well as how a drug's effects are influenced by the processes of absorption, metabolism, reabsorption, and excretion. Drug allergies and anaphylactic reactions must be kept in mind because some patients will experience them, causing potentially permanent damage to body organs or even death.

LEARNING GOALS
These learning goals correspond to the objectives at the beginning of the chapter, providing a clear summary of the chapter's most important points.
1. Every drug has a unique affinity for a target receptor (cell recipient). When the drug binds to its receptor, either an agonist or antagonist reaction is produced. An agonist is a drug that binds to a specific receptor, producing a stimulatory response. An antagonist is a drug that prevents an agonist from binding to its specific receptor.
2. A patient's response to drug therapy may be influenced by age, gender, weight, the drug's half-life, diurnal body rhythms, and certain diseases.
3. Drug metabolism occurs primarily in the liver, followed by the kidneys, nerve cells, and plasma. Metabolism converts molecules of drugs and biodegrades foreign substances. The process of drug conversion is known as biotransformation.

Microsomal enzymes convert most drugs into metabolites during metabolism.

4. Anaphylactic reactions commonly cause a sharp loss of blood pressure, urticaria (skin rash), diaphragm paralysis, and oropharynx swelling. The end result of an anaphylactic reaction can be cardiac collapse. Therefore, these reactions signify a true medical emergency. They can occur very rapidly. As a result, a thorough history of previous allergic reactions to drugs, serum, blood transfusions, or vaccines must be obtained from every patient before use of a medication.

5. An adverse effect is one that is harmful and undesired. A side effect is one that is unintended and may be either harmful or beneficial. Adverse drug reactions may affect pediatric or geriatric patients more dangerously due to the way their systems metabolize substances and also because of the lack of pediatric drug studies.

6. The four components of pharmacokinetics are absorption, distribution, metabolism, and excretion (elimination). Absorption depends on a drug's ability to cross cellular membranes and resist stomach, liver, or intestinal breakdown. Distribution rates are initially affected by the rate of blood flow to certain organs. Metabolism converts molecules of drugs and biodegrades foreign substances. Excretion removes drugs from the body.

7. Drug allergies are abnormal responses to drugs that occur in a small number of individuals. Allergic reactions may be characterized by previous exposure to the same or a chemically-related drug with rapid development of an allergic reaction after reexposure. The term *hypersensitivity* is often used synonymously with the term *allergy*.

8. Many drugs bind to circulating proteins, such as acid drugs, hormones, lipoproteins, and acid glycoproteins. Changes in protein binding can affect rates of drug distribution. Drugs that are lipid soluble enter the central nervous system (CNS) rapidly. Some drugs are more poorly distributed to the CNS because they must pass through the blood–brain barrier.

9. Idiosyncratic reactions are strange, unique, unpredicted drug reactions. They may be caused by enzyme deficiencies due to genetics and hormone imbalances. An example is the drug carisoprodol, which may cause transient quadriplegia, dizziness, and temporary vision loss.

10. Excretion is the last stage of pharmacokinetics. Because the kidneys are most important in this process, diseases of the kidneys can greatly affect drug excretion. Other routes of excretion include the lungs, breast milk, sweat, tears, urine, feces, bile, and saliva. Increased intake of fluids helps drugs to be excreted more readily. Diet and physical activity also influence excretion.

CRITICAL THINKING QUESTIONS

1. Explain why a drug's plasma half-life is important.
2. Explain why drugs that are metabolized through the first-pass effect may need to be administered by the parenteral route.

WEB SITES

REVIEW QUESTIONS

Multiple Choice

Select the best response to each question.

1. Which of the following organs is the major site of drug excretion?
   A. liver
   B. spleen
   C. gallbladder
   D. kidneys

2. Which of the following terms means the action of drugs within the body?
   A. pharmacology
   B. pharmacodynamics
   C. pharmacokinetics
   D. pathophysiology

3. The process of converting drugs to metabolize derivatives during metabolism is called
   A. excretion
   B. ionization
   C. binding
   D. biotransformation

4. What is the reason that sedatives are more effective if they are administered before bedtime?
   A. diurnal body rhythms
   B. nocturnal body rhythms
   C. pathophysiology
   D. adaptation

5. Which of the following is the process whereby a drug passes into body fluids and tissues?
   A. biotransformation
   B. elimination
   C. distribution
   D. absorption

6. The last stage of pharmacokinetics involves which of the following body organs?
   A. liver and stomach
   B. lungs
   C. kidneys
   D. small intestine and brain
7. Which of the following drugs may be excreted via the lungs?
   A. morphine
   B. digitoxin
   C. aspirin
   D. alcohol
8. Administration of corticosteroids may be more effective if administered during what time of the day?
   A. early evening
   B. early morning
   C. at noon
   D. at bedtime
9. The half-life of a drug is the major determinant of which of the following?
   A. the duration of elimination of a drug after administration of multiple doses
   B. the duration of action of a drug after a single dose
   C. the adverse effects of a drug after a single dose
   D. the interaction with another single dose
10. Which of the following factors may influence the intensity of drug effects?
   A. tolerance
   B. drug allergy
   C. drug price
   D. metabolism
11. Hypersensitivity is often used synonymously with which of the following terms?
   A. allergen
   B. antigen
   C. allergy
   D. immunogen
12. The body's slow adaptation to a drug, which results in higher doses required to achieve the same effect, is called
   A. tolerance
   B. synergism
   C. overdose
   D. toxicity
13. Any response to a drug that is unintended and occurs at doses normally used in patients is known as
   A. drug interaction
   B. idiosyncratic reaction
   C. anaphylactic shock
   D. adverse drug reaction
14. When a patient experiences a unique, strange, or unpredicted reaction to a drug, it is called
   A. idiosyncratic reaction
   B. tolerance
   C. potentiation
   D. synergism
15. Which of the following drugs are affected by diurnal body rhythms?
   A. antibiotics
   B. antacids
   C. sedatives
   D. serotonin antagonists

CASE STUDY

A 65-year-old man who has hepatitis C and cirrhosis of the liver has been hospitalized for a myocardial infarction. After treatment and discharge, he was prescribed warfarin. Three days later, he was unable to sleep normally so he took a high-dose phenobarbital, which had been left over from an earlier prescription. He was soon brought back to the hospital with signs of a stroke.

1. Why could stroke-like symptoms have developed after taking the phenobarbital while on warfarin therapy?
2. How might his age be related to potential drug toxicity?

Dosage Forms and Drug Sources

OBJECTIVES

Upon completion of this chapter, the reader should be able to the following:
1. Explain the classification of drug sources.
2. List three animal sources of drugs.
3. Describe the various dosage forms of drugs.
4. Explain plant and mineral sources of drugs.
5. Distinguish between engineered and synthetic sources of drugs.
6. Describe the various dosage forms of drugs.
7. Distinguish between creams and ointments.
8. Explain buffered tablets.
9. Distinguish between suspensions and syrups.
10. Distinguish between elixirs, emulsions, and fluidextracts.

KEY TERMS

Caplets	Ointment
Capsules	Pill
Creams	Solution
Elixirs	Sustained-release
Emulsion	Tablets
Gelcaps	Vaporize
Lotion	

INTRODUCTION

Respiratory care practitioners must be familiar with many different forms of medications. Drugs are derived from varieties of different sources. A thorough knowledge of drug forms and sources will help the respiratory care professional understand how drugs are used and administered.

Drug Forms

The science of formulating drugs into different types of preparations is known as pharmaceutics. This science also focuses on how different drug forms influence pharmacokinetics and pharmacodynamics. Each drug form is designed for the intended effects of the drug. It is important to determine whether a drug will be more effective in a solid, semisolid, liquid, or gaseous form. Some substances can undergo a change of state (phase) from solid to liquid (melt) or from liquid to gas (**vaporize**). Certain drugs are soluble in water. Some are soluble in alcohol, and others are soluble in a mixture of liquids.

> **POINT TO REMEMBER**
> Expiration dates should be checked carefully before a drug is administered.

Solid Drugs

Solid drugs are popular forms of medications (see **Figure 5–1**). They include pills, tablets, capsules, sustained-release tablets and capsules, enteric-coated tablets and capsules, caplets, gelcaps, powders, granules, and lozenges (troches). Some plasters are considered to be solid drugs, but they are usually classified as semisolid drugs.

Pills

A **pill** is a single-dose medication that is made by mixing a powdered drug with a liquid (often a syrup) and rolling it into a round or oval shape. An example of a pill is the contraceptive Ortho-Novum.

Tablets

Tablets are made by compressing or molding a powdered drug with bulk-filling material under high pressure. They may be of a variety of sizes, shapes, and colors and are available with special coatings for certain required uses (see Figure 5–1). In many cases, tablets are scored so they can easily be broken at the scored area. This allows one-half or one-quarter of the tablet to be taken. Unless a tablet is scored, it should never be broken because doing so could result in inaccurate dosage. Most tablets are made to be swallowed whole, though some are dissolved in the mouth, in water, or inserted into the vagina or rectum. Tablets are commonly referred to as pills, although this is not correct. Various forms of tablets include buccal, buffered, chewable, enteric coated, and sublingual. Buffered tablets are resistant to changes in body pH. An example is buffered aspirin, which is coated with a substance that neutralizes acid. Chewable tablets are commonly used for children, as are antacid and antiflatulent medications for adults. Sublingual tablets are dissolved under the tongue (an example is nitroglycerin, which is used for angina pectoris). Buccal tablets are placed between the cheek and gum until they are dissolved.

Capsules

Capsules are dosage forms in which the drug is encased in an external shell, usually made of hard or soft gelatin. They are most commonly cylindrical in shape. The drug inside may either be powdered, granulated, liquid, or a combination of any of these. Liquids with an unpleasant taste or odor are often encased in soft gelatin capsules. Hard gelatin capsules can be pulled apart, and the contents can be sprinkled onto food if the patient cannot easily swallow the capsule. Controlled-release capsules are used when the medication must be absorbed over a longer time period. It is important to remember that these types of capsules should never be crushed or dissolved; they should be swallowed whole to take advantage of their timed-release action. An example of a capsule is the calcium channel blocker verapamil.

> **POINT TO REMEMBER**
> Capsule sizes range from number 5 (the smallest) to number 000 (the largest).

Sustained-Release Tablets and Capsules

Sustained-release tablets and capsules contain several drug doses inside special coatings that dissolve at different rates. Sustained-release (also called controlled-, delayed-, prolonged-, or timed-release) tablets or capsules release their medications slowly over an extended period, rather than rapidly like conventional tablets or capsules. Diltiazem is an example of a sustained-release medication.

Enteric-Coated Tablets and Capsules

Enteric-coated tablets and capsules have a special coating that keeps them from dissolving in the stomach. This layer resists the acidic environment of the stomach. These types of oral drugs pass through the stomach to be dissolved in the intestine, which means that their action

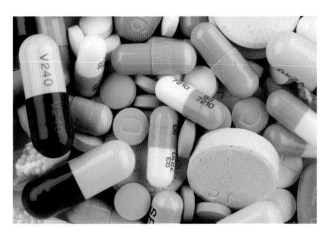

FIGURE 5–1 Solid drug forms.

is delayed until they reach the small intestine. Enteric coatings may be used to protect drugs that are easily broken down by stomach acid, to provide a sustained-release dose, or to guard against local adverse effects from a drug. Enteric coatings can prevent the nausea and vomiting that some drugs may induce if they dissolve in the stomach. Examples of enteric-coated medications include Ecotrin, penicillin G, and erythromycin.

Caplets

Caplets are shaped like capsules, but they are in the form of tablets. They are designed for easy swallowing due to their shape and film-coated covering. Examples of drugs in caplet form include many multiple vitamins.

Gelcaps

Gelcaps are oil-based medications enclosed in soft gelatin capsules. An example of a gelcap is the pain medication Aleve.

Powders

Powders are drugs that are dried and then ground into fine particles. Potassium chloride is an example of a common powdered medication.

Granules

Granules are many small pills, all of which are encased in gelatin capsules. Usually, these capsule-enclosed granules are specially coated so that they release medication over an extended period of time. An example of a granular medication is the asthma medicine Singulair.

Lozenges

Lozenges (troches) are usually solid, but sometimes semisolid, drugs designed for local application in the mouth or throat. They are usually flattened disks that are placed on the tongue or between the cheek and gum, where they are kept until they dissolve. Cough suppressants and sore throat treatments are commonly administered in the form of lozenges.

Semisolid Drugs

Semisolid drugs include dry powder aerosols such as Advair, creams, ointments, gels, and most plasters (see **Figure 5–2**).

Creams

Creams are usually white and contain a medication in a water–oil base. Creams are usually applied topically and may or may not contain medication. They are dispensed in a tube or a jar. Creams differ from lotions in that lotions contain more water and are more fluid. An example of a cream is Clearasil, which is used to treat acne.

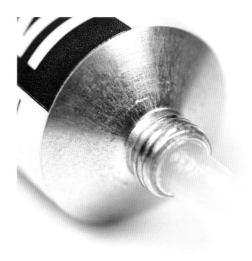

FIGURE 5–2 Semisolid dosage forms.

Ointments

An **ointment** is a greasy pharmaceutical product intended for external application. Ointments have either water or oil bases and are used for local skin protection, soothing, or as an astringent. They are sometimes applied transdermally for systemic effects. Ointments can also be used as anti-inflammatory drugs, topical anesthetics, and antibiotics. An example of an ointment is zinc oxide.

Gels (Jellies)

A gel is a jellylike substance that may be used as a vehicle to administer a topical medication. Gels contain fine particles of medications in a nonfatty base and are commonly applied to the skin. Some gels have a high alcohol content and can sting if applied to broken skin. An example of a gel or jelly is betamethasone, which is used for skin inflammation and itching.

Plasters

A plaster is a combination of a liquid and a powder that hardens as it dries. It is usually a semisolid drug but may also be solid. An example of a semisolid plaster is salicylic acid.

Liquid Drugs

Liquid drugs contain medications that are suspended or dissolved. They are very popular for use in children and infants due to their ease of use in comparison with solid drugs. Liquid drugs include solutions (which include elixirs, fluidextracts, sprits, and tinctures), mixtures and suspensions, syrups and linctuses, emulsions, liniments, gels (jellies), lotions, most aerosols, and magmas (see **Figure 5–3**).

Solutions

A **solution** contains one or more drugs dissolved in an appropriate solvent. It is usually a fluid, homogenous

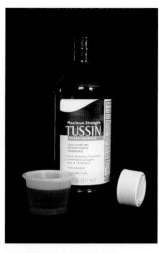

FIGURE 5-3 Liquid dosage forms.

(smooth and consistent) mixture. Elixirs, fluidextracts, spirits, and tinctures are highly concentrated solutions. Lugol iodine is an example of a medication available as a solution.

Elixirs

Elixirs consist of alcohol, sugar (for sweetening), water, and a flavoring agent. They may or may not contain medical substances. When the contained medication is not water soluble, it is first dissolved in alcohol, and the sugar and water are added later. All elixirs contain alcohol, although some pharmaceutical manufacturers advertise certain products as alcohol-free elixirs. This is a misuse of the term that may confuse the public. These so-called alcohol-free elixirs are usually either syrups or solutions. Elixirs are similar to tinctures except that tinctures are not sweetened. An example of an elixir is acetaminophen with codeine.

Fluidextracts

Fluidextracts are concentrated solutions of a drug removed from a plant source by mixing ground parts of the plant with a suitable solvent (usually alcohol). The plant parts are then separated from the solvent. Usually, a 1 mL fluidextract contains approximately 1 gram of medication. Fluidextracts are not administered directly to patients; they are prescribed as a drug source for the manufacture of final dosage forms. Only drugs from vegetable sources are used in fluidextracts. An example of a fluidextract is cascara, which is used in laxatives.

Spirits

Spirits (essences) contain alcohol and are used pharmaceutically as solvents. Examples of spirits or essences include peppermint and heptanals.

Tinctures

A tincture is usually derived from a plant source that contains alcohol and sometimes water. An example of a tincture is iodine, which is used as an antimicrobial agent.

Mixtures and Suspensions

In mixtures and suspensions, the medication is mixed with a liquid but is not dissolved. Therefore, they must be shaken well before administration. Examples of medications used in these forms include chlorpheniramine–pseudoephedrine (mixture) and betamethasone (suspension).

Syrups and Linctuses

Syrups and linctuses are aqueous drug forms that contain strong concentrations of various types of sugar and may or may not contain medical substances. Ipecac syrup is an example of a syrup that does not contain any medical substance but is used to induce vomiting. An example of medicated syrup is meperidine, which is used to treat pain. An example of a medicated linctus is codeine.

Emulsions

An emulsion is a pharmaceutical preparation that contains two agents that ordinarily cannot be mixed. The typical emulsion disperses an oil in water (oil-in-water emulsion), although some disperse water in oil (water-in-oil emulsion). Most creams and lotions are actually emulsions. An example of an emulsion is the anti-inflammatory metronidazole.

Liniments

A liniment is a liquid medication intended for external application. Most liniments are counterirritants intended to treat muscle or joint pain. An example of a liniment is camphor, which is used for many different skin conditions.

Lotions

A lotion is a pharmaceutical preparation intended for external application that typically contains water and an oil. Lotions may or may not contain medication. Lotions are patted onto the skin rather than being rubbed in. Because lotions that settle in their containers are actually suspensions, they should be shaken before use. An example of a lotion is calamine, which is used to treat itching.

Aerosols

An aerosol is a liquid or fine powder that is sprayed in a fine mist. In pharmacy, aerosols are frequently used as medication delivery systems. Aerosols are usually administered via devices such as oral inhalers and nebulizers. Aerosols that contain dry powders are classified as semisolid drugs. The most commonly used aerosols are respiratory treatments for asthma and skin sprays. An example of an aerosol is the bronchodilator albuterol.

Magmas

Magmas contain particles in a liquid suspension and are pasty in comparison with other suspensions. An example of a magma is milk of magnesia, which is used for many stomach conditions.

Gaseous Drugs

Gaseous drugs include anesthetic agents such as halothane and nitrous oxide. Inhalation medications can be administered via handheld nebulizers or metered-dose inhalers (see **Figure 5–4**).

Drug Sources

There are basically five sources from which drugs are derived: plants, animals (including humans), minerals, synthetic sources, and engineered sources.

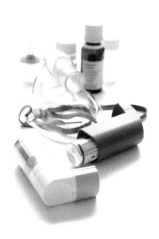

FIGURE 5–4 Gaseous dosage forms.

Plant Sources

Plant sources are organized by their chemical and physical properties. Alkaloids are bitter, alkaline compounds that contain nitrogen combined with acids to make a salt. Examples of alkaloids include nicotine and morphine sulfate. A popular cardiac glycoside is digoxin, which is made from digitalis, which in turn is derived from the foxglove plant.

Animal Sources

The body fluids of animals and humans are used as drug sources, including hormones, such as adrenaline and insulin, and enzymes, such as pancreatin and pepsin.

Mineral Sources

Mineral sources come from the earth and are used as they naturally occur. Examples of minerals include sodium, iodine, iron, gold, and potassium. Table salt is a common product that is actually sodium chloride. Severe rheumatoid arthritis is treated with gold, and certain skin conditions, such as psoriasis, are treated with coal tar.

Synthetic Sources

> **POINT TO REMEMBER**
>
> Synthetic drugs have evolved from the application of chemistry, biology, and computer technology.

Synthetic drugs are also known as manufactured drugs because they come from artificial sources. Examples of drugs derived from synthetic sources include Demerol, oral contraceptives, and sulfonamides. Some drugs are called semisynthetic because they are natural substances that are altered. An example of this type of drug is penicillin.

Engineered Sources

Genetic engineering is a new area of drug origin. New types of insulin have been made using gene splicing, as has tissue plasminogen activator, which is used to treat heart attack patients. Other types of drugs produced from engineered sources include growth

> **POINT TO REMEMBER**
>
> The first successful gene therapy was used in 1990 to treat an immune system defect in children.

hormones. Gene therapy is a new type of genetic engineering in which a missing or incorrectly acting gene is replaced by a healthy gene. Gene therapy has been used to treat immune system defects. Engineered products with modified DNA are now used for malignant brain tumors, HIV, and cystic fibrosis.

Patient Education

Respiratory therapists should explain to patients the form of their medication and exactly how it should be administered. Patients must understand if their medication is to be swallowed, chewed, placed under the tongue or in the cheek until dissolved, or administered in any other manner besides via the mouth.

SUMMARY

The science of formulating drugs into different types of preparations is known as pharmaceutics. Each drug form is designed for the intended effects of the drug. It is important to determine whether a drug will be more effective in a solid, semisolid, liquid, or gaseous form. There are basically five sources from which drugs are derived: plants, animals, minerals, synthetic sources, and engineered sources.

LEARNING GOALS

These learning goals correspond to the objectives at the beginning of the chapter, providing a clear summary of the chapter's most important points.

1. Drug sources include plants, animals (including humans), minerals, synthetic sources, and engineered sources. Minerals come from the earth. Synthetic drugs are also known as manufactured drugs. Engineered drugs come from genes and may be referred to as genetically engineered drugs.

2. The body fluids of animals and humans are used as drug sources, including hormones, such as adrenaline and insulin, and enzymes, such as pancreatin and pepsin.

3. Dosage forms include the following:
   - Solid drugs: pills, tablets, capsules, sustained-release tablets and capsules, enteric-coated tablets and capsules, caplets, gelcaps, powders, granules, lozenges (troches), and some plasters
   - Semisolid drugs: dry powder aerosols, creams, ointments, gels, and most plasters
   - Liquid drugs: solutions (elixirs, fluidextracts, spirits, tinctures), mixtures and suspensions,

syrups and linctuses, emulsions, liniments, gels (jellies), lotions, most aerosols, and magmas

▪ Gaseous drugs: inhaled drugs

4. Plant sources are organized by their chemical and physical properties and include alkaloids and glycosides. Mineral sources are used as they naturally occur in the earth, and they include sodium, iodine, iron, gold, and potassium.

5. Synthetic drugs are manufactured from artificial sources and include oral contraceptives and sulfonamides. Some drugs are called semisynthetic because they are natural substances that are altered, such as penicillin. Engineered drugs are the newest area of drug development, including gene splicing and hormone replacement. Engineered drugs include new types of insulin, tissue plasminogen activator, and drugs used for malignant brain tumors, HIV, and cystic fibrosis.

6. Each drug form is designed for the intended effects of the drug. It is important to determine whether a drug will be more effective in a solid, semisolid, liquid, or gaseous form. Some substances can undergo a change of state (phase) from solid to liquid (melt) or from liquid to gas (vaporize). Certain drugs are soluble in water, alcohol, or a mixture of liquids. Solid drugs are popular forms of medications. Liquid drugs contain medications that are very popular for use in children and infants due to their ease of use in comparison with solid drugs. Inhalation medications are administered via handheld nebulizers or metered-dose inhalers.

7. Creams are usually white and contain a medication in a water–oil base. They may or may not contain medication. Ointments are greasy products with either water or oil bases. Creams and ointments differ mostly in their consistencies, with creams being smoother and less greasy.

8. A buffered tablet is one that has a coating that makes it resistant to changes in pH. An example is buffered aspirin, which is coated with a substance that neutralizes acid.

9. Suspensions are medications mixed with a liquid but not dissolved. They must be shaken well before they are administered. Syrups are aqueous drug forms that contain strong concentrations of sugars and may or may not contain medical substances.

10. Elixirs consist of alcohol, sugar, water, and a flavoring agent, and they may or may not contain medications. Emulsions mix two agents that ordinarily cannot be mixed. They are usually composed of oil in water or water in oil. Fluidextracts are concentrated solutions of a drug that are removed from a plant source by mixing ground parts of the plant with a solvent (usually alcohol). They are not administered directly to patients, but instead are prescribed as a drug source for the manufacture of final dosage forms.

CRITICAL THINKING QUESTIONS

1. What are the advantages of enteric-coated tablets or capsules?
2. Why do practitioners prescribe sustained-release tablets or capsules?

WEB SITES

http://www.drugs.com/drug-classes.html
http://www.ifr.ac.uk/Materials/fractures/emulsions.html
http://www.mapharm.com/drug_sources.htm
http://www.naturodoc.com/library/nutrition/food.htm
http://www.nd.gov/cte/programs/health-careers/ppt/drug-forms.ppt
http://www.nlm.nih.gov/medlineplus/ency/article/002581.htm
http://www.people.vcu.edu/~asneden/alkaloids.htm

REVIEW QUESTIONS

Multiple Choice

Select the best response to each question.

1. Milk of magnesia is an example of a(n)
   A. emulsion
   B. magma
   C. suspension
   D. elixir

2. Which of the following are drugs that are dissolved in a solution of sugar and water and then flavored?
   A. elixirs
   B. syrups
   C. tinctures
   D. fluidextracts

3. Demerol is an example of a
   A. drug derived from a mineral source
   B. drug derived from an engineered source
   C. drug derived from a synthetic source
   D. drug derived from an animal source

4. Severe rheumatoid arthritis is treated with which of the following mineral sources?
   A. iodine
   B. gold
   C. potassium
   D. sodium

5. Which of the following medications may be absorbed over a longer time period?
   A. controlled-release capsules
   B. controlled substance drugs
   C. plasters
   D. lozenges

6. Which of the following dosage forms are usually solid drugs designed for local application via the mouth?
   A. granules
   B. troches
   C. gelcaps
   D. enteric-coated tablets

7. Which of the following is an example of a sublingual tablet?
   A. diltiazem
   B. verapamil
   C. zinc oxide
   D. nitroglycerin

8. Which of the following does *not* contain any medical substance?
   A. ipecac syrup
   B. codeine syrup
   C. meperidine syrup
   D. valproate sodium syrup

9. Which of the following is an example of a semi-solid drug?
   A. gelcap
   B. gel
   C. granule
   D. caplet

10. Aqueous solutions that contain high concentrations of sugar are called
    A. syrups
    B. elixirs
    C. spirits
    D. tinctures

11. Which of the following is an example of a drug derived from genetic engineering?
    A. coal tar
    B. pepsin
    C. new types of insulin
    D. morphine

12. Which of the following drug forms are derived from a plant source and contain alcohol?
    A. magmas
    B. tinctures
    C. liniments
    D. lotions

13. An example of a gel is
    A. betamethasone
    B. calamine
    C. metronidazole
    D. camphor

14. Which of the following are also known as manufactured drugs?
    A. mineral sources
    B. plant sources
    C. animal sources
    D. synthetic sources

15. Which of the following dosage forms are cylindrical in shape?
    A. pills
    B. capsules
    C. granules
    D. lozenges

CASE STUDY

A 56-year-old woman received a prescription for vaginal suppositories for a yeast infection. After 2 weeks, she returned to her physician with no change in her signs and symptoms. The physician asked her how she was using the suppositories, and she replied that she put one suppository under her tongue every 12 hours, the same way that she took another of her regular medications.

1. What is the responsibility of the physician in this case?
2. If the drug labeling was insufficient, who would be to blame?

Routes of Drug Administration

OBJECTIVES

Upon completion of this chapter, the reader should be able to do the following:

1. Describe parenteral drug administration types and locations.
2. Identify which routes of drug administration are the most dangerous, and explain why.
3. Describe various types of inhalation therapy.
4. Differentiate between sublingual and buccal drug administration.
5. Explain topical applications and differentiate them from transdermal methods.
6. Identify equipment and supplies required for parenteral administration of medication.
7. List the seven rights of drug administration.
8. Explain the differences between a nasogastric tube and a gastrostomy.
9. List the three most common sites for intramuscular administration.
10. Give four examples of drugs administered via transdermal delivery.

KEY TERMS

Aseptic technique	Lumen
Bevel	Needlesticks
Capillaries	Parenteral
Eustachian tubes	Reconstitute
Gastric reflux	Septicemia
Gauge	Shaft
Hilt	Sterility
Hub	Universal precautions
Lancet	

INTRODUCTION

Drug administration is important in providing complete care to patients. Safe delivery of prescribed medications is vital for respiratory therapists. Healthcare providers must be familiar with the general principles of drug delivery when administering drugs, supervising medication use, or providing assistance. This is a difficult task because of the large number of different drugs available, as well as the potential consequences of medication errors. Drugs can be administered via several methods or routes. Each route has its advantages and disadvantages. The best route to use depends on the type of medication, dosage form, and the desired effects.

Principles of Drug Administration

Respiratory care practitioners must be familiar with the principles of drug administration because different routes of administration can be dangerous or life threatening. Practitioners must understand the importance of medication errors (which are discussed more fully in Chapter 8). Therefore, practitioners have to follow the seven rights of drug administration. They are as follows:

1. The right patient: Ask the patient his or her name, and call the patient by name before administering the drug.
2. The right drug: Check the drug three times to confirm it is correct, and compare the written order with the label.
3. The right dose: Make sure that if calculations are required to determine the accurate dose, they are done correctly and are checked by another person.
4. The right route: Verify the physician's order to determine the correct route, and make sure this route is right for the patient.
5. The right time: Check the physician's order to determine exactly when the drug should be administered and how frequently.
6. The right technique: Make sure you are familiar with the technique required for correct administration, and ask for help if needed.
7. The right documentation: Immediately after administration, document the date and time, drug name, strength, dose, route, patient reactions, and details concerning patient education. Also chart the exact site of administration and any visible changes in the site.

Some administrations require aseptic technique and sterility because microorganisms may invade the patient and cause severe infection. Also, it is very important to understand how to prevent needlesticks and dispose of waste materials properly.

Routes of Drug Administration

> **POINT TO REMEMBER**
>
> Routes of administration are classified as enteral or parenteral.

The common routes of drug administration include enteral, sublingual, buccal, parenteral, topical (via the skin or mucous membranes), and transdermal delivery systems. Other routes of administration include inhalation, rectal, vaginal, and via the eye or ear. It is important that respiratory care practitioners are familiar with all of these various routes due to the many medications that they may be required to work with.

Enteral Route

The enteral route involves the use of the gastrointestinal (GI) tract for the administration and absorption of drugs. Of the enteral types of drugs, oral drugs in particular

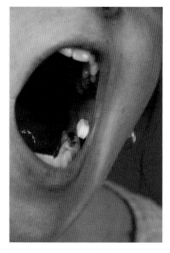

FIGURE 6–1 Buccal administration.

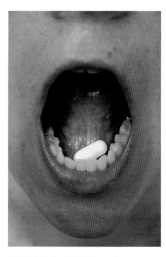

FIGURE 6–2 Sublingual administration.

are manufactured in a variety of forms, including capsules, liquid syrups, tablets, and elixirs. The oral route of administration is the most common type of enteral route. Oral medications are convenient, easy to use, and economical. Although most oral drugs are given to achieve a systemic effect, some of them (such as antacids and laxatives) are given for their local effect in the GI tract. Most oral drug forms can be used safely by patients to self-medicate for a variety of conditions.

Buccal and Sublingual Routes

Buccal and sublingual drugs are placed into specific areas of the mouth and are not absorbed by the GI

> **POINT TO REMEMBER**
>
> Any route other than oral, sublingual, buccal, and rectal is considered a parenteral administration route.

tract. They dissolve and are absorbed by the capillaries inside the mouth. Buccal medications are placed between the cheek and gum (see **Figure 6–1**), and sublingual medications are placed under the tongue (see **Figure 6–2**). These medications are absorbed via the capillary-rich tissues in these areas and enter the bloodstream directly. Because these drugs do not pass into the stomach or intestines before absorption, they produce a quicker therapeutic effect than do oral drugs that are swallowed.

Nasogastric Route

Patients who cannot swallow but still have a functioning GI tract may be fed via a tube inserted through the nose or directly through the stomach (see the next section). A nasogastric tube is a soft, flexible tube that is passed through a nostril into the stomach (see **Figure 6–3**). It is used to administer food, fluids, and drugs. This route of administration is normally used for only a short period of time. Nasogastric tubes may cause a risk for aspiration

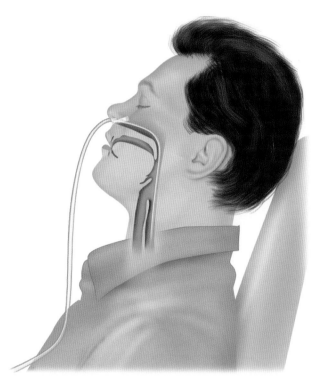

FIGURE 6–3 Nasogastric route.

due to **gastric reflux** because the tube prevents the gastroesophageal sphincter from closing. Drugs administered through either type of tube should be liquid or crushed and dissolved in a liquid vehicle. Liquid drugs are preferred because they cause less clogging of tubes than the crushed and dissolved types of drugs.

Gastrostomy

A gastrostomy tube is surgically inserted into the stomach for the administration of food, fluids, and drugs. These tubes are designed for long-term feeding. Gastrostomy tubes are preferred over nasogastric tubes because they leave the gastroesophageal sphincter intact and able to close normally.

Parenteral Drug Administration

Parenteral administration involves administering a drug by injection, using a needle and syringe. This method allows much more rapid absorption and distribution than oral administration. The three most commonly used parenteral routes are the subcutaneous, intramuscular, and intravenous routes. The intradermal route is also a form of parenteral drug administration. Parenteral drug administration is especially useful in emergencies, when the effects of a drug are required immediately.

There are several disadvantages, however. All injection equipment and medicines must be sterile (free of microorganisms). Parenteral medications may be expensive, occasionally painful, and often risky for patients to self-administer. Great care must be taken to inject a drug correctly to avoid serious harm and even death.

Medicines for injection must be in liquid form. They are commonly prepared as suspensions, beginning with a powdered form that is reconstituted in distilled water.

The seven rights of drug administration must be followed with great care during parenteral administration. Because of potential needlesticks, parenteral administration increases the risk of potential exposure to bloodborne pathogens. **Universal precautions** must be followed during the injection process. To avoid puncture wounds, never force a needle, **lancet**, or syringe into a sharps container, and never let a sharps container become more than two-thirds full before proper disposal.

Equipment

Appropriate needles, syringes, and drug forms must be selected for each type of parenteral administration. A needle consists of parts known as the hub, hilt, **shaft**, **lumen**, point, and **bevel**. The **hub** fits onto the syringe at the **hilt**. The tip of the needle's shaft is beveled (sloped), which helps the needle to cut through the skin, minimizing skin trauma. The inside diameter of the needle is called the **gauge** (see **Figure 6–4**). Needles are available in various gauge sizes and lengths. Interestingly, the smaller the number of a needle's gauge, the larger its size (an 18-gauge needle is larger than a 25-gauge needle). The type of injection to be administered and the thickness (viscosity) of the drug determines the correct gauge to select. The needle's length must be sufficient to penetrate the desired tissues without going in too deep. The patient's body size and amount of fatty tissue also influences the correct needle selection.

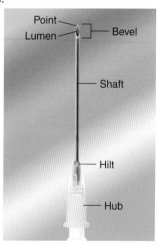

FIGURE 6–4 Parts of a needle.

The syringe consists of a barrel and a plunger. The barrel holds the drug to be administered and has calibrations on its exterior surface to indicate various amounts that it can hold. The plunger is pushed through the barrel to force the drug out of the hollow needle and into the patient's body (see **Figure 6–5**). Common 3-mL syringes are used for most drugs. Tuberculin syringes hold only 1 mL of medication. Insulin syringes are calibrated in units instead of mL and usually hold either 50 or 100 units per syringe. Insulin syringes have needles that are permanently

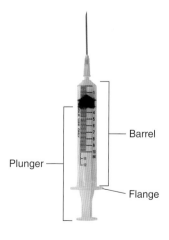

FIGURE 6–5 Parts of a syringe.

attached, unlike other types. They have no remaining space inside them after the plunger is fully depressed, allowing very accurate self-administration of the insulin.

Parenteral drugs are supplied in ampules, vials, or cartridges. Ampules are small glass or plastic containers that are sealed until just before use. They must be broken open. Vials are small bottles with rubber diaphragms that are easily punctured by needles. They contain either a liquid or a powdered medication that must be reconstituted with a specific liquid (diluent) to dilute and dissolve the powdered drug. Vials can contain either single or multiple doses (see **Figure 6–6**).

To reconstitute a powdered medication, a needle–syringe set must be used to instill the diluent into the powdered medication in the vial. Then a fresh needle–syringe set must be used to withdraw the mixed contents of the vial outward so that it can be administered to the patient. A cartridge is a small barrel that is prefilled with a sterile drug. The cartridge is slipped onto a special reusable syringe assembly so that its contents can be administered.

POINT TO REMEMBER

An effort must be made to eliminate needlestick injuries and the possible transfer of bloodborne diseases.

Intradermal Route

Intradermal injections are given within the upper layers of the skin. Intradermal injections usually require a tuberculin syringe attached to a 25- or 26-gauge needle that is between ⅜ and ½ inch in length. Usually, the inner forearm is the site of injection because it has less body hair and test results may easily be seen. The upper back is sometimes used instead. The angle of insertion is 15 degrees, nearly parallel to the skin. Absorption is slow. Only a small amount of medication may be injected (0.01 to 0.2 cc) to form a small bubble (wheal) under the skin (see **Figure 6–7**). Intradermal injections are commonly used for tuberculin and allergy tests. When the reaction is positive, a reddened, hardened, or raised area appears between 48 and 72 hours after injection. The injected drug is absorbed slowly with this type of injection.

Subcutaneous Route

Subcutaneous injections are given into a layer of fatty tissue directly below the skin. The amount administered is approximately 1 to 2 mL. Hormones, insulin, a few vaccines, and local anesthetics are commonly administered by subcutaneous injection. Examples of vaccines that are administered via subcutaneous injections include measles, mumps, and rubella (MMR) and varicella (chickenpox). Subcutaneous injections usually require a 23- to 27-gauge needle that is between ½ and ¾ inch in length. The needle should be inserted at a 45-degree angle to the skin (see **Figure 6–8**).

Intramuscular Route

Intramuscular injections are administered deep into a muscle. Because the body's muscles are well supplied with blood, absorption is faster in this method than absorption from the skin layers. Because muscles can also absorb more fluid without discomfort, the amount administered is usually between

POINT TO REMEMBER

When administering heparin subcutaneously, do not aspirate. Aspiration can damage surrounding tissues and cause bleeding and bruising.

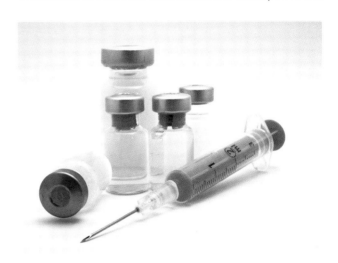

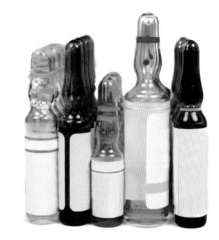

FIGURE 6–6 Single and multiple dose vials.

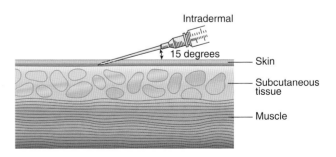

FIGURE 6–7 Intradermal injection.

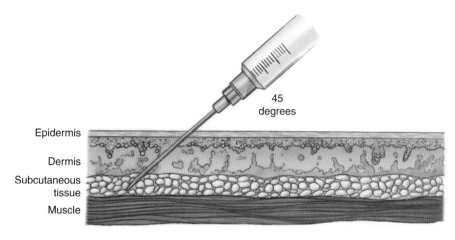

FIGURE 6–8 Subcutaneous injection.

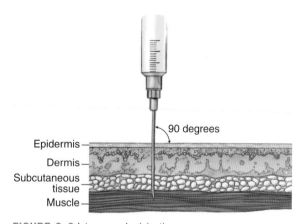

FIGURE 6–9 Intramuscular injection.

Intravenous Route

Intravenous injections are given directly into a vein. It is the best method of injection when a medication is needed quickly, as in an emergency situation. Intravenous injections are potentially the most dangerous method of administering medications. Therefore, great care must be taken when using this method because there is no quick way to correct errors. For example, if a dosage calculation is in error or an incorrect medication is administered, it will quickly affect the entire body. Intravenous injections must be sterile because they are invasive procedures, and contamination can cause several complications, including **septicemia** and other infections.

Intravenous infusion (also called IV drip) differs mainly because the speed of drug action is slower than when intravenous injections are given by pushing the solution into a vein. The term *infusion* describes a tube or needle inserted into a vein that allows fluids to slowly enter the bloodstream over a period of time. It is often used to maintain fluid level balances or to ensure a continuous drug effect. Medications may also be injected into an existing IV tube that already leads to a vein. Only physicians, registered nurses, paramedics, respiratory therapists, and a few other specifically trained individuals should administer drugs via the intravenous route. IV injections are usually used in emergency situations for an immediate effect. The disadvantage is that a painful infection may result. The needles used for IV injections are 1 to 1.5 inches in length, with gauges usually between 20 and 21.

Topical Drug Administration

Topical routes of drug administration involve the application of drug preparations to the skin or mucous membranes. This includes the eyes, ears, nose, respiratory tract, urethra, vagina, and rectum. Many topical drugs produce a local effect, such as corticosteroids, which are commonly used to treat skin inflammation. Local topical delivery of a drug produces fewer side effects than oral or parenteral forms of the same drug. This is primarily due to the extremely slow absorption of topically applied drugs and the fact that only minimal amounts of these drugs reach the general circulation. Examples of drugs applied topically to mucous membranes include antibiotic creams (such as those applied to the conjunctiva of the eyes) or hemorrhoidal creams applied to the rectum.

POINT TO REMEMBER

In an intramuscular injection, the reason for aspirating after the needle has pierced the muscle but before the medication has been injected is to ensure that the needle is not in a blood vessel.

1 and 3 mL. Common sites for intramuscular administration include the deltoid, vastus lateralis, and ventrogluteal (gluteus medius) muscles. Intramuscular injection is also the preferred method for substances that can irritate skin layers, such as penicillin. Because the injection enters deeply into a muscle, the danger of causing tissue damage is reduced (see **Figure 6–9**).

However, there is a risk of injecting the drug directly into a vein, which, in the case of penicillin, could cause serious adverse effects or even be fatal. During intramuscular administration, only large, healthy muscles should be utilized for injection, avoiding major bones, blood vessels, and nerves. Intramuscular injections usually require an 18- to 23-gauge needle that is between 1 and 3 inches in length.

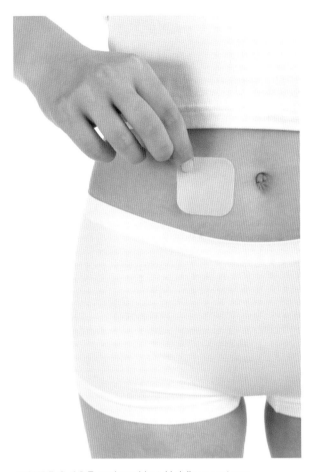

FIGURE 6–10 Transdermal (patch) delivery systems.

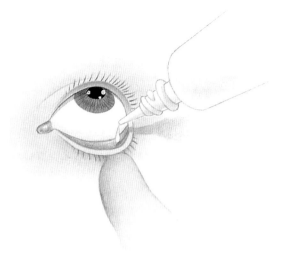

FIGURE 6–11 A figure showing the opthalmic route.

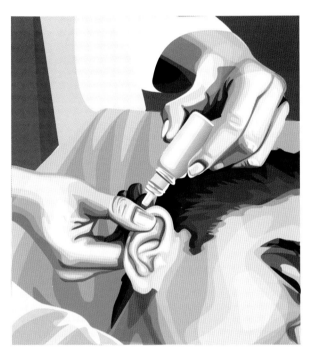

FIGURE 6–12 A figure showing the otic route.

Transdermal Delivery System

Some topical drugs are intended specifically for slow release and absorption in the general circulation and are administered for their systemic effects. An example is nitroglycerin that is applied via a transdermal patch to treat a systemic condition (such as coronary artery disease) instead of a local skin condition. Other examples of medications applied via transdermal delivery systems include scopolamine (Transderm-Scop) for motion sickness, estrogen (Vivelle-Dot) for menopausal symptoms, and nicotine (NicoDerm CQ) to help a patient quit smoking. The rate of delivery of a transdermal patch's medication may differ, and the actual dose can vary. The sites of application of transdermal patches should be regularly rotated to avoid adverse effects. Drugs applied via transdermal delivery systems avoid the first-pass effect in the liver and bypass digestive enzymes (see **Figure 6–10**).

Other Routes of Drug Administration

Other routes of drug administration include the eyes, ears, nose, rectum, or vagina, as well as by inhalation into the nose or mouth.

Ophthalmic Route

The ophthalmic route is used to treat local and surrounding eye conditions, such as excessive dryness, glaucoma, and infections, as well as dilating the pupils during examinations. Ophthalmic medications may be formulated as drops, irrigations, and ointments. Ophthalmic medications should be sterile (see **Figure 6–11**).

Otic Route

The otic route is used for local ear infections and to remove soft blockages of the ear canal. Eardrops and irrigations are often used to clean out the ears (see **Figure 6–12**).

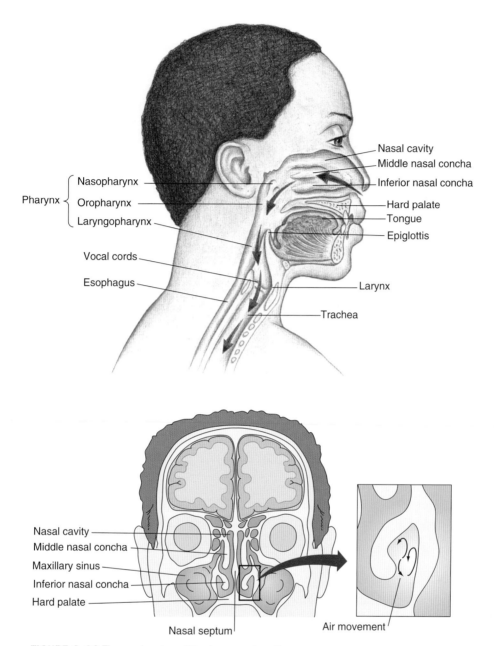

FIGURE 6–13 The nasal route and its sinuses and cavities.

Nasal Route

The nasal route is used for local and systemic drug administration. Advantages of this extremely absorptive route include the simplicity of using nasal sprays and drops, as well as avoidance of the first-pass effect and digestive enzymes. The only real disadvantage of the nasal route is the potential for mucosal irritation and damage to the nasal cavity's cilia. The astringent (shrinking) effects of many drops and sprays allow immediate relief of nasal congestion. The nasal sinuses and even the eustachian tubes of the ears may be reached by using the nasal route (see **Figure 6–13**).

Inhalation Therapy

Inhalation therapy is a very effective method of drug administration because the bronchioles and alveoli have a rich blood supply as well as a large surface area. Most inhaled medications begin their effects immediately. An aerosol consists of droplets or tiny particles suspended in a gas. Aerosol therapy delivers the medication to the immediate site of action, with few systemic adverse effects. Examples of medications given via aerosol therapy include those for bronchospasm and to loosen mucus.

Because they are absorbed across pulmonary capillaries, inhaled medications can produce systemic effects.

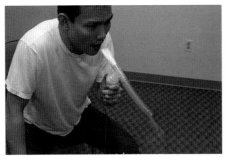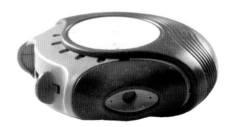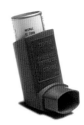

FIGURE 6–14 Nebulizers, dry powder inhalers, and metered dose inhalers.

Although most inhaled medications have few systemic effects, those that may be dangerous for inhalation include halothane and nitrous oxide. Other substances, such as glues and paint thinners, may also cause adverse systemic effects.

Nebulizers are devices that vaporize liquid medications into a mist that can be inhaled via a face mask or handheld device. The most common form of nebulizer is referred to as a jet nebulizer or atomizer. Types of nebulizers include the following:

- Blow-by nebulizers disperse medication in mist form. The nebulizer tube must be directed very close to the patient's mouth.
- Mask nebulizers cover the face to disperse medication without any spillage.
- Portable nebulizers provide a course of medication within 5 minutes of use and offer much smaller particles of medication than other devices.

Dry powder inhalers (DPIs) administer finely powdered drugs into the bronchial tree. They do not use a chemical propellant to push the medication out of the inhaler. The drug is instead released by breathing in a fast, deep breath. Types of DPIs include the following:

- Dry powder tube inhalers are straight tubes of medication that allow each dose to be easily loaded by turning the base.
- Dry powder disk inhalers are round discs of medication that allow each dose to be easily loaded by moving a switch.
- Single-dose dry powder inhalers are empty tubes or disks that require a prepackaged single dose of medication to be loaded prior to use.

Metered dose inhalers (MDIs) deliver specifically measured doses of medications into the lungs by using an enclosed propellant substance (see **Figure 6–14**). Types of MDIs include the following:

- Standard metered dose inhalers are pressurized boot-shaped containers that deliver medication by either pushing on the container, or they work automatically when the patient inhales. They may or may not include dose counters.
- Metered dose inhalers with spacers include spacers that hold the medication in place so the full dose

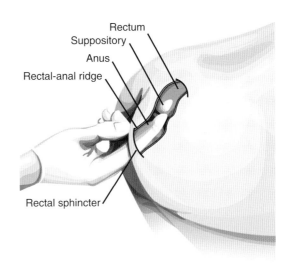

FIGURE 6–15 Rectal route.

may easily be inhaled. The patient can therefore inhale more slowly, increasing the amount of medication that is delivered into the lungs. The spacers may be built-in or insertable.

Patients must be careful when using inhaled medications to ascertain that each dose is as accurate as possible. If an inhaled drug does not move deeply enough into the respiratory tract, it may remain in the pharynx where it could be swallowed. This means that it could reach the GI tract and cause systemic complications. Oxygen is administered via inhalation for various conditions and disorders.

POINT TO REMEMBER

Patients may use metered dose inhalers (MDIs) at home. The respiratory therapist should train patients about the correct use of MDIs.

Rectal Route

The rectal route is used for both local and systemic drug effects (see **Figure 6–15**). Prochlorperazine (Compazine) suppositories are an example of a topical type of administration that is inserted rectally to alleviate nausea, not for local effects in the rectum. The rectal route is commonly used for patients who are unconscious or unable to take

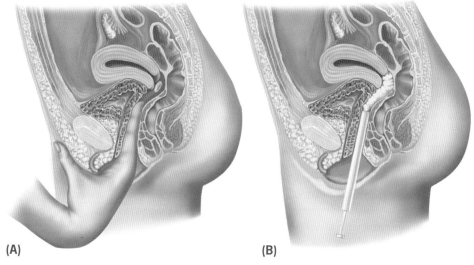

FIGURE 6–16 Vaginal route.

medications orally (such as when nausea or vomiting exists). Rectal drugs may also be in the form of enemas. Absorption is slower via this route than by others, and the first-pass effect, as well as digestive enzymes, are avoided.

Vaginal Route

The vaginal route is used to deliver medications for local pain or itching (see **Figure 6–16**). Dosage forms for vaginal use may be creams, jellies, foams, or suppositories. The patient should empty her bladder before vaginal drugs are inserted. After administration, a pad that covers the perineal area (between the vagina and anus) should be worn for absorption of any excess medication.

Documentation of Drug Administration

When administering medication, it is essential to document all procedures. Proper documentation assures that all procedures were done correctly and by whom. Documentation is also important in the case of subpoenas or other legal action. Correct documentation records lot numbers, dates of expiration, individuals who ordered medication administration, and many other types of information. Respiratory therapists should understand how to properly document every aspect of their job duties.

Patient Education

Patients should be instructed to call their healthcare provider if they develop a rash, itching, hives, an elevated temperature, or other complications after medication administration. Other complications may include redness, swelling, or pain at an intravenous site and swelling of the legs or feet.

SUMMARY

Each respiratory therapist should be familiar with the principles of drug administration and various routes or methods of drug administration. Medications can be administered by routes such as enteral, buccal, sublingual, nasogastric, and gastrostomy. They also can be administered through injection, such as via intradermal, subcutaneous, intramuscular, and intravenous routes. Other methods of drug administration are topical, transdermal, ophthalmic, otic, nasal, inhalation, rectal, and vaginal. There is a variety of equipment that the respiratory therapist should be familiar with, including needles, syringes, ampules, vials, and cartridges.

LEARNING GOALS

These learning goals correspond to the objectives at the beginning of the chapter, providing a clear summary of the chapter's most important points.

1. Parenteral drug administration includes the following:
    -   Intradermal injections are given within the upper layers of the skin and are injected so that the medication forms a small bubble (wheal) under the skin.
    -   Subcutaneous injections are given into a layer of fatty tissue directly below the skin.
    -   Intramuscular injections are administered deep into a muscle. Common sites for intramuscular administration include the deltoid, vastus lateralis, and ventrogluteal muscles. During intramuscular administration, only large, healthy muscles should be utilized for injection, avoiding major bones, blood vessels, and nerves.

Intravenous injections are given directly into a vein. The term *infusion* describes a tube or needle inserted into a vein that allows fluids to slowly enter the bloodstream over a period of time. Medications may also be injected into an existing IV tube that already leads to a vein.

2. Intravenous injections are potentially the most dangerous method of administering medications. Therefore, great care must be taken when using this method because there is no quick way to correct errors. For example, if a dosage calculation is in error or an incorrect medication is administered, it will quickly affect the entire body. Intravenous injections must be sterile because they are invasive procedures, and contamination can cause several complications, including septicemia and other infections.

3. Inhalation therapy includes aerosol therapy, vaporized liquids, dry powder inhalers, and metered dose inhalers. An aerosol consists of droplets or tiny particles suspended in a gas. Aerosol therapy delivers the medication to the immediate site of action, with few systemic adverse effects. Examples of medications given via aerosol therapy include those for bronchospasm and to loosen mucus. Nebulizers are devices that vaporize liquid medications into a mist that can be inhaled via a face mask or handheld device. Dry powder inhalers (DPIs) administer finely powdered drugs into the bronchial tree. Metered dose inhalers (MDIs) deliver specifically measured doses of medications into the lungs by using an enclosed propellant substance.

4. Sublingual medications are placed under the tongue. Buccal medications are placed between the cheek and gum. Both of them are dissolved for absorption by the capillaries in the mouth and bypass the GI tract for faster absorption into the systemic circulation.

5. Topical medications are commonly supplied in creams, ointments, and other liquid or semisolid forms that are applied to the skin. They are often rubbed in until they disappear and are usually intended for local effects. Transdermal patches administer a drug directly through the skin for slow absorption into the systemic circulation over time.

6. Equipment and supplies for parenteral drug administration include needles, syringes, ampules, vials, and cartridges. A needle consists of parts known as the hub, hilt, shaft, lumen, point, and bevel. Needles are available in various gauge sizes and lengths. The syringe consists of a barrel and a plunger. Various syringes are available. Common 3-mL syringes are used for most drugs. Tuberculin syringes only hold 1 mL of medication. Insulin syringes are calibrated in units (U) instead of mL and usually hold either 50 or 100 units per syringe. Parenteral drugs are supplied in ampules, vials, or cartridges. Ampules are small glass or plastic containers that are sealed until just before use. They must be broken open. Vials can contain either single or multiple doses. A cartridge is a small barrel that is prefilled with a sterile drug. The cartridge is slipped onto a special reusable syringe assembly so that its contents can be administered.

7. The seven rights of drug administration are the right patient, right drug, right dose, right route, right time, right technique, and right documentation.

8. A nasogastric tube is a soft, flexible tube that is passed through a nostril into the stomach. It is used to administer food, fluids, and drugs and is intended for short-time use. A gastrostomy tube is surgically inserted into the stomach for similar administration and is intended for long-term use.

9. The three most common sites for intramuscular administration are the deltoid, vastus lateralis, and ventrogluteal muscles.

10. Four examples of drugs administered via transdermal delivery include nitroglycerin, scopolamine, estrogen, and nicotine.

CRITICAL THINKING QUESTIONS

1. Explain why some patients need a gastrostomy tube and others require a nasogastric tube.

2. A physician orders a medication for an elderly patient. She must take a capsule every 8 hours. The patient has difficulty swallowing the capsules, and you are not able to administer the medication. What would you do?

WEB SITES

http://emedicine.medscape.com/article/80925-overview

http://www.drugtext.org/library/books/needle/routesm.html

http://www.enotes.com/nursing-encyclopedia/intravenous-medication-administration

http://www.merck.com/mmhe/sec02/ch011/ch011b.html

http://www.pulmonaryreviews.com/09jun/CCU1.html

http://www.surgeryencyclopedia.com/A-Ce/Aseptic-Technique.html

http://www.wrongdiagnosis.com/medical/topical_drug_administration.htm

REVIEW QUESTIONS

Multiple Choice

Select the best response to each question.

1. Which of the following is the preferred site for intramuscular injections in infants and children?
   A. deltoid muscle
   B. vastus lateralis
   C. ventrogluteal site
   D. dorsogluteal site

2. Which of the following needle gauges is most appropriate for the intramuscular administration of very thick penicillin?
   A. 16
   B. 18
   C. 21
   D. 25

3. A correctly administered intradermal injection will produce a
   A. wheel
   B. wheal
   C. wen
   D. pustule

4. A syringe marked with U100 will be used for which of the following medications?
   A. chemotherapy
   B. allergy testing
   C. tuberculin testing
   D. insulin

5. When giving a subcutaneous injection, a nurse should *not* inject more than how much into the subcutaneous tissue?
   A. 3 cc
   B. 2 cc
   C. 1 cc
   D. 1.5 cc

6. The sharpened end of the needle is called the
   A. hub
   B. point
   C. bevel
   D. lumen

7. The body areas used for intradermal injections are the
   A. deltoid muscle or gluteal muscle
   B. inner forearm or middle of the back
   C. outer forearm or middle of the back
   D. thigh or middle of the back

8. The point at which the shaft of a needle attaches to the hub is called the
   A. lumen
   B. shaft
   C. hilt
   D. flange

9. A small adhesive patch or disc that may be applied to the body near the treatment site is an example of the
   A. intradermal system
   B. subcutaneous system
   C. dermal system
   D. transdermal system

10. Insulin syringes are calibrated in
    A. cubic centimeters
    B. milliliters
    C. units
    D. minims

11. A prefilled syringe is known as a
    A. flange
    B. cartridge
    C. plunger
    D. vial

12. Which of the following is the route of administration of a drug that is placed between the gums and the cheek?
    A. buccal
    B. oral
    C. sublingual
    D. transdermal

13. Which of the following is the most dangerous route of drug administration?
    A. intramuscular
    B. intradermal
    C. intravenous
    D. subcutaneous

14. Short needles are used for which of the following routes of drug injections?
    A. intramuscular and subcutaneous
    B. intravenous and intradermal
    C. intradermal and subcutaneous
    D. intramuscular and intravenous

15. Which of the following routes is an enteral route of drug administration?
    A. topical
    B. intradermal
    C. intramuscular
    D. gastrointestinal tract

CASE STUDY

An 8-year-old girl was ordered to be tested for tuberculosis at the local health department clinic. An inexperienced nurse gave her a tuberculin test by intradermal injection. During the procedure, the nurse inserted the needle too deeply into the subcutaneous region. After 3 weeks, the patient returned to her physician with a large abscess and drainage of pus from her forearm.

1. What should the physician do in this situation?
2. What type of treatment should be given?

Drug Dosage Calculations

OUTLINE

OBJECTIVES

Upon completion of this chapter, the reader should be able to do the following:

1. Identify measurements included in the metric, apothecary, and household systems.
2. List the basic units of weight, volume, and length of the metric system.
3. Calculate equivalent measurements within the metric system.
4. Describe the international unit.
5. Define the most accurate method of calculating a child's dose.
6. Explain how the fraction proportion method is used to calculate the amount to administer.
7. Explain why the household system is not commonly used in medicine.
8. Describe the use of units and milliequivalents in dosage calculation.
9. Explain the rules for changing grams to milligrams and milliliters to liters.
10. Compare apothecary and household equivalents.

KEY TERMS

Desired dose	Milliliter
Diluent	Nomogram
Dosage ordered	Ounces
Dose	Unit
Metric system	Unit–dose

INTRODUCTION

Respiratory care therapists are responsible for assuring that all medications are prepared and administered to the patient exactly according to the prescriber's order. Often, drugs are delivered by a pharmacy or supplied by pharmaceutical representatives in unit–dose packs. It is important to understand that in these packs, the dosage ordered may differ from the dosage on hand. When this occurs, the respiratory care practitioner must be able to accurately calculate the correct dose before medication is dispensed and administered. There is no margin of error in drug calculations. Even a minor mistake may result in serious complications for the patient. Therefore, respiratory care practitioners must take great care in calculating all drug dosages.

Measurement Systems

Respiratory care practitioners who deal with medication administration must ensure the accuracy and correctness of drug dosages. They must have a thorough knowledge of the weights and measures used in drug administration. Three systems of measurement are used in pharmacology and the calculation of drug dosages: metric, apothecary, and household. The metric system is the predominant system used today, although household and apothecary measures, such as teaspoons and ounces, are still used less frequently. The metric system is the most accurate and safest system of measurement, and it is used throughout the world. It is based on the decimal system.

The metric system is commonly used for three parameters of measurement: weight, volume, and length. However, length is not used as a parameter in medication administration and dosage calculations. Weight and volume are the parameters used for these purposes. Weight is the most commonly used parameter, and it is essential as a dosage unit. The measurement of volume is the next most common parameter, and it is used to measure liquids.

TABLE 7-1   Basic Metric Units of Measurement

Parameters	Units	Abbreviations	Equivalencies
Weight	Gram (basic unit) Milligram Kilogram Microgram	g mg kg mcg	1 g = 1000 mg 1 mg = 0.001 g 1 kg = 1000 g 1 mcg = 0.000001 g
Volume	Liter (basic unit) Milliliter	L mL	1 L = 1000 mL 1 mL = 0.001 L
Length	Meter (basic unit) Centimeter Millimeter	m cm mm	1 m = 1000 mm 1 cm = 0.01 m 1 mm = 0.001 m

TABLE 7-2   Latin and Greek Prefixes

Origin	Prefix	Value
Latin	micro- (mc) milli- (m) centi- (c) deci- (d)	0.000001 0.001 0.01 0.1
Greek	deca- (da) hecto- (h) kilo- (k) mega- (M)	10 100 1000 1,000,000

Metric System

In the metric system, units are based on the number 10, the same as in the decimal system. The basic units of measurement in the metric system are listed in **Table 7-1**.

Metric units of measurement were standardized throughout the world when the International System of Units (abbreviated SI, from the French term *Système International d'Unités*) was established in 1960.

It is common to modify the basic units of weight and volume by adding Latin and Greek prefixes. These prefixes modify the amount described by each basic unit. For example, the prefix milli- means one-thousandth, so a milliliter is equivalent to one-thousandth of a liter. **Table 7-2** shows Latin and Greek prefixes used in medicine.

> **POINT TO REMEMBER**
>
> The abbreviation for microgram (mcg) is preferred over the abbreviation mg because it may be mistaken for the abbreviation for milligram, which is always mg.

> **POINT TO REMEMBER**
>
> An amount such as 0.5 L should always be written in this way, rather than as ⁵/₁₀ L or ½ L. This is because in the metric system, quantities are written as decimal numbers instead of fractions.

Apothecary System

The apothecary system originated in England and has been almost completely replaced by the metric system. It uses a variety of English measures (see **Table 7-3**) and even utilizes Roman numerals to indicate amounts of drugs. Apothecary measures are still used for acetaminophen, aspirin, and phenobarbital.

> **POINT TO REMEMBER**
>
> Ounces used for weight should not be confused with ounces used for volume.

Household System

The household system is used by most people in their homes with measurement devices that are not precisely accurate. This system is not used in medical settings. It utilizes only units of volume. **Table 7-4** shows common household measurements.

> **POINT TO REMEMBER**
>
> Because the volume of ordinary household spoons, cups, and glasses may vary, medications should not be administered using ordinary household utensils.

Milliequivalents and Units

Certain drugs are measured in milliequivalents and units to indicate their strength. Milliequivalents are defined as expressions of the number of grams of equivalent weight of a drug contained in 1 mL of a normal solution. Examples of substances measured in milliequivalents include potassium chloride and sodium bicarbonate.

Units are used to measure the potency of substances such as heparin, insulin, penicillin, and certain vitamins. A unit is defined as the amount of a substance required to produce a specific effect, and unit sizes differ for each drug. International units are used to measure many vitamins. They are not used to measure substances in terms of their physical weight or volume. Neither units nor milliequivalents can be directly converted into measurements of the apothecary, household, or metric systems.

Dosages and Doses

Prescriptions and verbal orders describe exact amounts of medication that the prescriber has ordered and how often it is to be administered. An exact amount of medication is described as the **dosage ordered**. A **dose** is the strength of a drug present in one dosage unit. Usually, this is the amount of drug on hand at the pharmacy to prepare the dosage ordered. The dosage and dose must be identified when the physician's order is received. Determine the dosage ordered and the dose on hand for the following prescription order:

Dosage ordered: Zocor 160 mg p.o. h.s.
Dose on hand: Zocor 80 mg tablets

The ordered dosage is one 160 mg tablet at bedtime by mouth. The dose on hand is 80 mg tablets, as the label in **Figure 7–1** shows.

The Desired Dose

The amount of medication to be administered to a patient is known as the **desired dose**. Two methods are used to calculate desired doses: the conversion factor method and the ratio and proportion method.

Conversion Factor Method

When the desired dose is unknown, the conversion factor method allows you to determine the amount of medication that the dose should contain.

Example 1
Dosage ordered: 1.5 mg
Dose on hand: listed in mcg

$$\frac{\text{Dosage ordered}}{\text{Desired dose}} = \frac{1.5 \text{ mg}}{x(\text{conversion factor})}$$

TABLE 7–3	Basic Apothecary Units of Measurement		
Parameters	**Units**	**Abbreviations**	**Equivalencies**
Weight	Grain (basic unit)	gr	$1 \text{ gr} = \frac{2}{1000} \text{ oz}$
	Dram	dr	$1 \text{ dr} = \frac{1}{8} \text{ oz}$
	Ounce	oz	1 oz = 480 gr
	Pound	lb	1 lb = 12 oz
Volume	Minim (basic unit)	M	$1 \text{ M} = \frac{1}{60} \text{ fl dr}$
	Fluidram	fl dr	$1 \text{ fl dr} = \frac{1}{8} \text{ fl oz}$
	Fluidounce	fl oz	$1 \text{ fl oz} = \frac{1}{16} \text{ pt}$
	Pint	pt	$1 \text{ pt} = \frac{1}{8} \text{ gal}$
	Quart	qt	1 qt = 2 pints
	Gallon	gal	1 gal = 4 quarts

TABLE 7–4	Basic Household Units of Measurement	
Units	**Abbreviations**	**Equivalencies**
Drop	gtt	$1 \text{ gtt} = \frac{1}{15} \text{ mL}$
Teaspoon	t (tsp)	1 tsp = 5 mL
Tablespoon	T (tbsp)	1 tbsp = 3 tsp
Fluid ounce	oz	1 oz = 2 tbsp
Cup	cup	1 cup = 8 oz
Pint	pt	1 pt = 2 cups
Quart	qt	1 qt = 2 pt
Gallon	gal	1 gal = 4 qt

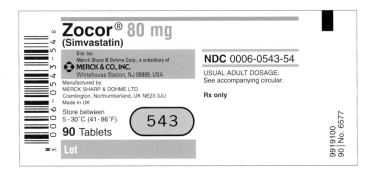

FIGURE 7–1 Zocor 80 mg. © Merck Sharp & Dohme Corp. Used with permission.

To determine the conversion factor, you must understand that milligrams (mg) relate to micrograms (mcg) as follows: 1 mg = 1000 mcg. Therefore,

$$\frac{1 \text{ mg}}{1000 \text{ mcg}} = \frac{1.5 \text{ mg}}{x}$$

This gives the following result:

$$1.5 \times 1000 = x \times 1$$

which means that

$$x = \frac{1.5 \times 1000}{1}$$

So

$$x = 1.5000 = 1500 \text{ mcg}$$

Ratio and Proportion Method

The ratio and proportion method is based on the understanding that two equal ratios that are equivalent to each other results in an equation known as a proportion. The term *ratio* is defined as the relationship between two quantities, usually expressed as the quotient of one divided by the other. All measures used in this method must be in the same system, and all units are the same. The terms of the ratios in a proportion must be written in the following order:

milligrams (mg):tablet (tab)::mg:tab

or

mg:milliliter (mL)::mg:mL

or

milligrams (mg) ÷ tablet (tab) = mg ÷ tab

Another way to express this is

$$\frac{h}{q} = \frac{d}{x}$$

where h = dose on hand; q = quantity on hand (number of tablets, capsules, or milliliters); d = desired dose; and x = unknown quantity.

Example 2

Dosage ordered: 2 g of amoxicillin

Dose on hand: amoxicillin 500 mg capsules

How much is to be given per dose?

$$\frac{1 \text{ g}}{1000 \text{ mg}} = \frac{2 \text{ g}}{x \text{ mg}}$$

$$x \text{ mg} = \frac{2 \text{ g} \times 1000 \text{ mg}}{1 \text{ g}}$$

$$x = 2000 \text{ mg}$$

Therefore,

$$\frac{500 \text{ mg}}{1 \text{ capsule}} = \frac{2000 \text{ mg}}{x}$$

$$x = \frac{2000 \text{ mg} \times 1 \text{ capsule}}{500 \text{ mg}} \quad 4 \text{ capsules}$$

Example 3

If 200 g of a drug costs $5.00, how much will 20 g cost? Using proportions, this appears as follows:

200 g:20 g::5.00:x

$$x = \frac{20 \text{ g} \times 5.00}{200 \text{ g}}$$

Therefore,

$$x = \frac{100}{200} = 0.50$$

So 20 g of this drug would cost $0.50.

> **POINT TO REMEMBER**
>
> Respiratory therapists should always check the answers to proportion problems by substituting the answer into the proportion, cross-multiplying, and seeing if the products are equal.

Calculating the Amount to Administer

It is necessary to calculate the amount to administer to a patient when calculating the related desired dose. Either the ratio and proportion method or the formula method can be used. Percentages also are discussed later in this chapter to aid in understanding their use in drug dosage calculations.

Ratio and Proportion Method

The dosage strength does not change based on the amount to be administered. For example, consider that

$$\frac{\text{Dose on hand}}{\text{Dosage unit}} = \frac{\text{Desired dose}}{\text{Amount to administer}}$$

So if a patient needs 100 mg of medication, and you have 50 mg tablets on hand, you would calculate the amount to administer as follows:

$$\frac{50 \text{ mg}}{1 \text{ tablet}} = \frac{100 \text{ mg}}{x}$$

Therefore,

$$50x = 1 \times 100$$

So

$$x = \frac{100}{50} = 2 \text{ tablets}$$

Example 4

Dosage ordered: Lopressor 100 mg p.o. bid
Dose on hand: Lopressor 50 mg

$$\frac{50 \text{ mg}}{1 \text{ tablet}} = \frac{100 \text{ mg}}{x}$$

$$50x = 100 \times 1$$

$$x = \frac{100}{50}$$

$$x = 2 \text{ tablets}$$

Example 5

Dosage ordered: diltiazem 120 mg p.o. once a day
Dose on hand: diltiazem 30 mg

$$\frac{30 \text{ mg}}{1 \text{ tablet}} = \frac{120 \text{ mg}}{x}$$

$$3x = 120 \times 1$$

$$x = \frac{120 \times 1}{30}$$

$$x = 4 \text{ tablets}$$

Formula Method

The formula method is based on the ratio and proportion method. Remember the following ratio:

$$\frac{h}{q} = \frac{d}{x}$$

Cross-multiply and simplify as follows:

$$\frac{d \times q}{h} = x$$

Remember the following:

d is the desired dose or ordered dosage

h is the dose on hand

q is the dosage unit or quantity on hand

x is the amount to administer

Example 6

Dosage ordered: Biaxin 500 mg
Dose on hand: Biaxin 250 mg

$$\frac{500}{250} \times 1 \text{ capsule} = x$$

Therefore,

$$2 \times 1 = 2$$

capsules would be administered to provide a total of 500 mg of medication.

Example 7

Dosage ordered: Calan 80 mg p.o. t.i.d.
Dose on hand: Calan 40 mg

$$\frac{d \times q}{h} = x$$

$$\frac{80 \times 1 \text{ tablet}}{40} = x$$

$$x = 2 \text{ tablets}$$

Percentages

Percentages are commonly used in drug dosage calculations and must be understood by respiratory care therapists. A percentage expresses a ratio of a certain number to 100. The symbol used to express a percentage is %. For example, the ratio of 25 to 100 is 25 percent, expressed as 25%. This is equivalent to 25 hundredths, which can be expressed as the decimal 0.25. Percentages may be expressed as fractions, decimals, or ratios. Twenty-five percent, therefore, is equivalent to the ratio 25:100.

Percentages are often used to show the strength of intravenous solutions. They are also used to indicate the strength of certain medications, such as ointments and solutions. For example, a 3% ointment means that the medication in the ointment constitutes 3 parts out of 100 parts. A 0.9% solution means that the medication in the solution constitutes less than 1 part out of 100 parts.

Conversions Between Systems

Although most drug doses are measured in metric units, sometimes you may be required to convert drug dosages between the various systems. It is important to understand the relationship between various measures of each system and their equivalencies. You also must be able to convert measurements within a given system. **Table 7–5** shows approximate equivalents for volume and weight between the measurement systems.

Oral Drug Calculations

Oral medications include solid and liquid forms, with tablets being the most common form of solid oral medication. Tablets may be swallowed, sublingual (dissolved under the tongue), buccal (dissolved between the cheek and gum), chewable, or made to be dissolved in water. It is important to always check a drug's label to find out how it should be correctly administered. Calculations of the exact amount of a drug that needs to be administered are critical in providing patients with safe and effective treatment.

TABLE 7–5 Approximate Equivalents Between Measurement Systems

Metric Unit	Apothecary Unit	Household Unit
5 mL	1 dr	1 tsp
15 mL	4 dr	1 T
30 mL	1 fl oz	2 T
240 mL	8 fl oz	1 cup
480 mL	16 fl oz	1 pt
960 mL	32 fl oz	1 qt
1 mg	gr ⅟₅₀ (¹/₅₀ grain)	3/100,000 oz
15 mg	gr ¼ (1/4 grain)	5/10,000 oz
30 mg	gr ss (1/2 grain)	1/1000 oz
60 mg	gr i (1 grain)	1/500 oz
0.5 g	gr viii (8 grains)	2/100 oz
1 g (1000 mg)	gr xv (15 grains)	2/1000 lb
1 kg (1000 g)	15,432 grains	2.2 lb

Solid Doses

When a tablet is scored (notched), it may be broken along the score line. Unscored tablets should never be broken because the dose will be incorrect. Before a solid dose is administered, the desired dose must be calculated in terms of how many tablets or capsules are required for the correct amount of medication. It may be necessary to convert the dosage ordered to the desired dose by using the same unit of measurement as the dose on hand. The fraction proportion method is then used to calculate the amount to administer:

$$\frac{\text{Dose on hand }(h)}{\text{Dosage unit }(q)} = \frac{\text{Desired dose }(d)}{\text{Amount to administer}}$$

Another way to calculate this is as follows:

$$\text{Desired dose }(d) \times \frac{\text{Dosage unit }(q)}{\text{Dose on hand }(h)}$$
$$= \text{Amount to administer}$$

So if 400 mg of ibuprofen was ordered for a patient to take over a 4-hour period, then as needed, for headache, and only 200 mg tablets of ibuprofen were on hand, use the previous formula to calculate the amount to administer for the first dose:

$$400 \text{ mg }(d) \times \frac{\text{Tablet }(q)}{200 \text{ mg }(h)}$$
$$= \text{Administer 2 tablets of 200 mg each}$$

Example 8
Dosage ordered: Aldomet 250 mg p.o. bid
Dose on hand: Aldomet 125 mg

$$\frac{d \times q}{h} = x$$
$$\frac{250 \times 1}{125} = x$$

$x = 2$ tablets

Example 9
Dosage ordered: Coumadin 5 mg p.o. q.d.
Dose on hand: Coumadin 2 mg scored tablets

$$\frac{d \times q}{h} = x$$
$$\frac{5 \times 1}{2} = x$$

$x = 2.5$ tablets

Liquid Doses

Due to the ability of liquid medications to be measured in small units of volume, a large range of doses can be administered. Liquid medications are very popular for use in children, the elderly, and for patients who have trouble swallowing solid doses. Liquid drug preparations may sometimes be supplied as powdered drugs that must be liquefied by using a diluent. Liquid drugs can be administered orally or by injection. Oral liquid medications are measured by using either calibrated measuring cups, medicine droppers (also called oral syringes), or calibrated spoons (see **Figure 7–2**).

It is important when calculating liquid doses to know the quantity of the prescribed medication. If a liquid medication contains 125 mg of medication per 5 mL of fluid, and the physician prescribes 375 mg of medication, how many mL of the mixture must be administered? Use the following formula:

$$\frac{5 \text{ mL}}{125 \text{ mg}}$$

$$375 \times \frac{5}{125} = \frac{1775}{125}$$
$$= \text{Administer 15 mL of the liquid medication}$$

Parenteral Dosage Calculations

Drugs for administration by injection contain medications that are dissolved in an appropriate liquid. These injectable medications may be prescribed in grams, milligrams, micrograms, units, or grains. They can be packaged as

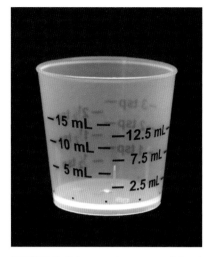 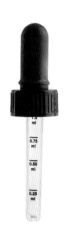 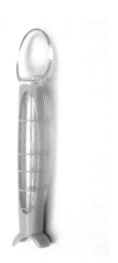

FIGURE 7–2 A measuring cup, medicine dropper, and calibrated spoon.

solvents (solutions) or in a powdered form, which needs to be diluted with a specific diluent solution. Many liquid drugs for injection are premixed commercially and available in ampules and vials for immediate use.

Subcutaneous Injection

Because there are fewer blood vessels in the subcutaneous layer of skin (also known as fatty tissue), drugs injected subcutaneously are absorbed slowly. Subcutaneous (SC) injections are administered at a 45-degree angle, and between 0.5 mL and 1 mL is injected. Either tuberculin (1 mL) syringes or 3-mL syringes are used for subcutaneous injections. Calculating dosages for subcutaneous injections may be done by using the following basic formula:

$$\frac{d}{h} \times v$$

Therefore, if the desired medication is available as 100 mg in 2 mL of solution, and the prescriber orders 75 mg to be administered, the calculation for administration would be as follows:

$$\frac{d}{h} \times v = \frac{75}{100} \times 2 = \frac{150}{100} = 1.5 \text{ mL}$$

Intramuscular Injection

Intramuscular (IM) injections are calculated using the same formula as for subcutaneous injections. These types of injections are absorbed more quickly than by subcutaneous or intradermal injections. Intramuscular injections usually contain between 0.5 mL and 3 mL of medication.

Example 10

Dosage ordered: Duramorph 50 mg/mL IM
Dose on hand: Duramorph 10 mg/mL

$$\frac{d}{h} \times v = x$$

$$\frac{50}{10} \times 1 = x$$

$$x = 5 \text{ mL}$$

Intravenous Injection

Intravenous (IV) injections and IV fluid therapy are used to administer medications, dextrose, vitamins, electrolytes, and water. Usually these medications are available in small vials, which are mixed into large-volume solutions at a compounding pharmacy before they are ready to be administered. The amount of medication in a parenteral solution is stated on the package label, and practitioners must be aware of how many milliliters are required to be administered based on how many milligrams of medication they contain. IV medications and fluids may be given by either continuous or intermittent infusion.

Example 11

Dosage ordered: Dilantin 200 mg IV stat
Dose on hand: Dilantin 250 mg/5 mL

$$\frac{d \times v}{h} = x$$

$$\frac{200 \text{ mg}}{250 \text{ mg}} \times 5 = x$$

$$\frac{200 \times 5}{250} = 4 \text{ mL}$$

Pediatric Dosage Calculation

Dosages for children of all ages are usually less than the adult dosages of a specific medication. Because their body mass and metabolism are different than adults, dosage calculations for children must be precise. Although the best way to assure accuracy when calculating pediatric dosages is the use of the child's weight and body surface area, it is important to understand the older methods, such as Young's rule, Clark's rule, and Fried's rule. Each medication contains information in its packaging that describes whether it is safe for use in children.

Young's Rule

Young's rule is used for children who are older than 1 year of age. The rule is based on only their age, not their body size or weight. The formula is as follows:

$$\text{Pediatric dose} = \frac{\text{Child's age (in years)}}{\text{Child's age (in years)} + 12} \times \text{Adult dose}$$

So if the adult dose of a medication is 500 mg, and the child who needs the medication is 7 years old, the dosage calculation would be as follows:

$$\text{Pediatric dose} = \frac{7 \text{ years}}{7 + 12 \text{ years} = 19 \text{ years}} \times 500 \text{ mg}$$

Therefore, the child's dose of this medication should be 184 mg.

Clark's Rule

Clark's rule is based on a child's weight and is more accurate than Young's rule and Fried's rule. It uses the average adult weight (150 lb) as its basis for calculation, as follows:

$$\text{Pediatric dose} = \frac{\text{Child's weight (in pounds)}}{150 \text{ pounds}} \times \text{Adult dose}$$

So if an adult dose of a drug is 200 mg, and the child in question weighs 45 pounds, the calculation of dosage would be as follows:

$$\text{Pediatric dose} = \frac{45 \text{ pounds}}{150 \text{ pounds}} \times 200 \text{ mg}$$

Therefore, the child's dose of this medication should be 60 mg.

Fried's Rule

Fried's rule is used for children (infants) who are younger than 1 year of age. The rule is based on both the child's age as well as the average adult dosage for a 150-lb adult. The formula is as follows:

$$\text{Pediatric dose} = \frac{\text{Child's age (in months)}}{150 \text{ pounds}} \times \text{Average adult dose}$$

So if the average adult dose of a drug is 300 mg, and the child is 6 months old, the calculation of dosage would be as follows:

$$\text{Pediatric dose} = \frac{6 \text{ months}}{150 \text{ pounds}} \times 300 \text{ mg}$$

Therefore, the infant's dose of this medication should be 12 mg.

Calculating Dosage Based on Body Surface Area

A nomogram is a chart that shows numeric relationships and is used to calculate a child's body surface area. This information is then used to calculate the correct dose of a medication for a child. A standard nomogram utilizes body weight and height to calculate body surface area. **Figure 7–3** shows a nomogram. For example, if a child is

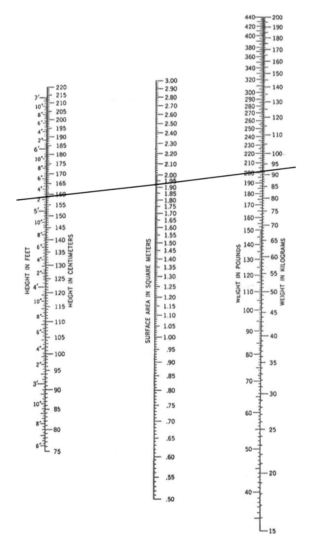

To calculate an adult's BSA, draw a straight line from the height (left column) to the weight (right column). The point at which the line intersects the surface area column is the BSA.

FIGURE 7–3 Nomogram.

35 inches in height and weighs 15 pounds, his or her body surface area would be approximately 0.6 square meters.

Patient Education

It is extremely important that patients receive instructions on how to take a prescribed drug and that they understand the medication's purpose. Each patient should fully understand the type of medication, its route of administration (if it is to be administered by the patient), the desired effect, and adverse effects that need to be reported if they occur. Patients must be instructed to take the medication exactly as directed and not to discontinue the medication until the date indicated. They should be told not to increase or decrease a drug's dosage without being instructed to do so by the prescriber.

SUMMARY

The metric system is the predominant system used in dosage calculations and prescriptions, although the apothecary and household systems are still in use for some medications. Respiratory care practitioners must be able to calculate dosages and convert between equivalents within each system and among the units of each system. Medication dosages are calculated using specific formulas for each type of form. Dosages for children are most accurately calculated by using a nomogram that utilizes a child's height and weight to determine his or her body surface area. Other calculations for children's doses include Clark's rule, Young's rule, and Fried's rule.

LEARNING GOALS

These learning goals correspond to the objectives at the beginning of the chapter, providing a clear summary of the chapter's most important points.

1. The metric system uses measurements such as grams, milligrams, kilograms, micrograms, liters, and milliliters. The apothecary system uses measurements such as grains, drams, ounces, pounds, and minims. The household system uses measurements such as drops, teaspoons, tablespoons, fluid ounces, cups, pints, quarts, and gallons.

2. In the metric system, the basic unit of weight is the gram, the basic unit of volume is the liter, and the basic unit of length is the meter.

3. In the metric system, 1 gram is equal to 1000 milligrams, $\frac{1}{1000}$ kilogram, and 1,000,000 micrograms.

4. International units are standardized throughout the world and are used to measure many vitamins. They indicate the amount required to produce a certain effect. International units do not measure substances in terms of their physical weight or volume.

5. The most accurate method of calculating a child's dose is by using a nomogram to determine the child's body surface area.

6. The fraction proportion method uses the following formula to calculate the amount to administer:

$$\frac{\text{Dose on hand } (h)}{\text{Dosage unit } (q)} = \frac{\text{Desired dose } (d)}{\text{Amount to administer } (x)}$$

7. The household system is not commonly used in medicine because it is not precisely accurate. Also, it utilizes only units of volume with measurement devices that may differ in size, such as spoons and droppers.

8. Certain drugs are measured in milliequivalents and units to indicate their strength. Milliequivalents are expressions of the number of grams of equivalent weight of a drug contained in 1 mL of a normal solution. A unit is defined as an amount of a substance required to produce a specific effect. Unit sizes differ for each drug. Units and milliequivalents cannot be directly converted into measurements of the apothecary, household, or metric systems.

9. To change grams into milligrams, multiply the number of grams by 1000. To change milliliters to liters, divide the number of milliliters by 1000.

10. The following are equivalencies between the apothecary and household systems:
    - 1 grain = 2/1000 ounce
    - 1 dram = 1/8 ounce
    - 1 ounce = 480 grains
    - 1 pound = 12 ounces
    - 1 minim = 1/60 fluid dram
    - 1 fluid dram = 1/8 fluid ounce
    - 1 fluid ounce = 1/16 pint
    - 1 pint = 1/8 gallon
    - 1 quart = 2 pints
    - 1 gallon = 4 quarts
    - 1 tablespoon = 3 teaspoons
    - 1 ounce = 2 tablespoons
    - 1 cup = 8 ounces
    - 1 pint = 2 cups

CRITICAL THINKING QUESTIONS

A physician orders Ceclor 125 mg per 5 mL p.o. q.i.d.
1. How much Ceclor should be given orally four times a day?
2. If the order for Ceclor was 250 mg per 5 mL p.o. t.i.d., how much should be given orally each time per day?

WEB SITES

http://lamar.colostate.edu/~hillger/common.html

http://www.bioscience.org/atlases/clinical/nomogram/
  nomochil.htm

http://www.dmacc.org/medmath1/HOUSEHOLD/
  hhold_pt.html

http://www.drugguide.com/ddo/ub/
  view/Davis-Drug-Guide/109514/0/
  Pediatric_Dosage_Calculations

http://www.mapharm.com/dosage_calc.htm

http://www.merck.com/mmpe/appendixes/ap1/
  ap1a.html

http://www.rncalc.com/drug_dosage_tablet/dosage_
  tablet.php

http://www.testandcalc.com/quiz/index.asp

http://www.tostepharmd.net/pharm/clinical/
  measurement.html

REVIEW QUESTIONS

Fill in the Blank

Identify the correct numeric values for each of the following measurements.

1. 1 L = _____ mL
2. 1 kg = _____ g
3. 1 cm = _____ m
4. 1 m = _____ mm
5. 1 mg = _____ g
6. 1 mL = _____ L
7. 1 mm = _____ m
8. 1 mcg = _____ mg
9. 1 mcg = _____ g
10. 1 pt = _____ pints
11. 1 oz = _____ gr
12. 1 lb = _____ oz
13. 1 gal = _____ quarts
14. 1 pt = _____ cups
15. 1 gtt = _____ mL
16. 1 tsp = _____ mL
17. 1 cup = _____ oz
18. 1 oz = _____ tbsp
19. 1 tbsp = _____ tsp
20. 1 cup = _____ mL
21. 1 qt = _____ mL
22. 1 T = _____ mL
23. 1 kg = _____ lbs
24. 1 qt = _____ pt
25. 1 gr = _____ mg

CALCULATE THE AMOUNT TO ADMINISTER

Calculate the desired dose and then calculate the amount to administer in the following exercises.

1. Dosage ordered: ampicillin 0.25 g p.o. q.i.d.
    Dose on hand: ampicillin 125 mg capsules
    Amount to administer: _____ capsule(s)
2. Dosage ordered: cloxacillin 500 mg p.o. t.i.d.
    Dose on hand: cloxacillin 125 mg per 5 mL
    Amount to administer: _____ mL
3. Dosage ordered: Covera-HS 480 mg p.o. b.i.d.
    Dose on hand: Covera-HS 240 mg tablets
    Amount to administer: _____ tablet(s)
4. Dosage ordered: Lopid 0.6 g p.o. b.i.d.
    Dose on hand: Lopid 600 mg tablets
    Amount to administer: _____ tablet(s)
5. Dosage ordered: Lorabid oral suspension 150 mg p.o. b.i.d.
    Dose on hand: Lorabid oral suspension 100 mg per 5 mL
    Amount to administer: _____ mL

CALCULATE THE AMOUNT FOR A SINGLE DOSE

Calculate the amount to prepare for a single dose.

1. Dosage ordered: Garamycin 40 mg IM q8h
    Dose on hand: Garamycin 80 mg/2 mL
    Administer: _____ mL
2. Dosage ordered: heparin 8000 U SC q12h
    Dose on hand: heparin 10,000 U/mL vial
    Administer: _____ mL
3. Dosage ordered: Adrenalin 0.2 mg SC stat
    Dose on hand: Adrenalin 1:2000 solution
    Administer: _____ mL
4. Dosage ordered: Cleocin 300 mg IM q.i.d.
    Dose on hand: Cleocin 0.6 g/4 mL
    Administer: _____ mL
5. Dosage ordered: Robinul 0.15 mg IM stat
    Dose on hand: Robinul 0.2 mg/mL
    Administer: _____ mL

CASE STUDY

Amanda is 11 months old, weighs 28 pounds, and is 33 inches tall. The adult dose of erythromycin is 400 mg every 6 hours by mouth.

1. What is the calculated dose of erythromycin that Amanda should receive based on her size, using Clark's rule to calculate?
2. If a nurse wants to use Fried's rule, what would Amanda's dose be? Show the steps needed to calculate.

Medication Errors

OBJECTIVES

Upon completion of this chapter, the reader should be able to the following:

1. Explain the importance of medication errors.
2. Identify factors that affect medication errors.
3. Describe how medication errors can be reduced.
4. Explain why documentation of medication errors is essential.
5. Identify factors related to patient errors.
6. Explain the importance of reporting medication errors.
7. List organizational and environmental methods that can reduce human error.
8. Define therapeutic duplication and explain how it can affect a patient.
9. Explain factors that can cause medication errors during the prescribing process.
10. Describe the potential for errors during medication administration.

KEY TERMS

Administration errors
Commission errors
Dispensing errors
Manufacturing errors
Medication error
National Drug Code
Omission errors
Patient error
Prescribing errors
Therapeutic duplication

INTRODUCTION

The National Coordinating Council for Medication Error Reporting and Prevention (NCCMERP) describes a medication error as "any preventable event that may cause or lead to inappropriate medication use or patient harm while the medication is in the control of the health-care professional, patient, or consumer."

Medications must be prescribed, prepared, dispensed, and administered to patients safely and appropriately. Despite healthcare providers' expertise and commitment, errors and other adverse events can occur, causing medications to potentially harm patients. For example, the wrong drug, strength, or dose can be administered. A sound-alike or look-alike drug can be mistaken for another. Medication can be given via the incorrect route of administration. Doses can be miscalculated. Medical equipment can be misused. The wrong medication can be prescribed or transcribed. The wrong patient can be chosen from a list on a computer screen. Errors happen every day in every healthcare setting.

The large number of new drugs and technologies introduced annually further complicate medication use. Another factor is the growing elderly population. Many older adults have chronic or acute conditions that require complex treatment strategies. Every error has the potential to be tragic and costly in both human and economic terms.

Factors Influencing Medication Errors

A medication error may be anything that has the potential to cause patient harm or lead to incorrect use of a medication. Medication errors can be made by anyone in the healthcare profession, as well as by patients. They also can be made by those involved in risk management, legal capacities, and manufacturing. Manufacturing errors may include the following:

- contamination
- mislabeling
- incorrect drug
- incorrect concentration
- incorrect dose

Factors that can influence medication errors include the following:

- miscommunication
- handwriting
- look-alike and sound-alike drugs
- misuse of zeroes and decimal points
- confusion of dosing units
- use of dangerous abbreviations and symbols
- lack of complete information
- omission errors

The most common type of medication error involves the drug's dosage.

The Significance of Medication Errors

Nearly 100,000 United States citizens experience permanent harm or death each year because of preventable medical errors. Approximately 7000 deaths are caused each year in the United States by medication errors. Those who survive the effects of a medication error may miss work and lose income, pay more medical expenses, and experience prolonged illnesses as they recover.

Reducing Medication Errors

There are many ways to reduce medication errors in the medical setting. Prescriptions with similar drug names should always be verified, including their spelling and strength. Warning labels must be affixed to prescription vials when required.

Unfamiliar abbreviations must be verified; use the Do Not Use list published by The Joint Commission or the Dangerous Abbreviations list published by the NCCMERP. Common abbreviations that should not be used according to The Joint Commission include the following:

- U: write out unit
- IU: write out International Unit
- Q.D., QD, q.d., qd: write out daily
- Q.O.D., QOD. q.o.d., qod: write out every other day
- MS, MSO$_4$, MgSO$_4$: write out morphine sulfate or magnesium sulfate
- @: can be mistaken for the number 2; write out at

The Joint Commission also advises that trailing zeroes should be avoided so that decimal points cannot be missed. An example is 3.0 mg, which should be written as 3 mg. If the decimal point were missed, the practitioner might think it says 30 mg, which is 10 times more than 3 mg. Also, leading zeroes must always be used. An example is .5 mg, which should be written as 0.5 mg. If the lack of a leading zero caused the decimal point to be missed, the practitioner might think it says 5 mg, which is 10 times more than 0.5 mg. The Joint Commission also advises that the symbols > (greater than) and < (less than) should be avoided. The greater than symbol can be mistaken for the number 7, and the less than symbol can be mistaken for the letter L (the abbreviation for liter). Instead, the terms greater than and less than should be written out. Common abbreviations that should not be used according to the NCCMERP include the following:

- µg: write out micrograms
- SC or SQ: write out subcutaneous
- TIW, T.I.W., tiw, t.i.w.: write out three times a week
- D/C: write out discharge or discontinue
- HS: write out half strength or at bedtime
- cc: can be mistaken for U (units) if poorly written
- AU, AS, AD, OU, OS, OD: may be mistaken for each other; write out both ears, left ear, right ear, both eyes, left eye, or right eye

When you discover drug interactions or therapeutic duplications, alert the pharmacist. Never guess when prescriptions have illegible handwriting; always confirm the drug, its strength, and its dosing schedule. Avoid selecting the incorrect drug product by using the pull–dispense–review (PDR) system. Check the drug name and any identifying numbers, such as the National Drug Code (NDC) number, when taking the drug from the shelf. Check its name, strength, and dosage form against the medication order. When returning the drug to the shelf, confirm this information a third time. Memorize the generic and brand names of commonly dispensed drugs. Memorize the strengths, dosage forms, and dosing frequencies of commonly dispensed drugs. Verify the identification of every person who picks up a prescription. Check all labels to make sure they are accurate. Avoid distractions by developing a routine that helps keep you focused. Give out patient information sheets as required. Verify all calculations to make sure they are correct.

Other general recommendations for reducing medication errors include having a defined system for drug administration, ordering, and dispensing. Drug use reviews, complete medication histories and profiles, and verified allergy information are good ways to avoid these situations. Making sure that drugs can be prepared in safe, clean environments without undue distractions is a further step. Error-tracking systems, standardized measurement systems, and an adequate number of staff members combine to provide a setting that encourages the reduction of medication errors.

Prescribing Errors

Prescribing errors involve physicians, nurse practitioners, dentists, pharmacists, and other healthcare professionals who are allowed to prescribe medications. Errors made by these individuals are often due to miscommunication or misinformation. Care must be taken to assure that all handwriting is clear and legible. A badly written prescription or medication order can cause confusion about drugs, quantities, and other information. Some drugs are marketed with names that are closely similar to other drugs. Poor handwriting may cause the wrong drug to be dispensed simply because the ordered drug's name was misread.

Another danger is the misuse of zeroes and decimal points. A poorly written number, such as 5.0, could be mistaken for 50 if the decimal point is not noticed. Because 50 is 10 times more than 5.0 (or 5), patient harm is a potential reality. For decimal values that are less than 1, a zero before the decimal point is always necessary to avoid medication errors. For example, eight-tenths of a milligram should always be written as 0.8 mg, never as simply .8 mg. This is because it is relatively easy to misread the number if the decimal point is not seen, causing the administered amount to be 8 mg, which is 10 times the intended amount. The use of symbols, such as apothecary symbols for dram or ounce, may easily be mistaken for various numbers and other terms. Symbols that can easily be mistaken should be avoided at all costs, with the desired quantities and measurements written out in full. For example, there is no mistaking 3 milligrams for 3 micrograms if the measurement is written out, but 3 mg and 3 mcg can be misread much more easily.

Errors concerning misinformation occur when a patient's drug or medical history was not taken sufficiently. Many different items must be included in these histories, including the patient's complete allergy history, a list of all the medications (and supplements) the patient is taking, previous conditions that have been diagnosed, and all lab test results. Therapeutic duplication describes a situation in which a medication is prescribed that the patient is already receiving, even if it is not exactly the same medication, increasing the chance for a medication error to occur. Also, a drug may conflict with another condition that the patient is experiencing. If the condition is not included in the patient's history, a new medication can be prescribed for the immediate reason for the patient's visit, yet it might be contraindicated because of the undocumented other condition.

Commission errors are those that occur when a drug that has been discontinued for the patient is accidentally restarted or when a drug is added to the patient's medication history in error. Patients may sometimes be confused due to illness or other medications, and this can result in them giving incorrect information about the medications they are taking or have previously taken.

Dispensing Errors

Dispensing errors may be made by people involved in any part of the dispensing of medications. These individuals include pharmacists, pharmacy technicians, and pharmacy assistants (regardless of their job titles). Distractions in the pharmacy setting may play a large role in causing dispensing errors. Serious medication errors can be caused by confusing one abbreviation for another or for a completely different term. Abbreviations that should be avoided were discussed previously. Inaccurate transcribing of medication orders can cause incorrect information to be entered into the pharmacy computer, resulting in all sorts of medication errors.

When a pharmacist does not sufficiently monitor a patient's drug therapy, the ordered medication, dose, or dosing frequency may cause medication errors. Drug interactions may occur if the potential for these interactions is missed. When two therapeutically equivalent drugs are ordered for the same patient, at the same time or different times, the pharmacist must alert the prescriber. Refills of discontinued medication can also be stopped by sufficient drug therapy monitoring.

Pharmacy staff may also cause medication errors to occur when they use improper sterile technique during compounding. Parenteral medications must be completely sterile and must be mixed using the precise amounts of compatible ingredients that have been correctly calculated. Other factors that may occur during the dispensing process include improper labeling, choosing incorrect drug products, putting completed medication packages into the incorrect patient's bag, and handing another patient's bag to a different patient without identifying the patient by name.

New and improved technology has helped to reduce dispensing errors. Systems such as Pyxis, Diebold, Acu-Dose-Rx, and Omnicell are among the leaders in automated dispensing technology. These various systems offer automated drug dispensing, computer interfaces that connect pharmacies with other healthcare professionals and suppliers, and extreme accuracy in all functions. Along with the use of bar codes on medications and medication-related supplies, quick and easy procedures are now in place to help verify most medication dispensing functions and their accuracy.

Administration Errors

Errors involving administration are commonly made by healthcare providers and caregivers. Administration

> **POINT TO REMEMBER**
>
> High-alert medications are associated with an increased risk of patient harm when they are administered inappropriately.

errors include giving a drug to the wrong patient, giving the incorrect strength of a drug, giving medications too frequently or not frequently enough, and using the incorrect dosage form.

Patient Errors

Patients commonly make medication errors when self-administering because they may be unaware of the correct information about specific drugs. They are often confused by generic and trade names and may be unaware that a generic drug they are taking is the same as a brand name drug they get from a pharmacy. Sometimes a patient receives a medication from one physician then receives another similar medication from a different physician. If the patient takes both medications without a healthcare professional being aware of the situation, the potential for therapeutic duplication exists because no one has instructed the patient properly. Another possibility for **patient error** is when a patient refills one of his or her medications that has been discontinued by the healthcare provider because the patient is unaware of the discontinuation.

According to the U.S. Pharmacopeia's Safe Medication Use Expert Committee, warfarin is the drug most commonly involved in medication errors in the home, followed by insulin, morphine, and vancomycin. Most medication errors at home are caused by communication problems, followed by lack of knowledge and inadequate (or lack of) monitoring. Most errors involve improper dose, followed by omission errors. Most of the time the patient and his or her family member or other caregiver is at fault, followed by nurses, then by physicians or pharmacists.

Patients need to understand that the prescribed amount must be strictly adhered to. Taking double the amount of headache tablets for a severe headache may not be safe. Skipping a dose of certain medications makes them less effective in treating the condition they were prescribed for. Taking less than the prescribed dose of a medication because it is expensive, with the rationale that it will last longer and save money, may result in less than the therapeutic dosage and ineffectiveness.

> **POINT TO REMEMBER**
>
> A number of technologies that can help reduce medication errors exist today. These include computerized physician order entry, automated dispensing machines, bar coding, computerized medication administration records, and smart infusion pumps.

Documenting Medication Errors

Medication errors should be documented in a clear, factual manner, without blame or judgment. When an error occurs, follow-up documentation should include the measures that were taken to counteract the error. Procedures and medications given for this situation should be included. Names of all individuals involved in or notified of the error should be listed. Failure to document occurrences of medication errors can lead to charges of negligence and have potential legal outcomes. A patient's medication administration record (MAR) should be updated with any medication error situations that may have occurred.

Complete incident reports should be created to identify factors that may have contributed to the error. This document is separate from the patient's medical record. Both documents may be used for legal reasons and for improving the medication administration process. Today, many hospitals and other healthcare institutions utilize quality improvement programs that include monitoring for medication errors.

Reporting Medication Errors

It is the healthcare practitioner's responsibility to report any medication errors they discover. The Food and Drug Administration (FDA) utilizes its MedWatch program to encourage voluntary reporting of any type of medication error so that it can be included in the FDA database. This is used to help other healthcare professionals avoid similar mistakes. A toll-free number (1-800-23-ERROR) is provided for confidential reporting of medication errors. The Institute for Safe Medication Practices (ISMP) accepts consumer and healthcare provider reports that are related to medication safety. This organization publishes *Safe Medicine*, a newsletter focusing on medication errors. The ISMP may be contacted at 215-947-7797 or via its Web site, http://www.ismp.org/.

ISMP has compiled a list of specific medications and drug classes that are considered to be high alert. This list includes adrenergic agonists and antagonists (given intravenously), general anesthetic agents, antiarrhythmics (lidocaine and amiodarone), antithrombotic agents, and chemotherapy medications. The high-alert drug list also includes hypertonic dextrose solutions, oral antidiabetic agents, intravenous digoxin and milrinone, intravenous moderate sedatives, narcotics, and total parenteral nutrition solutions.

The U.S. Pharmacopeia's anonymous medication errors reporting program, MEDMARX, is used by hospitals. The program's toll-free number is 800-822-8772, and its Web site is www.medmarx.com. Also, the National Coordinating Council for Medication Error Reporting and Prevention (NCCMERP) was formed in 1995 to help standardize the medication error reporting system. This organization coordinates information and education concerning medication errors. Their telephone number is 1-800-822-8772.

> **POINT TO REMEMBER**
>
> The specific medications that have been labeled high alert are intravenous insulin, anticoagulants, narcotics, intravenous potassium concentrations, and hypertonic sodium chloride solutions.

> **POINT TO REMEMBER**
>
> The first step in preventing medication errors is to create a safety culture that encourages the reporting of errors.

Patient Education

Respiratory therapists should emphasize that patients can be responsible for medication errors when they self-administer. They must take only the exact dosages that have been prescribed and not increase or decrease them. They also must follow dosage guidelines from OTC and herbal drugs exactly as indicated on the packaging. Patients must notify their physician of all OTC and herbal drugs they are taking. Those who are on several medications must be especially careful because of the higher potential for drug interactions.

SUMMARY

Medication errors may occur in the processes of prescribing, transcribing, dispensing, and administering medications. Illegible prescriptions may cause confusion among drugs with similar names. Medication errors occur due to misplacement of zeroes and decimal points. Another factor is improper conversion between measurement systems. Other considerations include lack of familiarity with a prescribed drug, incorrect interpretation of a prescription's contents, improper product preparation, lack of prescription monitoring, product labeling, and inaccurate dispensing.

Medication errors made by patients can be minimized by proper education. They can be avoided by verifying prescriptions with similar drug names and unfamiliar abbreviations. Medication errors can be prevented by becoming familiar with brand and generic names, strengths, dosage forms, and dosing frequencies of commonly dispensed drugs. Verifying all calculations can also minimize medication errors. The FDA (MedWatch), ISMP, and U.S. Pharmacopeia (MEDMARX) are three agencies that track medication error types and levels of harm by allowing reporting from healthcare professionals and consumers.

LEARNING GOALS

These learning goals correspond to the objectives at the beginning of the chapter, providing a clear summary of the chapter's most important points.

1. Close to 100,000 US citizens experience permanent harm or death each year because of preventable medical errors. Approximately 7000 deaths are caused each year in the United States by medication errors. Those who survive may miss work, lose income, pay more medical expenses, and experience prolonged illnesses.

2. Factors that can influence or affect medication errors include miscommunication, handwriting, look-alike and sound-alike drugs, misuse of zeroes and decimal points, confusion of dosing units, inappropriate abbreviations, lack of complete information, and omission errors.

3. Medication errors can be reduced by verifying prescriptions with similar drug names, verifying spellings, and verifying drug strengths. Warning labels should be affixed when required, and all labels must be verified. Unfamiliar abbreviations must be verified. Drug interactions and therapeutic duplications must be watched for. The drug and its dosing schedule must be confirmed. The correct drug must be selected. NDC numbers must be verified. Other techniques to reduce medication errors include memorizing generic names, brand names, strengths, dosage forms, and dosing frequencies of commonly dispensed drugs; verifying patients' IDs; avoiding distractions; checking calculations; and giving out patient information sheets.

4. Medication errors should be documented so that clear, complete records of actions that were taken to counteract the error can be established. For legal reasons, the names of everyone involved in the error should be documented. Good documentation helps to identify factors that contributed to the error to improve the medication administration process.

5. Patients commonly make medication errors when self-administering because of being unaware of the correct information about specific drugs. They may not understand therapeutic duplication and therefore may take too many of the same or very similar drugs that have been prescribed by different physicians. Patients may be unaware that a medication has been discontinued by a healthcare provider and refill the medication in error. Most patient errors occur because of communication problems, lack of knowledge, and inadequate (or lack of) monitoring.

6. Good reporting of medication errors helps to expand the databases of information about these errors, with the goal of reducing future errors. Information can then be coordinated and education can be provided to potentially stop future errors from occurring. A standardized medication error reporting system is the best way to reduce medication errors as much as possible.

7. Organizational factors related to medication errors include having a defined system for drug administration, ordering, and dispensing, as well as utilizing drug use reviews, complete medication histories and profiles, and verifying allergy information. Environmental factors related to medication errors include safe, clean environments without undue distractions, as well as error-tracking systems, standardized measurement systems, and adequate numbers of staff members.

8. Therapeutic duplication describes a situation in which a medication is prescribed that the patient is already receiving, even if it is not exactly the same medication. It can increase the chance for

a medication error to occur. Also, a drug may conflict with another condition that the patient is experiencing. If a condition is not included in the patient's history, a new medication might be contraindicated because of the undocumented condition.

9. Prescription errors may be caused by miscommunication, misinformation, illegible handwriting, similar drug names, misuse of zeroes and decimal points, use of easily mistaken symbols and abbreviations, lack of complete information, therapeutic duplication, conflicting drugs, and contraindications.

10. The potential for administration errors exists whenever healthcare providers and caregivers administer medications. Administration errors include giving a drug to the wrong patient, giving the incorrect strength of a drug, giving medications too frequently or not frequently enough, and using the incorrect dosage form.

CRITICAL THINKING QUESTIONS

1. Why should you be concerned about medication errors?
2. Explain how medication errors can be prevented and reduced.

WEB SITES

http://www.ahrq.gov/qual/errorsix.htm
http://www.chcf.org/topics/hospitals/index
.cfm?itemID=12682
http://www.highlighthealth.com/healthcare/
pharmacy-errors-avoid-prescription-dispensing-
mistakes/
http://www.icn.ch/matters_errors.htm
http://www.ismp.org/
http://www.medscape.com/viewarticle/408567_4
http://www.pubmedcentral.nih.gov/articlerender
.fcgi?artid=1744016
http://www.pubmedcentral.nih.gov/articlerender
.fcgi?artid=2671971
http://www8.nationalacademies.org/onpinews/
newsitem.aspx?RecordID=11623

REVIEW QUESTIONS

Multiple Choice

Select the best response to each question.

1. When a drug has been discontinued for a patient and is accidentally restarted, this situation is referred to as a(n)
   A. dispensing error
   B. administration error
   C. manufacturing error
   D. commission error

2. Errors involving the failure to administer a prescribed medication are referred to as
   A. dispensing errors
   B. commission errors
   C. omission errors
   D. administration errors

3. Medication errors happen every day in
   A. hospitals
   B. clinics
   C. pharmacies
   D. every healthcare setting

4. Manufacturing errors may include all of the following except
   A. incorrect doses
   B. warning labels
   C. mislabeling
   D. contamination

5. The most common type of medication error involves
   A. drug dosages
   B. contamination
   C. mislabeling
   D. miscommunication

6. Which of the following organizations introduced Dangerous Abbreviations that should *not* be used?
   A. Department of Health (DH)
   B. The Joint Commission
   C. Department of Insurance (DOI)
   D. Drug Enforcement Agency (DEA)

7. A respiratory care technologist administers a medication to the wrong patient. He must then take all of the following steps except
   A. notifying the physician
   B. documenting the medication error in his notebook
   C. filling out a complete incident report
   D. checking the vital signs of the patient

8. Most medication errors that occur at home are caused by
   A. taking two or three drugs per day
   B. taking only herbal drugs
   C. self-administration of drugs by children
   D. communication problems

9. Which of the following factors may play a large role in causing dispensing errors?
   A. distractions in the pharmacy setting
   B. network difficulties
   C. looking at a reference book to verify a drug's trade name
   D. asking questions related to the dosage of drugs

10. The abbreviation NDC means
    A. National Dental Commission
    B. National Drug Code
    C. New Drug Control
    D. No Dangerous Code

11. Which of the following is a general recommendation for reducing medication errors?
    A. defining the responsibilities of a respiratory care therapist
    B. getting general information from a pharmacist
    C. having a defined system for drug administration
    D. both a and c

12. Approximately how many people in the United States die from medication errors every year?
    A. 3000
    B. 7000
    C. 24,000
    D. 98,000

13. Which of the following is the correct way to write a dosage order for digoxin?
    A. digoxin 25.0 mg
    B. digoxin .25 mg
    C. digoxin 0.25 mg
    D. digoxin 025 mg

14. Which of the following federal agencies established the MedWatch program for the reporting of medication errors?
    A. CMS
    B. DEA
    C. The Joint Commission
    D. FDA

15. Parenteral medications must be
    A. completely sterile
    B. administered by a nurse
    C. approved by the DEA
    D. inexpensive

CASE STUDY

Heparin is often administered to newborn babies to prevent clotting in both their bodies and IV lines. A newborn was ordered to receive heparin, but the nurse misread the correct dosage, and the baby received 10,000 units per mL instead of the desired dose of 10 units per mL. The baby developed a nosebleed and skin bruising, and the mistake was discovered after measuring her blood clotting factors. Steps were taken immediately to counteract the effects of the heparin, and luckily the baby survived.

1. What drug is commonly used to counteract heparin overdosage?
2. If the error had not been discovered, what other signs and symptoms would result from the overdosage?

Treatment of Cardiopulmonary Disorders

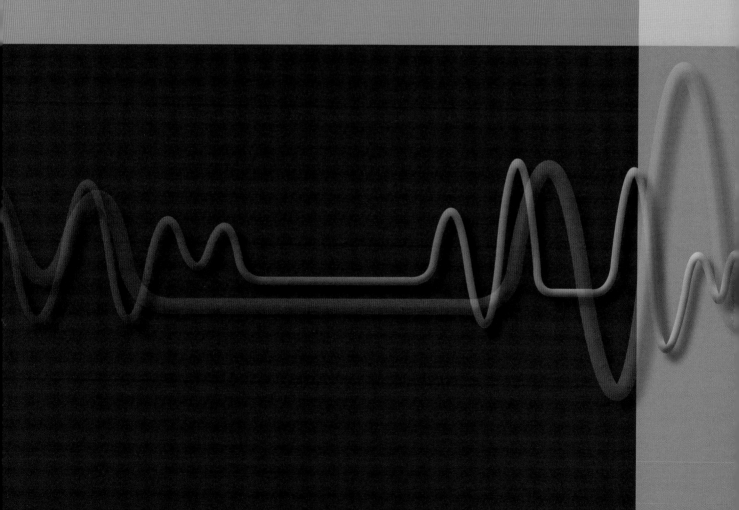

Antianginal Medications

OBJECTIVES

Upon completion of this chapter, the reader should be able to the following:

1. Define the pathophysiology of angina pectoris.
2. Name the mainstays of angina therapy.
3. Describe the method of action for each classification of drugs used to treat angina.
4. Identify the adverse effects of nitroglycerin.
5. Describe the contraindications of calcium channel blockers.
6. Explain the adverse effects of beta-adrenergic blockers.
7. Define bradycardia, tachycardia, vasodilation, and vasospasm.
8. Describe the adverse effects of calcium channel blockers.
9. List the routes of administration for nitroglycerin.
10. Define the terms sympathetic and prophylaxis.

KEY TERMS

Bradycardia	Tachycardia
Postural hypotension	Unstable angina
Prophylaxis	Variant angina
Reflex tachycardia	Vasodilation
Stable angina	Vasospasms
Sympathetic	

INTRODUCTION

Angina pectoris is a common form of ischemic heart disease and often precedes or accompanies myocardial infarction. Angina pectoris is defined as chest pain and as a squeezing pressure that can radiate to the jaw and arm. It caused by insufficient oxygen to an area of the myocardium. Angina pectoris affects patients who are older than age 55 years more than any other age group. The major risk factors associated with angina and coronary heart disease include cigarette smoking, elevated blood lipid levels, diabetes, and hypertension.

Anginal pain often is caused by physical exertion or emotional excitement. This is associated with increased myocardial oxygen demand, and episodes are usually of short duration. If physical rest and stress reduction occurs, the increased demands on the heart diminish. The discomfort then subsides within 5 to 10 minutes. There are several types of angina: classic (stable), unstable, and Prinzmetal (variant). In stable angina, oxygen requirements exceed the body's ability to supply oxygen. This may be caused by narrowing of the coronary arteries due to atherosclerosis (deposits of fat in the vessels) or from activities that increase physical exertion. Normally, this type of angina is reversed with rest. Stable angina is the most common form of angina.

Unstable angina is caused by severely decreased coronary blood flow. In this form, pain occurs when the patient is resting or sleeping. Unstable angina is accompanied by a high risk for myocardial infarction. Variant angina is caused by sudden coronary artery spasms that induce ischemia in the heart muscle. These spasms, if they occur over a long period of time, can lead to sudden death. However, variant angina is a relatively rare condition. Variant angina

POINT TO REMEMBER

Patients with angina develop ST segment elevation or depression on the electrocardiogram (ECG) during myocardial hypoxia. This can be induced diagnostically by the following:

» treadmill stress testing
» ergonovine, which induces coronary vasoconstriction
» dobutamine, which increases heart rate and contractility

may occur at the same time each day, and it can awaken a patient from sleep. It may intensify or worsen over a long period of time (often years) but does not carry the same concern as unstable angina.

Signs and symptoms include pressure or heaviness in the chest, which the patient may describe using other terms. It may be accompanied by sweating, light-headedness, hypotension, pulse changes (low or high), or indigestion. The pain may radiate to the arms, jaw, abdomen, or back.

Antianginal drugs are commonly used to dilate the coronary blood vessels. Organonitrates, beta-adrenergic blockers, and calcium channel blockers are the most commonly used antianginal medications (see **Table 9–1**). Nitrates and calcium channel blockers dilate the coronary arteries, which may improve their antianginal effects, primarily when they are used for vasospastic angina. Combination therapy with nitrates is often preferred in treating angina to reduce adverse effects.

Organonitrates

Organonitrates (also known as organic nitrates) are the oldest and most frequently used drugs for angina pectoris. They stop acute anginal attacks and may be administered as a lingual spray, sublingual tablets, buccal tablets, transdermal patches, and parenterally. Common organonitrates include nitroglycerin, erythrityl tetranitrate, isosorbide dinitrate, isosorbide mononitrate, and pentaerythritol tetranitrate.

Nitroglycerin

Initially the drug of choice for angina pectoris, nitroglycerin is effective, fast acting, and inexpensive. A variety of different nitroglycerin preparations are available. They range in how quickly they take effect and in how long their effect lasts. Sublingual nitroglycerin acts rapidly and lasts for about 1 hour.

Method of Action

Nitroglycerin dilates blood vessels by affecting vascular smooth muscle. In stable angina, it decreases cardiac oxygen demand, and in variant angina, it increases oxygen supply. Transdermal nitroglycerin patches are applied once daily, have a slower but longer-term effect, and are worn for only up to 12 hours per day. Nitroglycerin is also available as a topical ointment.

Clinical Implications

Sublingual nitroglycerin is ideal for treating acute anginal pain or to prevent angina, but no more than one tablet every 5 minutes, not to exceed three tablets, should be taken. If it is not effective, emergency medical attention should be sought. When administered intravenously, nitroglycerin is also used to reduce hypertension.

Adverse Effects

The most common adverse effect of nitroglycerin is headache caused by vascular dilation. Other adverse

TABLE 9–1 Antianginal Medications

Generic name	Brand name	Average adult dosage
Organonitrates:		
• isosorbide dinitrate	• Isordil, Isochron, Dilatate SR	• PO, SL: 5–40 mg q.i.d.
• isosorbide mononitrate	• Imdur, Ismo, Monoket	• PO: 5–10 mg b.i.d.
• nitroglycerin	• Nitrostat, NitroQuick, Nitro-Tab, Nitrolingual, Nitro-Time, Nitrogard, Nitro-Bid, Minitran, Nitrek, Nitro-Dur	• IV, SL, spray, PO, buccal, ointment, patch: varies widely from 5 mcg to 9 mg with administration based on form
β-adrenergic blockers:		
• atenolol	• Tenormin	• Injection, PO: 50–200 mg/day
• metoprolol	• Toprol XL, Lopressor, Betaloc	• Injection, PO: 50–450 mg b.i.d.
• nadolol	• Corgard (also generic versions)	• PO: 40–240 mg/day
• propranolol	• Inderal, Inderal-LA, InnoPran XL	• Injection, PO: 80–320 mg/day
Calcium channel blockers:		
• amlodipine	• Norvasc	• PO: 5–10 mg/day
• diltiazem	• Cardizem, Cardizem CD, Cardizem LA	• Injection, PO: 30–480 mg/day
• nicardipine	• Cardene, Cardene SR	• Injection, PO: 20–40 mg t.i.d.
• nifedipine	• Procardia, Procardia XL	• PO: 10–30 mg t.i.d.
• verapamil	• Calan	• Injection, PO: 80–480 mg/day

effects include syncope from postural hypotension and reflex tachycardia, which may occasionally induce an anginal attack. Additional adverse effects include apprehension, blurred vision, weakness, vertigo, and dizziness. Serious adverse effects include circulatory collapse and anaphylactoid reactions. Prolonged use of sublingual nitrates (such as nitroglycerin or amyl nitrate) often develops tolerance and withdrawal symptoms.

Contraindications

Contraindications include hypovolemia (decrease in circulating blood volume), myocardial infarction, raised intracranial pressure, and heart blockage. Nitroglycerin should never be used with alcohol or tobacco, and it should be avoided during pregnancy and lactation. It must be stored in a cool, dark place away from heat and light.

Precautions

It is important to note that nitroglycerine should be discontinued slowly over time because abrupt discontinuation may cause vasospasms. Nitroglycerin should be used with caution in severe liver or kidney disease, conditions that cause dry mouth, early myocardial infarction, and during lactation. Patients must be advised to avoid alcoholic beverages while they are taking nitroglycerin.

Isosorbide Dinitrate and Isosorbide Mononitrate

Isosorbide dinitrate and isosorbide mononitrate provide a longer duration of action than nitroglycerin. Isosorbide dinitrate is available as a sublingual tablet, and mononitrate is available as a chewable tablet.

Method of Action

Isosorbide mononitrate is preferred because it bypasses the first-pass metabolism. It decreases preload, left ventricular end volume, and diastolic pressure while reducing myocardial oxygen consumption. Isosorbide dinitrate relaxes vascular smooth muscle to dilate peripheral blood vessels. Both isosorbide mononitrate and isosorbide dinitrate are long-acting nitrates.

Clinical Implications

Isosorbide dinitrate and mononitrate effectively treat all types of angina pectoris. Isosorbide mononitrate is not indicated for acute attacks of angina. Isosorbide dinitrate relieves acute anginal attacks and manages long-term angina pectoris. These medications are also useful for prophylaxis.

POINT TO REMEMBER

Amyl nitrate is an inhaled vasodilator that is used for rapid relief of angina.

Adverse Effects

The most common adverse effects include headache, hypotension, facial flushing, and dizziness. Nausea, vomiting, fatigue, and weakness are additional adverse effects produced by isosorbide dinitrate and isosorbide mononitrate. Adhesives used in transdermal patches can produce allergic reactions. Sublingual dosage forms can cause burning or stinging under the tongue.

Contraindications

These medications must be used with caution in patients with glaucoma. Contraindications of isosorbide mononitrate include hypersensitivity, severe anemia, recent myocardial infarction, postural hypotension, and head trauma. Other contraindications include cerebral hemorrhage and pregnancy. Contraindications of isosorbide dinitrate are similar and also include GI disease.

Precautions

Tolerance to the use of nitrates may occur, with the effectiveness of these agents lessening over time. This is most common with long-acting nitrates. Patients must be free of nitrates for at least 10 to 12 hours per day.

Beta-Adrenergic Blockers

Beta-adrenergic blockers are also known as beta-blockers or β-blockers. Common beta-blockers include atenolol, metoprolol, nadolol, and propranolol.

Method of Action

Beta-blockers produce several beneficial effects. These agents reduce oxygen demand in the heart by decreasing the heart rate. This opposes sympathetic stimulation, which causes increased heart rate and force of contraction, as well as increased oxygen rate. This type of stimulation relates to the sympathetic nervous system and therefore the fight-or-flight response. Beta-blockers prevent myocardial ischemia and pain from developing.

Clinical Implications

Beta-adrenergic blockers are often used for angina pectoris in combination with nitrates. Persistent angina requires drugs from two or more classes. These include beta-adrenergic blockers combined with long-acting nitrates or calcium channel blockers. Beta-adrenergic blockers are ideal for patients who have both hypertension and coronary artery disease because of their antihypertensive action. They are considered the drugs of choice for the prophylaxis of chronic angina. Propranolol is used prophylactically for 1.5 to 3 years after an acute myocardial infarction to decrease ischemic damage.

Adverse Effects

Adverse effects include hypotension, bradycardia, insomnia (inability to sleep), bizarre dreams, diminished sex drive, impotence, and depression. Beta-adrenergic blockers may cause bronchospasm, so their use is contraindicated in patients with asthma.

Contraindications

These agents are contraindicated in patients with diabetes because their action of decreasing the heart rate masks hypoglycemia. Other contraindications include sinus bradycardia, greater than first-degree AV block, uncompensated heart failure, cardiogenic shock, and peripheral vascular disease. They are also contraindicated during pregnancy and lactation.

Precautions

Beta-adrenergic blockers should be used cautiously in patients with asthma and diabetes mellitus. Sudden discontinuation of beta-blockers should be avoided because this action can produce tachycardia. Propranolol should be used with caution in patients with variant (Prinzmetal) angina because it can increase the coronary spasm.

> **POINT TO REMEMBER**
>
> It is important with beta-blockers to avoid rapid withdrawal of treatment because they can induce anginal attacks and rebound hypertension.

Calcium Channel Blockers

Calcium channel blockers have a number of effects on the heart that are similar to those of beta-blockers. Calcium channel blockers are used for a number of cardiovascular conditions, including arrhythmias (see Chapter 10). These blockers are also used for treating all types of angina and may be used in combination with nitrates, beta-blockers, or both. They are effective in treating variant angina because they can reduce vasospasms that prevent the flow of blood and oxygen. Calcium channel blockers interfere with calcium ion movement through cell membranes, affecting the heart as well as the peripheral vasculature. Calcium channel blockers inhibit the transport of calcium into myocardial cells and also prevent contraction of vascular smooth muscle. This decreases vascular tone and causes vasodilation. Therefore, they are prescribed to treat hypertension. Calcium channel blockers are used to treat vasospastic angina, dysrhythmia, and hypertension. Bepridil (Vascor) is used specifically for angina pectoris.

Other Drug Classifications

Anticoagulants, antiplatelet drugs, and angiotensin-converting enzyme (ACE) inhibitors may be used in those who have angina, especially when it accompanies hypertension or myocardial infarction. These agents are discussed in Chapter 11.

Patient Education

Respiratory therapists should advise patients with a history of angina pectoris to carry sublingual nitroglycerin on a regular basis. Sublingual nitroglycerin works very quickly to alleviate the chest pain of angina pectoris. They should also educate patients about lifestyle modifications to reduce further progression of cardiovascular disease and angina. This includes: smoking cessation, regular exercise, stress management, maintaining a healthy body weight, and following a low-fat, low-sodium diet.

SUMMARY

Angina pectoris is a common form of ischemic heart disease. It often precedes or accompanies myocardial infarction. Angina is caused by insufficient oxygen to a part of the myocardium. Antianginal drugs dilate coronary blood vessels. Organonitrates, beta-adrenergic blockers, and calcium channel blockers are the most commonly used agents to treat angina pectoris. Organonitrates are the oldest and most frequently used drugs for angina pectoris. These agents dilate blood vessels and alter oxygen demand. Nitroglycerin was the initial drug of choice for this condition. Beta-adrenergic blockers (beta-blockers) work by decreasing the heart rate and oxygen demand. These agents are used for angina pectoris in combination with nitrates. They should be used cautiously in patients with asthma and diabetes mellitus. Calcium channel blockers lower blood pressure and inhibit heart contraction. Similar to beta-blockers, calcium channel blockers are used for a number of cardiovascular disorders, such as angina, hypertension, and arrhythmias.

LEARNING GOALS

These learning goals correspond to the objectives at the beginning of the chapter, providing a clear summary of the chapter's most important points.

1. Angina pectoris is a type of ischemic heart disease and usually precedes or accompanies myocardial infarction. It is defined as chest pain that can radiate to the jaw and arm. It is caused by insufficient oxygen to an area of the myocardium. It affects patients older than age 55 years more than any other group. Anginal pain is often caused by physical exertion or emotional excitement.

2. The mainstays of angina therapy include the organonitrates, beta-adrenergic blockers, calcium channel blockers, and cardiac glycosides.

3. The method of action of each of the antianginal drugs listed in this chapter is as follows:
   - Organonitrates: dilate blood vessels by affecting vascular smooth muscle
   - Beta-adrenergic blockers: reduce oxygen demand in the heart by decreasing oxygen rate
   - Calcium channel blockers: interfere with calcium ion movement to lower blood pressure

and inhibit contraction of vascular smooth muscle

4. The adverse effects of nitroglycerin include headache, hypotension, and tachycardia. Also, this drug should not be discontinued abruptly because doing so may cause vasospasms.

5. The contraindications of calcium channel blockers include allergy or hypersensitivity to these agents, hypotension, pregnancy, lactation, and congestive heart failure.

6. The adverse effects of beta-adrenergic blockers include: hypotension, bradycardia, insomnia (inability to sleep), bizarre dreams, diminished sex drive, impotence, and depression.

7. The definitions of bradycardia, tachycardia, vasodilation, and vasospasm are as follows:
   - Bradycardia: abnormally slow heartbeat
   - Tachycardia: abnormally fast heartbeat
   - Vasodilation: dilation of blood vessels
   - Vasospasm: spasms of the blood vessels

8. Common adverse effects of calcium channel blockers are dizziness, hypotension, fatigue, headache, and constipation.

9. Nitroglycerin is administered via IV or as sublingual tablets, lingual spray, oral tablets, buccal tablets, topical ointment, or a transdermal patch.

10. The definitions of sympathetic and prophylaxis are as follows:
    - Sympathetic: increasing heart rate, force, and oxygen; related to the actions of the sympathetic nervous system
    - Prophylaxis: prevention; commonly referred to as preventing disease

CRITICAL THINKING QUESTIONS

1. If a toddler finds his grandfather's nitroglycerin ointment in the bedroom and spreads it over his face and arms, what are the major risks and potential adverse effects that can occur?

2. A 56-year-old man suddenly feels severe chest pain that radiates to his left arm. Then he begins sweating. Because he is in a wheelchair, it is difficult for him to get to a phone quickly. His granddaughter, who is 5 years old, is aware that something is wrong, but she is unsure of what to do. What steps can she take to help her grandfather?

3. As women age, their risk of coronary artery disease increases, with the highest risk levels occurring after menopause. What is the primary cause of this?

WEB SITES

http://www.americanheart.org/presenter.jhtml?identifier=157
http://www.cedars-sinai.edu/patients/health-conditions/angina.aspx
http://www.mayoclinic.com/health/beta-blockers/HI00059
http://www.medicinenet.com/nitroglycerin/article.htm
http://www.nlm.nih.gov/medlineplus/ency/article/000165.htm
http://www.umm.edu/enc/article/002581.htm
http://www.webmd.com/hypertension-high-blood-pressure/treatment-calcium-channel

REVIEW QUESTIONS

Multiple Choice

Select the best response to each question.

1. Sublingual nitroglycerin is rapidly effective and lasts for approximately
   A. 5 minutes
   B. 15 minutes
   C. 30 minutes
   D. 60 minutes

2. Discontinuation of nitroglycerin should take place over time because the length of action of various nitroglycerin preparations can cause
   A. vomiting
   B. vasospasms
   C. hypertension
   D. bradycardia

3. Which of the following precautions is advisable for patients taking nitroglycerin?
   A. Discard unused tablets after 5 minutes.
   B. Avoid alcoholic beverages.
   C. Avoid food or liquids.
   D. Avoid coffee or green tea.

4. Which of the following is the most common adverse effect of nitroglycerin?
   A. headache
   B. diarrhea
   C. hypertension
   D. circulatory collapse

5. Which of the following is a disadvantage of using nitrates?
   A. renal impairment
   B. asthma
   C. glaucoma
   D. tolerance

6. Isosorbide mononitrate is *not* used for
   A. stable angina
   B. acute angina attacks
   C. unstable angina
   D. variant angina

7. Which of the following is the generic name of Norvasc?
   A. metoprolol
   B. verapamil
   C. amlodipine
   D. isosorbide

8. Beta-adrenergic blockers are ideal for patients who have
   A. only stroke
   B. only hypertension
   C. both hypotension and myocardial infarction
   D. both hypertension and coronary artery disease

9. Calcium channel blockers are used to treat all of the following except
   A. hypertension
   B. angina pectoris
   C. arrhythmia
   D. hyperlipidemia

10. Which of the following is an example of a beta-adrenergic blocker?
    A. diltiazem
    B. amlodipine
    C. metoprolol
    D. isosorbide

11. Administration of intravenous nitroglycerin is contraindicated in all of the following except
    A. hypovolemia
    B. hypertension
    C. myocardial infarction
    D. heart blockage

12. Which of the following is the generic name of Imdur?
    A. isosorbide mononitrate
    B. isosorbide dinitrate
    C. nitroglycerin
    D. amlodipine

13. What is the reason that combination therapy with nitrates is preferred in the treatment of angina pectoris?
    A. It increases blood volume.
    B. It is less expensive.
    C. It has fewer adverse effects.
    D. It is better tolerated.

14. Which of the following antianginal medications is a calcium channel blocker?
    A. nicardipine
    B. propranolol
    C. isosorbide
    D. metoprolol

15. Which of the following cannot be used as a route of administration for nitroglycerin?
    A. sublingual
    B. intravenous
    C. intramuscular
    D. topical

CASE STUDY

A 25-year-old male patient complains of chest pain on the left side of his chest near the lower ribs, radiating to the back and shoulder. He says the pain continues for several minutes.

1. What procedures should be taken to diagnose the cause of his chest pain?

2. If the physician determines that the patient has angina, what advice should the respiratory therapist give to the patient?

Antiarrhythmia Medications

OBJECTIVES

Upon completion of this chapter, the reader should be able to the following:

1. Describe the classifications of drugs for the treatment of various arrhythmias.
2. Explain the method of action of potassium and calcium channel blockers.
3. Define sodium channel blockers.
4. Describe the adverse effects of beta-adrenergic blockers.
5. Explain how cardiac glycosides affect the correction of tachycardia.
6. Describe defibrillators and why they play an important role in correcting arrhythmias.
7. Describe the clinical implications of sodium channel blockers.
8. List the adverse effects of calcium channel blockers.
9. Identify the most serious type of arrhythmia.
10. Identify the most powerful, yet least toxic, class of antidysrhythmics.

KEY TERMS

Acidosis	Fibrillation
Action potential	Flutter
Agranulocytosis	Pheochromocytoma
Automaticity	Sinus node
Bioavailability	Stevens-Johnson
Bradyarrhythmias	syndrome
Catecholamine	Stroke volume
Conduction velocity	Tachyarrhythmias
Defibrillation	Thromboembolism
Exfoliative dermatitis	

INTRODUCTION

The heart muscle is unique among the other muscles of the body because it can generate and rapidly conduct its own electric impulses or action potentials. These action potentials result in the excitation of myocardial muscle fibers. These impulses are recorded on an electrocardiogram. Disorders of cardiac impulse generation and conduction range from annoying, benign arrhythmias to those that can cause serious heart function disruption and sudden cardiac death. The heart normally beats between 60 and 100 times per minute. With each beat (contraction), blood is pumped throughout the body. The blood supplies oxygen and nutrients to cells and organs, including the heart. The term arrhythmia is defined as any deviation from the normal pattern of heartbeat. Arrhythmias are sometimes called dysrhythmias. Cardiac arrhythmias may result from disturbances in the pacemaker function of the sinoatrial node, from alterations in conduction pathways and velocity, or from activation of pacemakers outside the sinus node. Normal sinus rhythm conduction progresses as follows:

Sinoatrial (SA) node → atrioventricular (AV) node → bundle of His → bundle branches (right and left) simultaneously → Purkinje fibers

This process causes contractions of the atria and ventricles. Cardiac dysrhythmias may be benign or lethal. The patient's response to the rhythm determines the urgency of treatment. Cardiac dysrhythmias are often classified as tachyarrhythmias or bradyarrhythmias.

> **POINT TO REMEMBER**
>
> There are two major categories of dysrhythmias:
> » alteration in impulse formation, such as rate, rhythm, or ectopic beats
> » alteration in conductivity, such as heart blocks

Arrhythmias may result from internal or external forces. Internal forces include hypoxia, electrolyte disturbances, acidosis, diseases of the myocardium, and atherosclerosis. External forces include stress, exercise, pain, anemia, and hypovolemia. Atrial fibrillation is the most common type of arrhythmia, and although it is not usually life threatening, it is a risk factor for stroke. Ventricular fibrillation is the leading cause of sudden cardiac death in the United States.

Arrhythmia Classifications

Dysrhythmias originate as sinus, atrial, ventricular, or heart blocks. An arrhythmia is an irregular heart rhythm or heart rate that is too rapid or too slow. They can impair the ability of the heart to distribute blood. **Table 10–1** lists the various types of arrhythmias.

> **POINT TO REMEMBER**
>
> Complications of arrhythmias are sudden cardiac death, heart attack, heart failure, and thromboembolism.

Drug Therapy for Arrhythmias

Antiarrhythmic drugs are used to treat irregular heart rhythms and rate. There are five phases in the cardiac action potential:

1. Phase 0: upstroke due to sodium
2. Phase 1: peak due to inactivation of sodium channels
3. Phase 2: plateau due to inward calcium current balancing outward potassium current
4. Phase 3: repolarization due to potassium current after calcium channel close
5. Phase 4: diastolic depolarization due to gradual increase in sodium permeability (see **Figure 10–1**)

Antiarrhythmic drugs are categorized into four classes: I, II, III, and IV. Each class is determined according to the method of action and structural similarities of the drugs they contain. Class I antiarrhythmics are further

> **POINT TO REMEMBER**
>
> Holter monitoring, event monitoring, and loop recording (implantable recorders that can be placed close to the heart to continually record electric activity) can detect arrhythmias as well as the effectiveness of drug therapy during a patient's daily activities.

TABLE 10–1   Arrhythmia Classifications

Arrhythmia	Heart Rate	Comments
Atrial fibrillation	300–400 bpm	May be nonmodifiable, modifiable, or related to other diseases (especially coronary artery disease, heart failure, and hypertension); is defined as rapid, uncoordinated contractions; is the most common arrhythmia, affecting people more often as they age
Atrial flutter	160–350 bpm	Usually occurs in right atrium, which contracts more often than the ventricle contracts; treated by inserting a catheter into the atrium rather than with drug therapy
Sinus bradycardia	Less than 60 bpm	May be normal in trained athletes who maintain a large stroke volume and during sleep
Sinus tachycardia	More than 100 bpm	A normal response during fever, exercise, and in situations that incite sympathetic stimulation
Supraventricular tachycardia	Up to 200 bpm	Occurs in the heart above the area of the ventricles; may be intermittent or frequent; may last several seconds to a few hours
Ventricular fibrillation	More than 600 bpm	The most dangerous type of arrhythmia; may be life threatening due to inability of ventricles to fill with blood and ineffective blood pumping; can usually only be reversed with an electric shock to the heart via a defibrillator
Ventricular tachycardia	More than 200 bpm	May occur when electric impulses between heart chambers are impaired across scar tissue that has been caused by a previous heart attack

subdivided into class Ia, Ib, and Ic (see **Table 10–2**).

There are four primary mechanisms of antiarrhythmic action that correspond to the four major classes of antiarrhythmics. **Table 10–3** summarizes the antiarrhythmic agents and lists their method of action and uses.

Sodium Channel Blockers (Class I)

Class I sodium channel blockers are the largest class of antidysrhythmics. They are divided into three subgroups: Ia, Ib, and Ic. These subgroups are based on slight differences in their mechanisms of action. Sodium channel blockers act, in general, by reducing the maximal rate of contraction of the myocardium. They accomplish this by blocking sodium ion channels in myocardial cells. This slows the

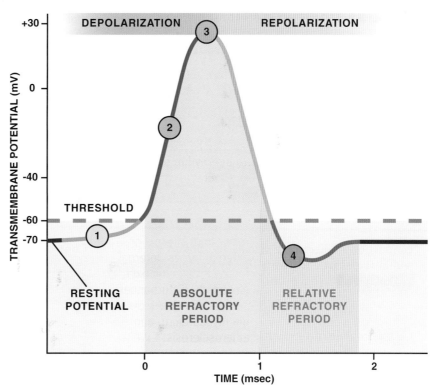

FIGURE 10–1 Action potential.

TABLE 10–2 Classes of Antiarrhythmics

Class	Generic Name	Trade Name	Dosage Strength
I: sodium channel blockers • Ia: intermediate effects	• disopyramide • procainamide • quinidine gluconate • quinidine sulfate	• Norpace, Norpace CR • Procanbid, Pronestyl • Quinadure • Generic only	• 100–150 mg • 250–1000 mg • Injection: 80 mg/mL; tablet: 324 mg • 200–300 mg
Ib: short effects	• lidocaine • mexiletine • phenytoin	• Xylocaine • Mexitil • Dilantin	• Injection: 0.5–4% • 150–250 mg • Injection: 10–15 mg/kg, then 300 mg/day in divided doses
Ic: prolonged effects	• flecainide • moricizine • propafenone	• Tambocor • Ethmozine • Rythmol, Rythmol SR	• 50–150 mg • 200–300 mg • 150–425 mg
II: beta-adrenergic blockers	• acebutolol • esmolol • propranolol	• Sectral • Brevibloc • Inderal, InnoPran XL	• 200–400 mg • 10–250 mg/mL • PO (tablet or capsule): 10–160 mg; injection: 1 mg/mL; PO (solution): 20 mg/5 mL
III: potassium channel blockers	• amiodarone • bretylium • dofetilide • ibutilide • sotalol	• Cordarone, Pacerone • Bretylium • Tikosyn • Corvert • Betapace, Betapace AF	• Injection: 50 mg/mL; PO: 100–400 mg • Injection: 5 mg/kg rapid IV injection; IM: 5-10 mg/kg0– • PO: 500 mcg bid, indivualized per patient • 0.01 mg/kg, individualized per patient • 240 mg
IV: calcium channel blockers	• diltiazem • verapamil	• Cardizem, Tiazac • Calan, Calan SR, Isoptin SR, Verelan, Verelan PM, Covera HS	• PO: 30–540 mg for angina and hypertension; IV: 0.25 mg/kg IV bolus over 2 min for atrial fibrillation • PO (extended release capsule): 180–360 mg; PO (tablet): 40–120 mg; PO (extended release tablet): 100–300 mg; injection: 2.5 mg/mL

TABLE 10–3 Summary of Antiarrhythmic Agents

Drug Class	Category	Method of Action	Uses
Ia	Sodium channel blocker	Slows phase 0 depolarization	SV, ventricular tachycardia
Ib	Sodium channel blocker	Shortens phase 3 repolarization	Ventricular tachycardia
Ic	Sodium channel blocker	Slows phase 0 depolarization	Refractory ventricular arrhythmias
II	Beta-blocker	Suppresses phase 4 depolarization	Atrial arrhythmias, SV tachycardia
III	Potassium channel blocker	Prolongs phase 3 repolarization	Atrial arrhythmias, ventricular tachycardia
IV	Calcium channel blocker	Shortens action potential	Atrial arrhythmias, SV tachycardia

conduction of electronic signals and action potential within the heart and across the myocardium, reducing automaticity.

Class Ia

Class Ia contains drugs with intermediate effects, including quinidine, procainamide, and disopyramide (see Table 10–2).

Method of Action

Quinidine depresses myocardial excitability, automaticity, conduction velocity, and contractility. Procainamide depresses myocardium excitability to electric stimulation, reducing conduction velocity in the atria, ventricles, bundles of His, and Purkinje fibers. This increases the duration of the refractory period, primarily in the atria. Disopyramide decreases myocardial conduction velocity and excitability in the atria, ventricles, and accessory pathways.

Clinical Implications

Quinidine is used for atrial fibrillation and flutter. Quinidine should be taken with food to avoid gastric upset, and patients should consume only small amounts of citrus fruits, vegetables, and milk. Procainamide is used for life-threatening ventricular dysrhythmias. The usual dosage is between 250 and 625 mg every 3 to 4 hours. Disopyramide is used to treat premature ventricular contractions and ventricular tachycardia that does not require cardioversion. Class Ia antiarrhythmic agents are also used to treat symptomatic ventricular tachyarrhythmias and for prophylactic control of supraventricular arrhythmias.

Adverse Effects

Procainamide may cause nausea, vomiting, headache, and abdominal pain. High doses may produce confusion or psychosis. Quinidine may cause dizziness, ringing in the ears, vertigo, headache, visual impairment, nausea, vomiting, diarrhea, and fever, as well as potentially decreased respiration. It reduces the renal elimination of digoxin, which can lead to an increase in digoxin toxicity. Procainamide can induce lupuslike syndrome. The adverse effects of disopyramide include constipation, dry mouth, urine retention, and visual disturbances.

Contraindications

Procainamide is contraindicated in patients with complete AV block, blood dyscrasias, myasthenia gravis, and severe congestive heart failure. Quinidine is not to be used in patients with myasthenia gravis, optic neuritis, or tinnitus. Quinidine sulfate is contraindicated in pregnant women. Disopyramide is contraindicated in cardiogenic shock, bundle branch block, certain forms of congestive heart failure, hypotension when not secondary to cardiac arrhythmia, hypokalemia, and pregnancy.

Precautions

When using quinidine, patients should be aware of any chest pain, diarrhea, or heart rhythm changes. Quinidine should be taken with food to avoid gastric upset, and patients should consume only small amounts of citrus fruits, vegetables, and milk. Procainamide must be used cautiously in patients with bone marrow suppression, hypotension, cardiac enlargement, congestive heart failure, coronary occlusion, myocardial infarction, ventricular dysrhythmia due to digitalis intoxication, hepatic or renal insufficiency, electrolyte imbalance, bronchial asthma, or history of systemic lupus erythematosus. Disopyramide must be used cautiously in cardiomyopathies, cardiac conduction abnormalities, hepatic or renal impairment, urinary tract diseases, diabetes mellitus, myasthenia gravis, narrow-angle glaucoma or family history of glaucoma, during lactation, and in the elderly.

Class Ib

Class Ib drugs are sodium channel blockers without anticholinergic activity. They include lidocaine, mexiletine, and phenytoin (see Table 10–2). Lidocaine can suppress ventricular arrhythmias to reduce primary ventricular fibrillation and is a very effective parenteral antiarrhythmic.

Method of Action

Lidocaine is rapidly metabolized in the liver with a high extraction ratio, and it has a low bioavailability. Thus, it is not used orally. It appears to block sodium channels, greatly affecting depolarized or ischemic tissues. Mexiletine is similar to lidocaine but has been modified for oral administration. It is more effective when used with another antidysrhythmic agent. Mexiletine shortens the action potential refractor period duration and improves resting potential.

Clinical Implications

Lidocaine is used for rapid control of ventricular arrhythmias during acute myocardial infarction, cardiac surgery, cardiac catheterization, and in digitalis intoxication-caused ventricular arrhythmias. Mexiletine is used for acute and chronic ventricular arrhythmias, recurrent cardiac arrests, and suppression of premature ventricular contractions due to ventricular tachyarrhythmias. Phenytoin is an anticonvulsant that also has antiarrhythmic effects.

Adverse Effects

There are a few adverse effects. At large doses it can produce convulsions, tremors, delirium, paresthesias, and drowsiness. The adverse effects of mexiletine include gastrointestinal and neurologic symptoms, as well as increased liver enzyme levels.

Contraindications

Lidocaine is contraindicated in a history of hypersensitivity to amide-type local anesthetics, in severe trauma or asepsis, blood dyscrasias, supraventricular arrhythmias, Adams-Stokes syndrome, untreated sinus bradycardia, and severe types of heart block. Lidocaine should be avoided when using cimetidine. Mexiletine is contraindicated in severe left ventricular failure, cardiogenic shock, severe bradyarrhythmias, heart block, and pregnancy. It should not be used concurrently with drugs that alter urinary pH.

Precautions

Lidocaine should be used cautiously in liver or kidney disease, congestive heart failure, hypoxia, respiratory depression, hypovolemia, shock, myasthenia gravis, elderly patients, family history of malignant hyperthermia, and during pregnancy. Mexiletine should be used cautiously in patients with sinus node conduction irregularities, intraventricular conduction abnormalities, hypotension, severe congestive heart failure, renal failure, and liver dysfunction.

Class Ic

Class Ic antiarrhythmic drugs include flecainide, propafenone, and moricizine (see Table 10–2). They have prolonged effects upon the body and induce marked reductions of sodium permeability changes.

Method of Action

Flecainide slows conduction velocity throughout the myocardial conduction system and increases ventricular refractoriness. Propafenone directly stabilizes myocardial membranes. Moricizine reduces the fast inward current carried by sodium ions and shortens phase I and phase II repolarization. This results in decreased action

potential duration and effective refractory period. It also has potent local anesthetic effects.

Clinical Implications

Flecainide is used for life-threatening ventricular dysrhythmias. Propafenone also is used for ventricular dysrhythmias. Moricizine is used for ventricular tachycardia and ventricular premature depolarization that may be life threatening.

Adverse Effects

The adverse effects of flecainide include dizziness, fatigue, chest pain, blurred vision, headache, constipation, changes in taste perception, and nausea. The adverse effects of propafenone include blurred vision, dizziness, fatigue, somnolence, headache, vertigo, hypotension, abdominal discomfort, constipation, nausea, dry mouth, taste alterations, and vomiting. The adverse effects of moricizine include dizziness, anxiety, euphoria, headache, lightheadedness, diarrhea, dry mouth, abdominal discomfort, and nausea.

Contraindications

Flecainide is contraindicated in hypersensitive patients, right bundle branch block, cardiogenic shock, hepatic impairment, congestive heart failure, acute myocardial infarction, electrolyte imbalance, and during pregnancy. Propafenone is contraindicated in uncontrolled congestive heart failure, cardiogenic shock, AV block without a pacemaker, cardiogenic shock, bradycardia, marked hypotension, bronchospastic disorders, electrolyte imbalance, hypersensitivity, non-life-threatening arrhythmias, chronic bronchitis, emphysema, pregnancy, and in children. Moricizine is contraindicated in hypersensitive patients, during AV block unless a pacemaker is present, in right bundle branch block when associated with left hemiblock unless a pacemaker is present, and in cardiogenic shock.

Precautions

Flecainide should be used with caution in atrial fibrillation, cardiac disease, elderly patients, sick sinus syndrome, renal impairment, and in children and infants. Propafenone should be used with caution in congestive heart failure, AV block, hepatic or renal impairment, during lactation, and in older adults. Moricizine should be used with caution in patients with new or increasing dysrhythmias, in coronary artery disease, history of myocardial infarction, history of congestive heart failure, history of cardiomegaly, conduction abnormalities, significant hepatic impairment, and in children.

Beta-Adrenergic Blockers (Class II)

Beta-adrenergic blockers may be the most powerful antidysrhythmic agents available, and they also have the least toxicity. They include propranolol, acebutolol, and esmolol (see Table 10–2). Sinus tachycardia may be slowed by beta$_1$-antagonists and cholinergics. Diagnosis of an arrested heart or certain types of heart block is often difficult because patients usually must be connected to an electrocardiograph while experiencing arrhythmias to determine the exact type of rhythm disorder that is occurring. Proper diagnosis and optimum pharmacotherapy can affect arrhythmia frequency and consequences quite significantly.

Method of Action

Beta-blockers act primarily by reducing the effects of the sympathetic nervous system on the myocardium. They act by decreasing heart rate and excitability. Nonselective beta-blockers of both cardiac and bronchial adrenoreceptors compete with epinephrine and norepinephrine for available beta-receptor sites. In higher doses, propranolol exerts direct quinidine-like effects, depressing cardiac function including contractility and arrhythmias. It lowers supine and standing blood pressures in hypertensive patients. Acebutolol decreases exercise-induced heart rates and decreases cardiac output. Esmolol inhibits the agonist effects of agents such as catecholamine by competitive binding at beta-adrenergic receptors.

Clinical Implications

Beta-blockers are often utilized to manage arrhythmias. Beta$_1$-antagonists are used to refresh an arrested heart and treat certain types of heart block. Propranolol is used to manage cardiac arrhythmias (paroxysmal supraventricular tachycardia, atrial flutter, and fibrillation) and prophylaxis after a myocardial infarction. This agent is also used for digitalis intoxication, anesthesia, thyrotoxicosis, angina pectoris due to coronary atherosclerosis, pheochromocytoma, and hereditary essential tremor. It may be used alone or in combination with thiazides and other antihypertensives. Acebutolol is used for mild to moderate hypertension and to manage recurrent, stable ventricular arrhythmias. Esmolol is used for supraventricular tachyarrhythmias during or after surgery, for short-term treatment of sinus tachycardia, and to control heart rate in myocardial infarction.

Adverse Effects

Propranolol may cause fever, pharyngitis, respiratory distress, weight gain, and cold extremities. Additional adverse effects include leg fatigue, arthralgia, impotence or decreased libido, erythematosus, and psoriasis-like eruptions. Some patients experience pruritus, erythema multiforme, and urticaria. Serious adverse effects of propranolol include anaphylactic or anaphylactoid reactions, Stevens-Johnson syndrome, and exfoliative dermatitis. It may also cause serious agranulocytosis and laryngospasm. Acebutolol may cause fatigue, dizziness, insomnia, drowsiness, confusion, and fainting. Serous adverse effects of acebutolol may include bradycardia, diarrhea, constipation, and agranulocytosis. Esmolol may cause headache, dizziness, somnolence, confusion, agitation, hypotension, cold extremities, bradyarrhythmias,

flushing, and myocardial depression. The most serious adverse effect of esmolol is bronchospasm.

Contraindications

Occasionally, beta-blockers may depress left ventricular function and are contraindicated in asthma. Propranolol is contraindicated in heart block, congestive heart failure, right ventricular failure secondary to pulmonary hypertension, ventricular dysfunction, and sinus bradycardia. Other contraindications include cardiogenic shock, significant aortic or mitral valvular disease, bronchial asthma, bronchospasm, and severe COPD. Additional contraindications include pulmonary edema, allergic rhinitis, major depression, peripheral vascular disease, and pregnancy. Acebutolol is contraindicated in severe bradycardia, cardiogenic shock, acute bronchospasm, pulmonary edema, during lactation, and in children younger than 12 years of age. Esmolol is contraindicated in hypersensitive patients, cardiac failure, heart block, sinus bradycardia, cardiogenic shock, decompensated congestive heart failure, bronchial asthma, acute bronchospasm, COPD, pulmonary edema, and pregnancy. Esmolol has not been established as safe for use in children.

Precautions

Propranolol is the most commonly used beta-blocker for antidysrhythmic effects. Patients should notify their physician if their pulse drops to less than 60 beats per minute while taking this drug. Patients should rise from a lying or sitting position to a standing position slowly. Acebutolol should be used with caution in impaired cardiac function, congestive heart failure, cerebrovascular disease, renal or hepatic impairment, diabetes mellitus, and with general surgical anesthesia. Acebutolol therapy should not be ceased abruptly. Esmolol should be used with caution in patients with history of allergy, congestive heart failure, diabetes mellitus, kidney function impairment, and during lactation.

Potassium Channel Blockers (Class III)

Potassium channel blockers alter the repolarization phase of the heart's contraction. Class III antiarrhythmics prolong the action potential by blocking potassium channels and prolonging phase 3 repolarization. This prolongation of potential contraction duration of the Purkinje and ventricle muscle fibers decreases the frequency of heart failure. Amiodarone and sotalol are examples of these blockers, with slightly different effects. Table 10–2 lists various potassium channel blockers.

Method of Action

Amiodarone blocks potassium as well as sodium ion channels. It has effects of all four major classes. Amiodarone acts at all sites in the myocardium, which is unusual for an antiarrhythmic. It effectively reduces almost any type of arrhythmia. Sotalol also has both class II and III properties. Its beta-blocking effects may appear more detectable than its potassium channel blocking effects.

Clinical Implications

Amiodarone is used for atrial dysrhythmias in patients with heart failure. Several weeks are required for the oral forms of this drug to take effect, but the effects can last up to 8 weeks after being discontinued due to its extended half-life. The IV form of amiodarone is typically used only for serious ventricular dysrhythmias. Sotalol is used for ventricular dysrhythmias that are considered life threatening.

Adverse Effects

Amiodarone may cause muscle weakness, numbness, tingling, fatigue, abnormal gait, dyskinesias, dizziness, and paresthesias. Other adverse effects of amiodarone include headache, bradycardia, hypotension, congestive heart failure, and arrhythmias. Serious adverse effects of this agent include sinus arrest, cardiogenic shock, and hepatotoxicity. Sotalol may cause AV block, hypotension, aggravation of congestive heart failure, bradycardia, dyspnea, chest pain, palpitation, and occasionally bleeding. The most serious adverse effects of sotalol include life-threatening ventricular arrhythmias, including polymorphous ventricular tachycardia.

Contraindications

Amiodarone is contraindicated in hypersensitive patients, cardiogenic shock, severe sinus bradycardia, advanced AV block unless with a pacemaker, bradycardia, and severe liver disease. Amiodarone should be avoided during pregnancy or lactation. Sotalol is contraindicated in hypersensitive patients, bronchial asthma, acute bronchospasm, cardiogenic shock, and uncontrolled congestive heart failure. Sotalol is not advised for chronic bronchitis, emphysema, hypokalemia, and low creatinine clearance.

Precautions

Patients must notify their physician if they experience coughing, changes in heart rate or rhythm, vision changes, or shortness of breath while taking amiodarone. This drug may cause dizziness when changing positions, so they should do this slowly. Elderly patients should be advised to protect their skin and eyes from the sun when taking this drug. Sotalol must be used cautiously in congestive heart failure, electrolyte disturbance, recent myocardial infarction, diabetes, renal impairment, pregnancy, excessive diarrhea, or profuse sweating.

Calcium Channel Blockers (Class IV)

Class IV antiarrhythmics are calcium channel blockers. Only two calcium channel blockers have been approved specifically as antiarrhythmics: verapamil and diltiazem (see Table 10-2). Because they relax smooth muscle and cause vasodilation, these agents are useful for angina and hypertension. The primary calcium channel blocker is verapamil, but diltiazem is also used (it is less potent but has increased vasodilation effects). Verapamil was the first calcium channel blocker ever used.

Method of Action

Calcium channel blockers decrease calcium entry into heart cells and blood vessels. Verapamil primarily slows conduction of the AV node, decreases the heart rate, and increases the effective refractory period. Its effects lead to decreased cardiac work and energy consumption in patients with vasospastic angina. This increases oxygen delivery to the myocardium. Diltiazem inhibits calcium ion influx to improve myocardial perfusion, reducing left ventricular workload.

Clinical Implications

Because calcium channel blockers relax smooth muscle and cause vasodilation, these agents are useful for angina pectoris and hypertension. Verapamil stabilizes dysrhythmias and is also used for hypertension and angina. Verapamil is used for atrial flutter and atrial fibrillation. It is available in oral, sustained-release, and IV forms. Diltiazem is used for vasospastic angina, chronic stable angina, and essential hypertension. The IV form is used for atrial fibrillation or flutter and supraventricular tachycardia.

Adverse Effects

Verapamil may cause dizziness, vertigo, headache, fatigue, constipation, sleep disturbances, depression, syncope, hypotension, congestive heart failure, bradycardia, severe tachycardia, and peripheral edema. The most serious adverse effect of verapamil is AV block and heart failure. Diltiazem may cause headache, fatigue, dizziness, asthenia, drowsiness, nervousness, insomnia, confusion, tremor, gait abnormality, edema, arrhythmias, angina, bradycardia, congestive heart failure, flushing, hypotension, syncope, or palpitations.

Contraindications

Verapamil is contraindicated in severe hypotension, cardiogenic shock, cardiomegaly, digitalis toxicity, severe congestive heart failure, and pregnancy. Extended-release forms of verapamil should not be used in children younger than 18 years of age. Diltiazem is contraindicated in hypersensitive patients, acute myocardial infarction, congestive heart failure, severe hypotension, and pregnancy. It should not be used in patients undergoing intracranial surgery, and it has not been established as safe for use in children.

Precautions

Patients should monitor their blood pressure before taking verapamil and notify their physician if it is below

90/60 mm Hg, if they have any difficulty breathing, or if they experience changes in their heart rhythm. Verapamil should be taken with food to avoid stomach upset. Because it causes constipation, patients should increase their intake of fiber. Diltiazem should be used with caution in right ventricular dysfunction, severe bradycardia, conduction abnormalities, renal or hepatic impairment, and in older adults. The effects of calcium channel blockers on the myocardium can be antagonized by digoxin, catecholamines, or calcium.

Miscellaneous Medications for Arrhythmia

POINT TO REMEMBER

Potassium and magnesium can be useful to decrease digoxin toxicity.

Miscellaneous medications for arrhythmia include digoxin and phenytoin (although phenytoin is not used as commonly). Digoxin is used for atrial fibrillation and flutter, reducing arrhythmias by slowing conduction velocity, and prolonging refraction in the Purkinje fibers and AV node. It may be administered orally or IV. It has a narrow therapeutic index, so digoxin doses must be carefully controlled. The first dose must equal one-half of the total daily dose. See Chapter 12 for more information on cardiac glycosides.

Nonpharmacological Treatments

Most medications to treat dysrhythmias are used when other nonpharmacological treatments will not be effective. Nonpharmacological treatments primarily include the use of external defibrillators and implantable cardioverter defibrillators. Pacemakers are devices that are implanted to correct dysrhythmias that cause the heart to beat too slowly. Other nonpharmacological treatments include destroying the myocardial cells that have caused the abnormal conduction. This is accomplished via catheter ablation, wherein a catheter is inserted into the myocardium for the procedure.

Defibrillators

Serious dysrhythmias may be corrected through defibrillation (also known as cardioversion), which involves electrically shocking the heart. This shock temporarily stops all electric impulses in the heart, whether normal or abnormal. This often causes the SA node to automatically correct the conduction so that a normal sinus rhythm is reestablished.

Implantable Cardioverter Defibrillators

Implantable cardioverter defibrillators (ICD) are inserted into patients to restore normal rhythm. They may either pace the heart properly or give it an electric shock when a dysrhythmia occurs. These devices can also store infor-

mation about the heart rhythm that can be evaluated by a healthcare practitioner at a later date.

Patient Education

Respiratory therapists should advise patients to be aware that fever, hypoxia, stress, infection, and drug toxicity may cause various types of arrhythmias. Most patients who have ischemic heart disease exhibit premature ventricular complexes, particularly if they have recently experienced myocardial infarction. Therefore, respiratory therapists should emphasize that if the physician ordered a Holter monitor for the patient, he or she must always wear it for the prescribed time period.

SUMMARY

Arrhythmias are irregular heart rhythms or heart rates that are too rapid or too slow. Antiarrhythmic drugs are categorized as class I (sodium channel blockers), class II (beta-adrenergic blockers), class III (potassium channel blockers), and class IV (calcium channel blockers). Miscellaneous medications for arrhythmias include digoxin and phenytoin. Other treatments include various types of defibrillators, pacemakers, and catheter ablation. Defibrillation involves electrically shocking the heart to allow the SA node to correct the heart rhythm.

LEARNING GOALS

These learning goals correspond to the objectives at the beginning of the chapter, providing a clear summary of the chapter's most important points.

1. Drugs for the treatment of arrhythmias include the following classes:
   - Class I: sodium channel blockers
   - Class II: beta-adrenergic blockers
   - Class III: potassium channel blockers
   - Class IV: calcium channel blockers
2. Potassium channel blockers block potassium ion channels in myocardial cells, which delays repolarization of the cells, lengthens the refractory period, and tends to stabilize dysrhythmias. Calcium channel blockers block calcium ion channels to slow conduction velocity, thus stabilizing certain dysrhythmias. Their action is similar to that of beta-adrenergic blockers, and they are safe medications that are well tolerated by most patients.
3. Sodium channel blockers are the largest class of antidysrhythmics. They block sodium ion channels to prevent depolarization, slowing the spread of action potential across the myocardium and suppressing the natural pacemaking activities of the heart. Adverse effects vary widely amongst these types of blockers, and special precautions should be taken when using these blockers in elderly adults.

4. The adverse effects of beta-adrenergic blockers include fatigue, bradycardia, hypotension, diminished libido, impotence, hypoglycemia, nausea, diarrhea, bronchospasm, dyspnea, heart failure or block, dizziness, abnormal vision, decreased concentration, hallucinations, insomnia, nightmares, depression, metabolism changes, and edema.

5. For tachycardia, the cardiac glycosides slow the cardiac rate, which is often the result of compensatory sympathetic reflexes (consequences of heart failure). When the failure is corrected, the heart does not need to compensate by experiencing tachycardia, so it returns to normal. This slowing down of the heart rate has also been attributed to the action of digitalis on the vagus nerve. This drug sensitizes the sinoatrial node, atrium, and atrioventricular node to impulses from this nerve.

6. Serious dysrhythmias may be corrected through defibrillation (cardioversion), which involves electrically shocking the heart. This shock temporarily stops all electric impulses in the heart, whether normal or abnormal. This often causes the SA node to automatically correct the conduction so that a normal sinus rhythm is reestablished. Implantable cardioverter defibrillators (ICD) are inserted into patients to restore normal rhythm. They may either pace the heart properly or give it an electric shock when a dysrhythmia occurs. These devices can also store information about the heart rhythm for evaluation by a healthcare practitioner at a later date.

7. The clinical implications of sodium channel blockers include atrial fibrillation, premature atrial or ventricular contractions, ventricular tachycardia, and severe ventricular dysrhythmias.

8. The adverse effects of calcium channel blockers include constipation, headache, hypotension, and bradycardia.

9. The most serious type of arrhythmia is ventricular fibrillation. It involves a heart rate of more than 600 bpm. This condition may be life threatening due to the inability of the ventricles to fill with blood, resulting in ineffective blood pumping. Ventricular fibrillation can usually only be reversed with an electric shock to the heart via a defibrillator.

10. The most powerful, yet least toxic, class of the antidysrhythmics is class II—the beta-adrenergic blockers.

CRITICAL THINKING QUESTIONS

1. If you, a respiratory care practitioner, find a patient unconscious on the hospital floor, what should you do for the patient? List the specific steps.

2. Explain and differentiate between defibrillators and implantable cardioverter defibrillators.

WEB SITES

http://yourtotalhealth.ivillage.com/calcium-channel-blockers.html

http://www.americanheart.org/presenter.jhtml?identifier=118

http://www.cvpharmacology.com/antiarrhy/sodium-blockers.htm

http://www.heartlibrary.com/heart-library-arrhythmia-drug-treatment.aspx

http://www.medicinenet.com/beta_blockers/article.htm

http://www.nlm.nih.gov/medlineplus/pacemakersandimplantabledefibrillators.html

http://www.quickmedical.com/defibrillator/faq.html

http://www.stereotaxis.com/Patients-Families/Arrhythmias/

REVIEW QUESTIONS

Multiple Choice

Select the best response to each question.

1. Which of the following arrhythmias is the most dangerous and life threatening?
   A. supraventricular tachycardia
   B. ventricular fibrillation
   C. ventricular tachycardia
   D. atrial fibrillation

2. Amiodarone (Cordarone) is included in which of the following classes of antiarrhythmics?
   A. sodium channel blockers
   B. calcium channel blockers
   C. beta-adrenergic blockers
   D. potassium channel blockers

3. Mexiletine (Mexitil) is included in which of the following classes of antiarrhythmics?
   A. sodium channel blockers—class Ia
   B. sodium channel blockers—class Ib
   C. sodium channel blockers—class Ic
   D. potassium channel blockers

4. Which of the following is a life-threatening adverse effect of potassium channel blockers, specifically sotalol?
   A. ventricular arrhythmias
   B. sleep disturbances
   C. peripheral edema
   D. headache

5. Which of the following statements is *not* true regarding sodium channel blockers?
   A. They reduce the maximal rate of contraction of the myocardium.
   B. They slow the action potential of the heart.
   C. They increase heart rate and excitability.
   D. They are the largest class of antidysrhythmics.

6. Which of the following is an indication of lidocaine?
   A. convulsions
   B. ventricular arrhythmias
   C. hypotension
   D. cardiogenic shock

7. Which of the following classes of antiarrhythmics is the most powerful, with the least toxicity?
   A. sodium channel blockers
   B. beta-adrenergic blockers
   C. potassium channel blockers
   D. calcium channel blockers

8. Adverse effects of lidocaine include
   A. convulsions, tremor, and drowsiness
   B. ventricular arrhythmias, abdominal pain, and visual impairment
   C. fever, constipation, and urine retention
   D. visual disturbances, hypertension, and urine retention

9. Which of the following is the generic name of Pronestyl?
   A. verapamil
   B. amiodarone
   C. procainamide
   D. propranolol

10. Quinidine is contraindicated in which of the following?
    A. pulmonary hypertension and atrial fibrillation
    B. severe congestive heart failure and myasthenia gravis
    C. acute myocardial infarction and electrolyte imbalance
    D. ventricular tachycardia and premature ventricular contractions

11. Which of the following is the most common type of arrhythmia and is *not* usually life threatening?
    A. ventricular fibrillation
    B. sinus bradycardia
    C. ventricular tachycardia
    D. atrial fibrillation

12. Which of the following is an example of a class II antiarrhythmic drug?
    A. esmolol
    B. digoxin
    C. quinidine
    D. verapamil

13. The generic name of Tambocor is
    A. propafenone
    B. moricizine
    C. flecainide
    D. mexiletine

14. Which of the following signs or symptoms should patients notify their physician about when taking beta-blockers for dysrhythmias?
    A. if their pulse drops to less than 100 beats per minute
    B. if their pulse drops to less than 60 beats per minute
    C. if their systolic blood pressure drops to less than 160 mm Hg
    D. if their systolic blood pressure drops to less than 120 mm Hg

15. Patients should monitor their blood pressure before taking verapamil and notify their physician if it is below
    A. 90/60 mm Hg
    B. 120/80 mm Hg
    C. 140/100 mm Hg
    D. 200/130 mm Hg

CASE STUDY

A 56-year-old woman is on telemetry monitoring. She has a normal sinus rhythm with a rate of 82 beats per minute. The alarm on the machine sounds, and the monitor shows chaotic activity on the screen. What should the respiratory therapist do?

Antihypertensive Medications

OBJECTIVES

Upon completion of this chapter, the reader should be able to do the following:

1. Discuss beta-blockers.
2. Describe the classifications of antihypertensives.
3. Discuss the angiotensin-converting enzyme.
4. Describe the mechanisms of action for each class of drugs used to treat hypertension.
5. Classify different types of diuretics.
6. Discuss the differences between the mechanisms of action of alpha$_1$- and beta-blockers.
7. List the precautions to be considered when using calcium channel blockers.
8. Describe the contraindications of angiotensin II receptor antagonists.
9. Discuss the differences between the mechanisms of action between centrally-acting and peripherally-acting agents.
10. List the risk factors for developing systemic hypertension.

KEY TERMS

Aldosterone	Peripheral
Asymptomatic	Prolapse
Bradykinin	Renin
Depolarization	Stenosis
Hypovolemia	Sympathetic nerves
Neurotransmitters	

INTRODUCTION

Hypertension can be defined as an elevation in systolic and/or diastolic blood pressure. Essential hypertension is defined as a chronic elevation in blood pressure that occurs without evidence of any other disease. Secondary hypertension is defined as an elevation of blood pressure that results from some other disorder, such as kidney disease.

Hypertension is a major cause of death in the United States. Nearly 60 million US citizens are estimated to be hypertensive. Currently, the diagnosis of hypertension is given when the diastolic pressure exceeds 90 mm Hg and/or the systolic pressure exceeds 140 mm Hg (in men older than 50 years of age) or when the systolic pressure exceeds 160 mm Hg (in women of all ages.) These values are associated with an increase in mortality of more than 50% (see **Table 11–1**).

Hypertension is essentially asymptomatic. Therefore, as many as one-third of people with hypertension are thought to be undiagnosed. The cause of primary hypertension (also called essential hypertension) is unknown. However, various risk factors are associated with an increased likelihood of developing primary hypertension. These include genetics, aging, race, obesity, high salt intake, smoking, stress, excess alcohol consumption, and other hard-to-define environmental factors. The roles of these factors are not greatly understood, but they play some direct or indirect part in the development of hypertension. A genetic factor is suggested by family history of hypertension. Race is important as well, especially considering that blacks have nearly double the occurrence of hypertension as whites.

Secondary hypertension may also be asymptomatic. However, when it is symptomatic, headache is the most common symptom. Severe hypertension may cause dizziness, nausea, vomiting, visual disturbances, renal insufficiency, and hypertensive crisis. Secondary hypertension involves multiple systems with a direct or indirect impact on the renal system. Chronic stress causes prolonged excess of catecholamines and cortisol.

Hypertensive crisis is a severe rise in blood pressure that has either already caused organ damage (hypertensive emergency) or has the potential to cause organ damage (hypertensive urgency). Hypertensive crisis may be caused by secondary mechanisms. If it is due to elevated catecholamines, a phentolamine test can be used for diagnosis. Phentolamine is an alpha-antagonist that rapidly reduces

blood pressure that has been elevated due to pheochromocytoma, monoamine oxidase inhibitors, cocaine, or clonidine withdrawal.

Uncontrolled hypertension produces increased demands on the heart. This can result in left ventricular hypertrophy and heart failure. Uncontrolled hypertension also causes atherosclerosis, kidney disease, and stroke.

Regulation of Blood Pressure

Blood pressure is regulated by the central nervous system (CNS), sympathetic nerves, heart, blood vessels, and kidneys. The heart regulates the amount of blood that is ejected from the ventricles. It does this by increasing or decreasing the rate of contractions. The CNS and sympathetic nerves control heart rate and blood flow through the arteries by releasing chemical substances called neurotransmitters. The kidneys' role in regulating blood pressure occurs when they detect a drop in renal blood supply, causing the release of renin, which plays a major role in controlling blood pressure. Reabsorption of water is primarily influenced by aldosterone, a hormone secreted by the adrenal cortex in response to low blood volume or low solute concentration in the kidneys' tubular fluid. Aldosterone causes the distal convoluted tubule cells to increase sodium and water reabsorption from the tubular fluid.

Drug Therapy for Hypertension

Lifestyle modifications are the first step in preventing and managing hypertension. If left untreated, hypertension may cause aneurysms of arteries in the abdomen, aorta, or brain, and it can even lead to blindness. It may also cause ischemic heart disease and stroke. Hypertension can damage arteries by causing the formation of thrombi that block blood supply to the heart and brain and by causing atherosclerosis. Medications used in the treatment of hypertension act at specific sites to control blood pressure: the kidneys, brain, sympathetic nerves, and blood vessels.

TABLE 11–1 Classification of Blood Pressure in Adults

Blood Pressure Classification	Systolic Blood Pressure (mm Hg)	Diastolic Blood Pressure (mm Hg)
Normal	Less than 120	Less than 80
Prehypertensive	120–139	80–89
Stage 1 hypertension	140–159	90–99
Stage 2 hypertension	Greater than or equal to 160	Greater than or equal to 100

Main Drug Therapy
Angiotensin-Converting Enzyme Inhibitors

Also known as ACE inhibitors, angiotensin-converting enzyme inhibitors lower blood pressure by blocking angiotensin-converting enzyme (ACE). This enzyme converts angiotensin I into angiotensin II, which raises blood pressure due to its potent vasoconstriction. Angiotensin-converting enzyme inhibitors are summarized in **Table 11–2**. They also cause the release of norepinephrine and aldosterone. ACE inhibitors are often used in combination with diuretics, such as hydrochlorothiazide.

> **POINT TO REMEMBER**
>
> Treatment of secondary hypertension focuses on correcting the underlying cause and controlling hypertensive effects.

Method of Action

ACE inhibitors block the conversion of angiotensin I to angiotensin II via angiotensin-converting enzyme. Angiotensin II causes direct vasoconstriction and the retention of salt and water. ACE inhibitors reduce angiotensin II and aldosterone levels by inhibiting ACE activity and decreasing sodium reabsorption in the renal tubules. ACE inhibitors also inhibit the degradation of bradykinin, which dilates the arteries to reduce peripheral resistance and lower blood pressure.

Clinical Implications

ACE inhibitors are powerful antihypertensive agents. ACE inhibitors are also indicated for the prevention of other cardiovascular disorders, prevention of nephropathy (in diabetics), and to treat congestive heart failure and left ventricular dysfunction. ACE inhibitors are especially effective in treating hypertension when used with a diuretic.

Adverse Effects

ACE inhibitors may cause dry cough, hyperkalemia, hypotension, loss of taste, diarrhea, lightheadedness, airway obstruction due to angioedema, and skin rash.

Contraindications

ACE inhibitors are contraindicated during pregnancy due to potentially harmful effects to the fetus. They are also contraindicated in patients with previous history of angioedema associated with ACE inhibitor therapy, as well as renal artery stenosis.

Precautions

To reduce the risk of hyperkalemia, salt and potassium substitutes should be avoided. ACE inhibitors should be used with caution in patients with impaired renal function, aortic valve stenosis, cardiac outflow obstruction, dehydration, hypovolemia, and in hemodialysis patients.

TABLE 11–2 Angiotensin-Converting Enzyme Inhibitors

Generic Name	Brand Name	Average Adult Dosage
benazepril	Lotensin	PO: 5–40 mg
captopril	Capoten	PO: 12.5–100 mg
enalapril	Vasotec	PO: 2.5–20 mg; injection: 1.25 mg/mL
fosinopril	Monopril	PO: 10–40 mg
lisinopril	Prinivil, Zestril	PO: 2.5–40 mg
moexipril	Univasc	PO (coated tablet): 7.5–15 mg
perindopril	Aceon	PO: 2–8 mg
quinapril	Accupril	PO: 5–40 mg
ramipril	Altace	PO: 1.25–10 mg
trandolapril	Mavik	PO: 1–4 mg

TABLE 11–3 Angiotensin II Receptor Blockers

Generic Name	Brand Name	Average Adult Dosage
candesartan	Atacand	PO: 4–32 mg
eprosartan	Teveten	PO: 400–600 mg
irbesartan	Avapro	PO: 75–300 mg
losartan	Cozaar	PO: 25–100 mg
olmesartan	Benicar	PO: 5–40 mg
telmisartan	Micardis	PO: 20–80 mg
valsartan	Diovan	PO: 40–320 mg

Angiotensin II Receptor Blockers

Angiotensin II receptor blockers (ARBs) are antagonists that lower blood pressure by blocking angiotensin II binding (see **Table 11–3**). They also inhibit angiotensin II stimulation of the growth of smooth muscle. They reduce hypertrophy of the atria and ventricles that are related to chronic hypertension. ARBs do not inhibit angiotensin II-stimulated repair and growth of tissues. ARBs are commonly used in conjunction with the diuretic hydrochlorothiazide.

Method of Action

Angiotensin II receptor blockers work similarly to ACE inhibitors, primarily blocking angiotensin II binding (see **Figure 11–1**). They do not increase bradykinin levels enough to produce the dry cough that is produced by ACE inhibitors, however.

Clinical Implications

Angiotensin II receptor blockers are indicated for the control of high blood pressure, treatment of heart failure,

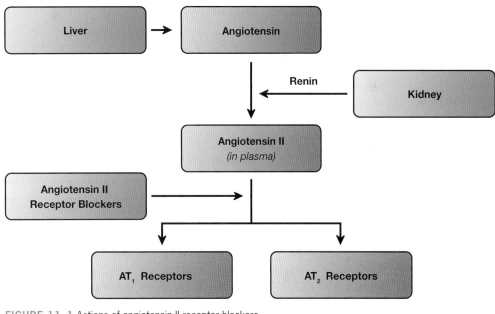

FIGURE 11–1 Actions of angiotensin II receptor blockers.

Method of Action

Overactivity of the sympathetic nervous system increases blood pressure primarily by increasing cardiac output. Beta-blockers may be selective or nonselective. Both types decrease blood pressure by decreasing the heart rate and peripheral resistance, but the selective types are not as likely to cause bronchospasm. Higher doses of beta-blockers eliminate this selectivity. Beta-blockers of all types also decrease the heart rate and the force of heart contractions, thereby lowering cardiac output by blocking beta-adrenergic receptors in the heart. They also decrease renin release and CNS sympathetic output. If used continually, vasodilation will occur due to decreased release of renin from the kidneys.

Clinical Implications

Beta-blockers are primarily indicated for hypertension, angina, mitral valve prolapse, cardiac arrhythmia, atrial fibrillation, congestive heart failure, myocardial infarction, glaucoma, prevention of migraines, control of anxiety and hyperthyroidism, essential tremor, and alpha-blocker-related pheochromocytoma (see Table 11–4). They are also used in combination with diuretics, such as bendroflumethiazide, hydrochlorothiazide, and chlorthalidone.

Adverse Effects

Beta-blockers may cause dizziness, lethargy, nausea, impotence, bradycardia, decreased exercise tolerance, bronchospasm, hypoglycemia, insomnia, and palpitations. More serious adverse effects include cardiac rhythm disturbance, congestive heart failure, and depression. Sudden withdrawal of beta-blockers can lead to exacerbation of angina and myocardial infarction.

Contraindications

Beta-blockers are contraindicated in patients with bronchial asthma, severe COPD, inadequate myocardial function, cardiac failure, and cardiogenic shock. They have not been established as safe for use in children younger than 18 years of age.

Precautions

Beta-blockers should not be discontinued abruptly due to potential arrhythmias or angina. They should be

and prevention of kidney failure in patients who have diabetes or high blood pressure. They are especially effective when used along with a diuretic. ARBs are the preferred antihypertensive agent for type 2 diabetes. They are preferred over beta-blockers for hypertensive patients. When a patient cannot tolerate an ACE inhibitor, ARBs are usually the next drugs of choice.

Adverse Effects

Unlike ACE inhibitors, which can produce a dry, persistent cough in patients, ARBs do not produce this complication to any great degree. ARBs may cause adverse effects, such as abdominal pain, dizziness, constipation, fatigue, impotence, hyperkalemia, and muscle cramping.

Contraindications

ARBs are contraindicated in pregnant patients, especially during the second and third trimester, due to potential harm to the fetus.

Precautions

Like ACE inhibitors, ARBs should be used with caution in patients with impaired renal function, aortic valve stenosis, cardiac outflow obstruction, dehydration, hypovolemia, and in hemodialysis patients.

Beta-Adrenergic Blockers

Beta-adrenergic blockers (also known as beta-blockers or β-blockers) lower blood pressure by decreasing the heart rate and peripheral resistance. Each type causes specific actions:

- Beta$_1$-receptor binding: cardiac stimulation
- Beta$_2$-receptor binding: bronchial relaxation

used with caution in patients taking cimetidine and salicylates. Beta-blockers should be used cautiously in patients with diabetes mellitus, hyperthyroidism, renal failure, and renal impairment.

Alpha₁-Adrenergic Receptor Blockers

Alpha₁-blockers produce vascular relaxation to reduce peripheral resistance and lower blood pressure.

Method of Action

Drugs such as prazosin, doxazosin, and terazosin lower blood pressure by blocking postsynaptic alpha-receptors in blood vessels. These agents relax blood vessels while reducing cholesterol levels. Some of these blockers also reduce urethral resistance and increase urine flow.

Clinical Implications

Alpha₁-blockers are indicated for the treatment of hypertension, ischemic heart disease, benign prostatic hyperplasia (with high blood pressure), to lower urinary tract symptoms, after transurethral procedures, and for noninflammatory chronic pelvic pain syndrome (see **Table 11–5**). Prazosin is sometimes used in combination with the diuretic polythiazide.

Adverse Effects

The most common adverse effects of these blockers include orthostatic hypotension, palpitations, lightheadedness, headache, dizziness, dry mouth, and fainting.

Contraindications

These blockers are contraindicated in renal impairment and those with hypotension or fainting. Certain alpha₁-blockers have not been established as safe to use during pregnancy or lactation or for pediatric patients. Others are contraindicated for use in patients with severe hepatic insufficiency or angina.

Precautions

Patients should be instructed to take the first dose of these blockers at bedtime so they will be recumbent (lying down and relaxed) during the initial adjustment to the drug. These blockers must be used with caution in patients with hypersensitivity, coronary artery disease, cardiac arrhythmias, benign prostatic hyperplasia, prostate cancer, hepatic or renal disease, hypertension with cerebral thrombosis, angina, sickle cell anemia, dizziness, lightheadedness, fainting, orthostatic hypotension, and during pregnancy or lactation. Caution must also be taken when giving these blockers to older adults.

TABLE 11–4 Beta-Adrenergic Blockers

Generic Name	Brand Name	Average Adult Dosage
acebutolol	Sectoral	PO: 200–400 mg
atenolol	Tenormin	PO: 25–100 mg
betaxolol	Kerlone	PO: 10–20 mg
bisoprolol	Zebeta	PO: 5–10 mg
carvedilol	Coreg	PO: 3–25 mg
metoprolol	Lopressor, Toprol XL	PO (immediate release tablet): 25–100 mg PO (extended release tablet): 25–200 mg; injection: 1 mg/mL (5 mL)
nadolol	Corgard	PO: 20–160 mg
penbutolol	Levatol	PO: 20 mg
pindolol	Generic only	PO: 5–10 mg
propranolol	Inderal, Inderal LA, InnoPran XL	PO (tablet): 10–120 mg PO (extended release capsule): 80–120 mg PO (sustained release capsule): 60–160 mg; oral solution: 4 mg/mL and 8 mg/mL; injection: 1 mg/mL
timolol	Generic only	PO: 5–20 mg

TABLE 11–5 Alpha₁-Adrenergic Receptor Blockers

Generic Name	Brand Name	Average Adult Dosage
doxazosin	Cardura, Cardura XL	PO: 1–8 mg PO (extended release): 4–8 mg
prazosin	Minipress	PO: 1–5 mg
terazosin	Hytrin	PO: 1–10 mg

Central Alpha₂-Adrenergic Agonists

Clonidine, guanabenz, and guanfacine are central alpha₂-adrenergic agonists that lower the heart rate and reduce blood pressure, and they reduce plasma concentrations of norepinephrine. They decrease systolic and diastolic blood pressure and the heart rate with mild and infrequent orthostatic effects (see **Table 11–6**). Clonidine is sometimes used in combination with the diuretic chlorthalidone, and methyldopa is sometimes used in combination with the diuretic hydrochlorothiazide.

Method of Action

Central alpha-adrenergic agents stimulate alpha₂-adrenergic receptors in the brain. This inhibits sympathetic outflow to the peripheral vessels. Methyldopa appears to lower blood pressure by forming methyl-norepinephrine, which displaces norepinephrine in the

TABLE 11-6   Central Alpha₂-Adrenergic Agonists

Generic Name	Brand Name	Average Adult Dosage
clonidine	Catapres, Catapres-TTS, Duraclon	PO: 0.1–0.3 mg; transdermal patch: 0.1–0.3 mg over 24 hours; epidural injection: 100 mcg/mL
guanfacine	Tenex	PO: 1–2 mg
methyldopa	Generic only	PO: 125–500 mg; injection: 50 mg/mL
reserpine	Generic only	PO: 0.1–0.25 mg

TABLE 11-7   Direct Vasodilators

Generic Name	Brand Name	Average Adult Dosage
diazoxide	Hyperstat IV	IV: 1–3 mg/kg push (max: 150 mg)
hydralazine	Apresoline	PO: 10–50 mg q.i.d. (max: 300 mg/day)
minoxidil	Loniten	PO: 5–40 mg/day single or divided doses (max: 100 mg/day)
nitroprusside	Nitropress	IV: 1.5–10 mcg/kg/min

CNS. These agonists work by stimulating the alpha₂-adrenergic receptors in the CNS to inhibit sympathetic vasomotor centers, thus lowering the heart rate and reducing blood pressure.

Clinical Implications

These agents are indicated as step 2 drugs for high blood pressure (along with diuretics), hot flashes, and drug or alcohol withdrawal treatment. They may also be administered epidurally as adjunct therapy for severe pain.

Adverse Effects

Centrally acting alpha₂-agonists may cause dry mouth, orthostatic hypotension, impotence, constipation, and sedation. Methyldopa may also cause depression, gastrointestinal upset, and nasal congestion, with less frequent adverse effects including galactorrhea (milk discharge), hemolytic anemia, and liver dysfunction.

Contraindications

These agonists are contraindicated during anticoagulant therapy, any clotting or bleeding disorder, polyarteritis nodosa (inflammatory destruction of medium-sized arteries), scleroderma (hardening of certain body tissues), and during pregnancy or lactation.

Precautions

These agonists should be used with caution in patients with severe coronary insufficiency, recent myocardial infarction, cerebrovascular disease, sinus node dysfunction, diabetes mellitus, chronic renal failure, Raynaud disease (reduced blood flow to the extremities), thromboangiitis obliterans (recurring inflammation and clotting related to tobacco use), and history of major depression. Older adults should also use them cautiously.

Direct Vasodilators

Direct vasodilators (peripherally acting blockers) are strong antihypertensives that are typically used only when a hypertensive patient is unresponsive to all other available types of medications. These agents can produce serious adverse effects.

Method of Action

Direct vasodilators act directly on arterial smooth muscle. These blockers interfere with the release of norepinephrine from the nerve endings, or they may block vascular smooth muscle receptors.

Clinical Implications

Peripherally acting blockers are indicated for hypertension, benign prostatic hypertrophy, and occasionally congestive heart failure, Raynaud disease, peripheral ischemia, and pheochromocytoma (see **Table 11-7**). Hydralazine may be used in combination with the diuretic hydrochlorothiazide.

Adverse Effects

These blockers may cause adverse effects such as orthostatic hypotension, edema, headache, vertigo, dizziness, somnolence, fatigue, nervousness, anxiety, abdominal pain, nausea, leukopenia, eczema, and pruritus.

Contraindications

Peripherally acting blockers are contraindicated in hypersensitive patients and those who have hypotension or fainting. They have not been established as safe for use in children or during pregnancy.

Precautions

These blockers should be used with caution in patients with hepatic conditions, renal conditions, hypertension with cerebral thrombosis, angina, sickle cell anemia, and during pregnancy or lactation.

Calcium Channel Blockers

Calcium channel blockers effectively lower blood pressure by relaxing blood vessels to decrease peripheral resistance. They act by blocking calcium channels, suppressing depolarization, and reducing heart muscle contraction strength. They also decrease heart rate and cardiac output. Calcium channel blockers were discussed in detail in Chapter 10.

Diuretics

Diuretics are particularly effective at potentiating the effects of other antihypertensives. Low doses of hydrochlorothiazide in combination with a beta-blocker or an ACE inhibitor is often used as first-line therapy. Loop diuretics and the aldosterone antagonist (potassium-sparing) diuretics also lower blood pressure. They accomplish this by first decreasing vascular volume (by suppressing renal reabsorption of sodium and increasing salt and water excretion) and by decreasing cardiac output. Diuretics are discussed in greater detail in Chapter 13.

Patient Education

It is essential for respiratory therapists to educate patients about preventing and controlling hypertension. Advice to patients must include the following:

1. A change in lifestyle is always recommended first, such as diet control, weight loss, increased activity, and decreased stress.
2. Low sodium consumption and medications that lower blood cholesterol are also recommended.

SUMMARY

Hypertension is a major cause of death in the United States, with nearly 60 million citizens estimated to be hypertensive. Hypertension is an elevation of the systolic and/or diastolic blood pressure, and it may be either primary (essential) or secondary. The actual cause of primary hypertension is unknown, although there are many risk factors for its development. These include aging, genetics, race, smoking, obesity, stress, and high salt intake. Blood pressure is controlled by the CNS, ANS, kidneys, heart, and blood vessels.

Lifestyle modifications are the first steps in preventing and managing hypertension. Drug therapy for hypertension includes combinations of ACE inhibitors, angiotensin II receptor blockers (ARBs), beta-adrenergic blockers, alpha$_1$-adrenergic receptor blockers, central alpha$_2$-adrenergic agonists, vasodilators, calcium channel blockers, and diuretics. ACE inhibitors and ARBs are often used in combination with diuretics.

Beta-blockers are mostly used for hypertension, angina, cardiac arrhythmia, congestive heart failure, mitral valve prolapse, glaucoma, myocardial infarction, and prevention of migraines. Alpha$_1$-adrenergic blockers are indicated for the treatment of angina, hypertension, and benign prostatic hyperplasia. Central alpha$_2$-adrenergic agonists are used as second-line agents for hypertension, hot flashes, and treatment of alcohol withdrawal.

LEARNING GOALS

These learning goals correspond to the objectives at the beginning of the chapter, providing a clear summary of the chapter's most important points.

1. Beta-blockers include those that bind to beta-receptors to cause cardiac stimulation and those that bind to beta-receptors to cause bronchial relaxation.
2. Antihypertensives are classified as ACE inhibitors, angiotensin II receptor blockers (ARBs), beta-blockers, alpha$_1$-blockers, centrally acting alpha$_2$-blockers, peripherally acting blockers, calcium channel blockers, and diuretics.
3. Angiotensin-converting enzyme (ACE) converts angiotensin I into angiotensin II, which raises blood pressure due to its potent vasoconstriction. It also causes the release of norepinephrine and aldosterone.
4. The mechanisms of action for each class of drug used to treat hypertension are as follows:
   - ACE inhibitors: reduce angiotensin II and aldosterone levels by inhibiting ACE activity, decreasing sodium reabsorption in the renal tubules
   - ARBs: work similarly to ACE inhibitors, primarily blocking angiotensin II binding; do not increase bradykinin levels enough to produce the dry cough that is produced by ACE inhibitors
   - Beta-blockers: decrease blood pressure by decreasing heart rate and peripheral resistance
   - Alpha$_1$-blockers: act by causing the relaxation of blood vessels while reducing cholesterol levels; some also reduce urethral resistance and increase urine flow
   - Centrally acting alpha$_2$-blockers: work by stimulating the alpha$_2$-adrenergic receptors in the CNS to inhibit sympathetic vasomotor centers, thus lowering heart rate and reducing blood pressure
   - Peripherally acting blockers: interfere with the release of norepinephrine from the nerve endings or may block vascular smooth muscle receptors
   - Calcium channel blockers: act by blocking calcium channels, suppressing depolarization, and reducing heart muscle contraction strength
   - Diuretics: act to increase the rate of urine flow; generally increase the excretion of sodium and lower blood volume
5. Diuretics are divided into four categories:
   - Thiazide diuretics: excrete water, sodium, chloride, and potassium
   - Loop diuretics: inhibit sodium and chloride reabsorption
   - Potassium-sparing diuretics: promote potassium retention
   - Osmotic diuretics: control the solubility of sodium in water

6. Alpha₁-blockers relax blood vessels and reduce cholesterol levels, and beta-blockers decrease heart rate and peripheral resistance, although they eventually cause vasodilation due to the release of renin.

7. Calcium channel blockers should be used with caution if patients experience any signs of hypotension; have upcoming surgeries; have severe heart conditions, aortic stenosis conditions, or congestive heart failure; use beta-blockers; are pregnant or lactating; or are hypersensitive.

8. Like ACE inhibitors, angiotensin II receptor blockers (ARBs) should be used with caution in patients with impaired renal function, aortic valve stenosis, cardiac outflow obstruction, dehydration, hypovolemia, and in hemodialysis patients.

9. Centrally acting agents work by stimulating the alpha₂-adrenergic receptors in the CNS to inhibit sympathetic vasomotor centers, thus lowering the heart rate and reducing blood pressure. Peripherally acting agents interfere with the release of norepinephrine from the nerve endings or may block vascular smooth muscle receptors.

10. Risk factors for systemic hypertension include genetics, aging, race, obesity, smoking, stress, and other hard-to-define environmental factors.

CRITICAL THINKING QUESTIONS

1. Which antihypertensive medications are safer and more popular than others?
2. Differentiate primary hypertension from secondary hypertension.

WEB SITES

http://users.rcn.com/jkimball.ma.ultranet/
    BiologyPages/C/Circulation2.html
http://www.aafp.org/afp/990600ap/3140.html
http://www.calciumchannelblockers.net
http://www.cardiologychannel.com/hypertension/
    pharm.shtml
http://www.cvpharmacology.com/diuretic/diuretics
    .htm
http://www.fpnotebook.com/CV/Pharm/
    PrphrlActngAdrnrgcAntgnst.htm
http://www.ionchannels.org/showabstract
    .php?pmid=10494492
http://www.medicinenet.com/ace_inhibitors/article.htm
http://www.medicinenet.com/beta_blockers/article.htm
http://www.vasg.org/alpha_2_agonists.htm

REVIEW QUESTIONS

Multiple Choice

Select the best response to each question.

1. Which of the following organs plays a major role in regulating blood pressure and is the site of action for diuretics?
    A. heart
    B. liver
    C. brain
    D. kidney

2. Which of the following agents inhibit sympathetic vasomotor centers to lower the heart rate and reduce blood pressure?
    A. calcium channel blockers
    B. central alpha-adrenergic agents
    C. angiotensin-converting enzyme inhibitors
    D. angiotensin II receptor blockers

3. Which of the following chemical substances is produced by the kidneys?
    A. renin
    B. aldosterone
    C. angiotensin II
    D. bradykinin

4. Benazepril and quinapril are examples of which class of antihypertensive drugs?
    A. beta-blockers
    B. ACE inhibitors
    C. ARBs
    D. alpha₂-agonists

5. Minoxidil and hydralazine are examples of which class of antihypertensive drugs?
    A. vasodilators
    B. alpha₁-blockers
    C. beta-adrenergic blockers
    D. angiotensin II receptor blockers

6. Avapro is the trade name for
    A. losartan
    B. sectoral
    C. irbesartan
    D. prazosin

7. Which of the following statements is true?
    A. ACE inhibitors are often used in combination with antituberculosis agents.
    B. ACE inhibitors block the conversion of angiotensin I to angiotensin II via angiotensin-converting enzyme.
    C. ACE inhibitors are especially effective in treating renal failure.
    D. ACE inhibitors may cause hypokalemia and hypertension.

8. The method of action of angiotensin II receptor blockers is similar to that of the
   A. direct vasodilators
   B. alpha₁-adrenergic blockers
   C. beta-adrenergic blockers
   D. ACE inhibitors
9. Peripherally acting blockers are *not* indicated for
   A. benign prostatic hypertrophy
   B. orthostatic hypotension
   C. hypertension
   D. pheochromocytoma
10. Inderal is the trade name for
    A. propranolol
    B. timolol
    C. losartan
    D. valsartan
11. Which of the following antihypertensive agents are contraindicated in patients with renal artery stenosis?
    A. alpha₁-adrenergic blockers
    B. direct vasodilators
    C. beta-adrenergic blockers
    D. angiotensin-converting enzyme inhibitors
12. Nadolol and penbutolol are examples of
    A. beta-adrenergic blockers
    B. alpha-adrenergic blockers
    C. angiotensin-converting enzyme inhibitors
    D. calcium channel blockers
13. Minipress is the trade name of
    A. labetalol
    B. doxazosin
    C. prazosin
    D. terazosin
14. Clonidine and guanfacine are examples of which class of antihypertensive drugs?
    A. direct vasodilators
    B. central alpha-adrenergic agents
    C. angiotensin II receptor blockers
    D. beta-adrenergic blockers
15. Which of the following is the cause of primary hypertension?
    A. the cause is unknown
    B. obesity
    C. excessive alcohol use
    D. chronic glomerulonephritis

CASE STUDY

A 55-year-old male is brought into the emergency department with severe headache, palpitations, sweating, nervousness, hyperglycemia, nausea, vomiting, and syncope. The diagnosis, after laboratory tests, is based on increased catecholamines and their metabolites in his urine. Intravenously injected histamine causes a sharp increase in blood pressure, and the administration of phentolamine produces a marked decrease.

1. What is the likely diagnosis for this patient?
2. What type of treatment should be started?

Heart Failure and Treatment

OBJECTIVES

Upon completion of this chapter, the reader should be able to do the following:
1. Identify factors that contribute to heart failure.
2. Explain core drug knowledge about cardiac glycosides.
3. Identify the significant adverse effects of cardiac glycosides.
4. Describe the effects of phosphodiesterase inhibitors.
5. Identify the best diuretic drugs to treat heart failure.
6. Explain the method of action of ACE inhibitors to treat heart failure.
7. Describe the adverse effects of phosphodiesterase inhibitors.
8. Explain how cardiac glycosides affect the myocardium in the treatment of heart failure.
9. Describe the rationale for polypharmacy in treating heart disease.
10. Differentiate between left- and right-sided heart failure.

KEY TERMS

Cardiotonic	Loading dose
Cor pulmonale	Phosphodiesterase
Diastolic heart failure	Pulmonary emboli
Foxglove plant	Stroke volume
Hepatosplenomegaly	Systolic heart failure

INTRODUCTION

Heart failure occurs when the heart's ability to pump blood becomes impaired. Congestive heart failure (CHF) is defined as a type of heart failure accompanied by congestion of body tissues. This type eventually becomes complicated by pulmonary or systemic venous congestion. An individual with heart failure has less tolerance to exercise, reduced quality of life, and a shortened life span. The incidence of heart failure increases with age. Nearly 700,000 people die of heart failure each year in the United States. Mortality from heart failure is highest for males, blacks, and elderly people.

Factors That Contribute to Heart Failure

The heart fails primarily from processes that cause it to work harder over many years or because of damage to the myocardium. Cardiac output decreases as a result. Systemic hypertension is the most common factor that causes left ventricular failure of the heart. When heart valves become narrowed, heart failure rates are higher than when the valves are normal. Increased cardiac workloads may also be the result of congenital defects. Heart muscle cells and contractility may be affected by cardiomyopathies, atherosclerotic coronary disease, and myocardial infarction. Ventricular filling may be reduced by tachyarrhythmias or atrial-ventricular dissociation and impaired by pericarditis. Contractility may also be affected by ventricular arrhythmias. Failure of the right side of the heart is most commonly caused by failure of the left side of the heart. Cor pulmonale is defined as right heart failure due to pulmonary hypertension. This can occur as a complication of hypoxemia due to various lung diseases. Acute right ventricular failure can be precipitated by pulmonary embolism.

Classifications of Heart Failure

Many forms of heart disease involve impairment of the left or right ventricle. Therefore, heart failure is classified as left heart failure or right heart failure.

Left-Sided Heart Failure

> **POINT TO REMEMBER**
>
> Shortness of breath due to congestion of the pulmonary circulation is one of the major manifestations of left-sided heart failure.

Left-sided heart failure is commonly called congestive heart failure. It can be categorized further as systolic heart failure (systolic ventricular dysfunction) or diastolic heart failure (diastolic ventricular dysfunction). These two types can occur individually or together. Left ventricular failure usually develops in coronary artery disease, hypertension, most forms of cardiomyopathy, and with congenital defects.

Right-Sided Heart Failure

Right-sided heart failure can be caused by left-sided heart failure. This is due to an increase in left ventricular filling pressure that is reflected back into the pulmonary circulation. The resistance to right ventricular emptying increases as pressure in the pulmonary circulation rises. Because the right ventricle is not able to compensate for this increased workload, it

> **POINT TO REMEMBER**
>
> Although the most common cause of heart failure is coronary artery disease, it also occurs in infants, children, and adults with congenital and acquired heart defects.

dilates and fails. As a result, the systemic venous circulation pressure rises, causing hepatosplenomegaly and peripheral edema. Right ventricular failure is usually caused by prior left ventricular failure. Other causes include multiple pulmonary emboli, primary pulmonary hypertension, pulmonary artery stenosis, or valve stenosis.

Drugs to Treat Heart Failure

When treating heart failure, the underlying problem should be treated first. The heart's workload must be reduced by avoiding excessive fatigue,

> **POINT TO REMEMBER**
>
> Acute complications of heart failure include pulmonary edema, acute renal failure, arrhythmias, and thromboembolism.

stress, and sudden exertion. This is important to prevent acute episodes of heart failure. To reduce stress on the heart, prophylactic measures should be undertaken. For example, the influenza vaccine is important to prevent respiratory infections, which can have serious effects on the heart.

Other common treatments include maintaining an appropriate diet. This entails the consumption of less sodium, less cholesterol, adequate iron and proteins, and sufficient amounts of fluids. Antianxiety drugs and sedatives may be useful in reducing stress to the heart. The advantage of using multiple different drugs for heart failure is that in combination they can strengthen the heart muscle while reducing swelling of tissues by removing excessive sodium and water. Thus, the use of polypharmacy to treat heart failure results in lowered blood pressure and better potential results.

In cases of right heart failure, congestion and edema of the lungs must be treated with drugs designed for these conditions. Therefore, there is no one single drug that can reduce all the signs and symptoms of heart failure because the left and right types of heart failure require different medications.

Common drugs prescribed for heart failure are summarized in **Table 12–1**. ACE inhibitors and ARBs were discussed in full detail in Chapter 11. Diuretics will be discussed in detail in Chapter 13.

Angiotensin-Converting Enzyme Inhibitors

ACE inhibitors reduce renin secretion and vasoconstriction. This decreases systemic vascular resistance. The ACE inhibitors are the mainstays for the treatment of hypertension and are also the drugs of choice to slow the progression of heart failure. ACE inhibitors are relatively safe to use. They have replaced digoxin as the drug of choice for treating chronic heart failure. Unless it is specifically contraindicated, all patients with heart failure should receive an ACE inhibitor. They are started in small doses and gradually increased. ACE inhibitors are discussed in detail in Chapter 11.

TABLE 12-1   Drugs to Treat Heart Failure

Generic Name	Trade Name	Average Adult Dosage
Beta-adrenergic blockers • carvedilol • metoprolol	• Coreg • Toprol-XL	• PO: 3.125 mg b.i.d. for 2 weeks • PO (extended release): 25 mg/day for 2 weeks
Cardiac glycosides • digoxin	• Lanoxin, Lanoxicaps	• PO: 0.125–0.5 mg/day
Phosphodiesterase inhibitors • inamrinone • milrinone	• Inocor • Primacor	• IV: 0.75 mg/kg bolus given slowly over 2–3 min, then 5–10 mcg/kg/min • IV: 50 mcg over 10 min, then 0.375–0.75 mcg/kg/min
Vasodilators • hydralazine • isosorbide dinitrate	• Apresoline • Isordil, Sorbitrate, Dilatate	• PO: 10–50 mg q.i.d. • PO: 2.5–30 mg q.i.d., with meals and at nighttime

Angiotensin II Receptor Blockers

Angiotensin II receptor blockers act similarly to ACE inhibitors. Recent drugs of this type that have been approved to treat heart failure include candesartan (Atacand) and valsartan (Diovan). Angiotensin II receptor blockers (ARBs) are discussed in detail in Chapter 11.

Cardiac Glycosides

Cardiac glycosides are obtained from various types of the foxglove plant and have the clinical name digitalis. Prior to ACE inhibitors, cardiac glycosides were the mainstays of heart failure treatment. Digoxin and digitoxin are the primary cardiac glycosides; they differ primarily in that digitoxin has a longer half-life. However, digitoxin is no longer used in the United States. These glycosides cause the heart to beat more forcefully, yet more slowly. Because ACE inhibitors are safer, cardiac glycosides are usually only used for advanced stages of heart failure in combination with other agents. It is important to understand that the margin of safety between therapeutic and toxic doses of digitalis is narrow. Frequent serum digoxin levels should be obtained as therapy with this agent progresses. The dosage should be adjusted based on the results of these levels and the patient's response to the drug.

Method of Action

The primary action of digitalis is a direct cardiotonic action on the myocardium. It exerts positive inotropic force through binding to sodium- and potassium-activated APT pumps. The term inotropic is defined as "affecting the force of muscle contraction." This process leads to increased intracellular sodium concentrations, and subsequently, more available intracellular calcium during systole. In congestive heart failure, stroke volume may be increased. This empties the ventricles more effectively and lowers diastolic ventricular pressures (and ultimately, pulmonary pressures) to diminish congestion.

Clinical Implications

Digoxin (Lanoxin) is the most commonly used digitalis preparation for congestive heart failure. Initial digitalization may be accomplished rapidly or slowly, depending on the urgency of the treatment. Sometimes digoxin requires a loading dose to determine what the maintenance dose should be. Digoxin is also used for various types of arrhythmias.

Adverse Effects

Common adverse effects of cardiac glycosides include fatigue, headache, muscle weakness, visual disturbances, nausea, and vomiting. More serious adverse effects include mental depression, arrhythmias (due to hypokalemia resulting from diuretics), and hypercalcemia.

Contraindications

Cardiac glycosides are contraindicated in hypersensitive patients, ventricular fibrillation, and ventricular tachycardia (unless it is caused by congestive heart failure).

Precautions

These drugs should be used with caution in patients with hypokalemia, renal insufficiency, acute myocardial infarction, advanced heart disease, and hypothyroidism. They should also be used cautiously during pregnancy or lactation and in older adults.

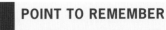

POINT TO REMEMBER

An antidote for digoxin toxicity is Digibind.

Beta-Adrenergic Blockers

Long-term therapy with beta-adrenergic blockers has been shown to reduce morbidity and mortality in congestive heart failure patients. Left ventricular dysfunction is associated with activation of renin–angiotensin–aldosterone and the sympathetic nervous system. Several beta-blockers (carvedilol, metoprolol, and bisoprolol) are used to treat heart failure. Beta-adrenergic blockers are discussed in detail in Chapter 11.

Phosphodiesterase Inhibitors

Cardiac glycosides were the drugs of choice for treating congestive heart failure for about 2 centuries. Later, dopamine and dobutamine were introduced due to their positive inotropic actions in managing decompensated heart failure. In 1977 amrinone was discovered, leading to an interest in drugs that combine both positive inotropic and vasodilator actions. These drugs are selective or nonselective phosphodiesterase inhibitors, also known as inodilator drugs.

Phosphodiesterase inhibitors became available in the 1980s. They block the enzyme phosphodiesterase in cardiac and smooth muscle. These agents are more toxic than others that are used for heart failure, and they are usually reserved for patients who do not respond to ACE inhibitors or cardiac glycosides. They are, therefore, usually used for only 2 to 3 days at a time.

Method of Action

These inhibitors block phosphodiesterase to increase the amount of calcium available for myocardial contraction. This results in positive inotropic action and vasodilation. Cardiac output increases because contractility is increased, and left ventricular afterload is decreased.

Clinical Implications

Inamrinone and milrinone are used for short-term management of congestive heart failure in patients who do not respond to traditional therapies (such as digitalis, diuretics, or vasodilators). Phosphodiesterase inhibitors may be used in conjunction with other drugs for the treatment of congestive heart failure.

Adverse Effects

Phosphodiesterase inhibitors may cause hypersensitivity, hypoxemia, ascites, jaundice, and pleuritis. Nephrogenic diabetes insipidus, nausea and vomiting, anorexia, and abdominal cramps are also common adverse effects of phosphodiesterase inhibitors. The most serious adverse effect of milrinone is ventricular arrhythmia.

Contraindications

Phosphodiesterase inhibitors are contraindicated in surgery, acute myocardial infarction, uncorrected hypokalemia, and dehydration. They are also contraindicated in women of childbearing age and during pregnancy or lactation.

Precautions

Phosphodiesterase inhibitors should be used with caution in cardiovascular disease, renal and hepatic impairment, and in patients with jaundice. They have not been established as safe for use in children younger than age 16 years.

Vasodilators

Vasodilators have hypotensive effects but play a minor role in the treatment of heart failure. They are discussed in detail in Chapter 11.

Diuretics

Diuretics are commonly prescribed in the treatment of heart failure. They reduce signs and symptoms of heart failure, such as pulmonary edema and swelling in the feet, ankles, and legs. Because elevated blood pressure may accelerate existing heart failure or cause it to occur, these actions are desirable to combat its symptoms. Diuretics are rarely prescribed alone; they are given in combination with other drugs used to treat heart failure. However, it is important to remember that potassium levels should be measured when using diuretics. Thiazides and loop diuretics, in particular, can cause hypokalemia. The loop diuretics (such as furosemide) are most frequently prescribed for heart failure because of their effectiveness in removing fluid from the body. See Chapter 13 for a detailed discussion of diuretics.

Patient Education

To reduce symptoms of heart failure, the respiratory therapist should advise patients of the following: limit alcohol intake, reduce fat intake, stop smoking, reduce stress, and develop an exercise program.

SUMMARY

Systemic hypertension is the leading cause of left ventricular failure of the heart. Left-sided heart failure is usually referred to as congestive heart failure. Failure of the right side of the heart is usually caused by failure of the left side of the heart. The treatment of heart failure involves reducing the heart's workload by decreasing fatigue, stress, and sudden exertion. An adequate diet is also important in maintaining a healthy heart. Drugs used to treat heart failure include beta-adrenergic blockers, cardiac glycosides, phosphodiesterase inhibitors, and vasodilators. Other agents that are used include ACE inhibitors, angiotensin II receptor blockers (ARBs), and diuretics.

LEARNING GOALS

These learning goals correspond to the objectives at the beginning of the chapter, providing a clear summary of the chapter's most important points.

1. The heart fails primarily from processes that cause it to work harder or because of myocardial damage. Systemic hypertension is the most common factor that causes left ventricular heart failure. Narrowing of the heart valves is also a contributing factor. Other factors include congenital defects, cardiomyopathies, atherosclerotic coronary disease, and myocardial infarction.

2. Cardiac glycosides are obtained from types of the foxglove plant and have the clinical name digitalis. Digoxin and digitoxin are the primary cardiac glycosides. They cause the heart to beat more forcefully, yet more slowly. The margin of safety between therapeutic and toxic doses of digitalis is narrow, so cardiac glycosides are used only for advanced stages of heart failure.

3. Significant adverse effects of cardiac glycosides include mental depression, anorexia, and diarrhea.

4. Phosphodiesterase inhibitors block the enzyme phosphodiesterase in cardiac and smooth muscle. This increases the amount of calcium available for myocardial contraction, resulting in positive inotropic action and vasodilation. The result is increased cardiac output, increased contractility, and decreased left ventricular afterload.

5. The best diuretic drugs used to treat heart failure are the loop diuretics. This is because of their effectiveness in removing fluid from the body.

6. ACE inhibitors work by reducing renin secretion and vasoconstriction, which decreases systemic vascular resistance.

7. Phosphodiesterase inhibitors may cause ventricular arrhythmia, hypersensitivity, hypoxemia, ascites, jaundice, pleuritis, nephrogenic diabetes insipidus, nausea, vomiting, anorexia, and abdominal cramps.

8. Cardiac glycosides affect the myocardium with a direct cardiotonic action to increase the force of contraction by inhibiting the membrane enzyme called ATPase, which is activated by sodium and potassium. This inhibition increases intracellular levels of calcium.

9. Polypharmacy is used for treating heart disease because there is no one single drug that can reduce the various signs and symptoms. Left and right types of heart failure require different medications. Some strengthen the heart muscle, and others remove excess sodium and water from the tissues.

10. Left-sided heart failure is commonly called congestive heart failure and usually develops in coronary artery disease, hypertension, most forms of cardiomyopathy, and with congenital defects. Right-sided heart failure can be caused by left-sided heart failure. Right ventricular failure is usually caused by prior left ventricular failure, with other causes including multiple pulmonary emboli, primary pulmonary hypertension, pulmonary artery stenosis, or valve stenosis.

CRITICAL THINKING QUESTIONS

1. Why are cardiac glycosides not as popular as they used to be in the treatment of congestive heart failure?
2. What are the current drugs of choice for the treatment of heart failure?

WEB SITES

http://www.abouthf.org/questions_stages.htm
http://www.americanheart.org/presenter
  .jhtml?identifier=118
http://www.hrspatients.org/patients/heart_disorders/
  heart_failure/risk_factors.asp
http://www.mayoclinic.com/health/
  high-blood-pressure-medication/hi00057
http://www.medicinenet.com/beta_blockers/article.htm
http://www.people.vcu.edu/~urdesai/car.htm
http://www.pubmedcentral.nih.gov/articlerender
  .fcgi?artid=1760738

REVIEW QUESTIONS

Multiple Choice

Select the best response to each question.

1. Which of the following are the drugs of choice for treating chronic heart failure?
   A. cardiac glycosides
   B. diuretics
   C. angiotensin-converting enzyme inhibitors
   D. phosphodiesterase inhibitors
2. The cardiac glycosides are usually used for which of the following conditions?
   A. malignant hypertension
   B. advanced stages of heart failure
   C. acute heart failure
   D. acute myocardial infarction
3. Which of the following statements is true regarding the use of beta-adrenergic blockers in congestive heart failure?
   A. Long-term therapy has been shown to reduce morbidity and mortality.
   B. Long-term therapy has been shown to cause renal failure.
   C. Short-term therapy has been shown to increase hypertension.
   D. Short-term therapy has been shown to produce severe liver impairments.

4. Which of the following statements is false regarding phosphodiesterase inhibitors?
   A. They increase the amount of calcium available for myocardial contraction.
   B. They increase the amount of phosphorus available for the blood.
   C. They decrease left ventricular afterload.
   D. They are used for the short-term management of heart failure.

5. Obstructions of blood vessels in the lungs, usually due to blood clots, are referred to as
   A. pneumoconiosis
   B. pulmonary edema
   C. pulmonary hypertension
   D. pulmonary emboli

6. Which of the following statements is true about mortality from heart failure?
   A. It is highest for females, whites, and elderly people.
   B. It is highest for males, blacks, and elderly people.
   C. It is highest for girls, blacks, and children.
   D. It is highest for boys, whites, and children.

7. Left-sided heart failure is commonly called
   A. cardiomyopathy
   B. congestive heart failure
   C. congenital heart failure
   D. cardiopulmonary failure

8. The trade name of carvedilol is
   A. Coreg
   B. Inocor
   C. Primacor
   D. Apresoline

9. Which of the following agents should be administered intravenously?
   A. digoxin (Lanoxin)
   B. metoprolol (Toprol-XL)
   C. inamrinone (Inocor)
   D. hydralazine (Apresoline)

10. The mainstays for the treatment of hypertension and the progression of heart failure include
    A. cardiac glycosides
    B. angiotensin-converting enzyme inhibitors
    C. angiotensin II receptor blockers
    D. calcium channel blockers

11. The primary action of digitalis is a direct
    A. cardiotonic action
    B. inhibition of increases in intracellular levels of potassium
    C. decreased stroke volume
    D. increased diastolic ventricular pressure

12. More serious adverse effects of cardiac glycosides include all of the following except
    A. mental depression
    B. congestive heart failure
    C. diarrhea
    D. anorexia

13. An example of a phosphodiesterase inhibitor is
    A. hydralazine
    B. digoxin
    C. metoprolol
    D. milrinone

14. Which of the following is a vasodilator?
    A. hydralazine
    B. inamrinone
    C. digoxin
    D. carvedilol

15. A first dose of a drug administered in excess of the maintenance dose to achieve therapeutic drug levels is referred to as a
    A. dosage regimen
    B. dose-effect relationship
    C. loading dose
    D. dose-response relationship

CASE STUDY

A 67-year-old man was admitted to a hospital. His signs and symptoms revealed dyspnea, orthopnea, fatigue, and nonproductive cough associated with pulmonary congestion. Twenty-four hours later, he had clinical manifestations of left-sided heart failure, including crackles from pulmonary congestion, hemoptysis (spitting up blood from the lungs), and restlessness and confusion from reduced cardiac output. The patient was given normal adult doses of an ACE inhibitor. Two days later, he had severe hypotension.

1. What was the cause of his severe hypotension?
2. What can be done to treat the severe hypotension?

Diuretics

OUTLINE

OBJECTIVES

Upon completion of this chapter, the reader should be able to do the following:

1. Explain the composition of the urinary system.
2. Describe the structure and function of the nephrons.
3. Explain the antidiuretic hormone and its effects on urine volume.
4. Explain the clinical implications for the use of diuretics in various conditions and disorders of the human body.
5. Classify the major types of diuretics.
6. Describe the method of action of thiazide diuretics.
7. List the major adverse effects of potassium-sparing diuretics.
8. Describe the contraindications of thiazide diuretics.
9. Explain the clinical implications of osmotic diuretics.
10. Describe the high-ceiling diuretics and to which types of diuretics they belong.

KEY TERMS

Antidiuretic hormone (ADH)
Collecting ducts
Collecting tubules
Diuresis
Diuretic
Endogenous
Erythropoietin
Exogenous
Filtrate
Filtration
Gynecomastia
Hepatic encephalopathy
Hilum
Homeostasis
Hyponatremia
Interstitial fluid
Juxtaglomerular apparatus
Juxtaglomerular cells
Major calyces

Minor calyces
Muscle cells
Nephron
Nephrotic syndrome
Primary hyperaldosteronism
Renal columns
Renal cortex
Renal medulla
Renal papilla
Renal pelvis
Renal pyramids
Renal sinus
Tubular fluid
Tubular reabsorption
Tubular secretion
Ureters
Urethra
Urinary bladder
Urine

INTRODUCTION

The fluid volume of the body is kept balanced by a self-regulating, homeostatic process known as diuresis, which increases urine production and the excretion of water and electrolytes. Any substance that causes diuresis is known as a diuretic. These substances decrease renal reabsorption of sodium and increase its excretion along with water. Other electrolytes may be excreted during this process as well. Various types of diuretics are used based on the individual patient's needs. Thiazide and thiazide-like diuretics, loop diuretics, and potassium-sparing diuretics decrease circulating volume and conditions related to excess volume. Osmotic diuretics decrease intraocular and intracranial pressure as well as treat renal failure. Carbonic anhydrase inhibitors decrease tubular hydrogen ion secretion and increase sodium and water excretion.

Structure and Functions of the Urinary System

The organs of the urinary system include the kidneys, ureters, urinary bladder, and urethra (see **Figure 13–1**). The kidneys filter waste products from the bloodstream. They then convert this filtrate into urine. The ureters, urinary bladder, and urethra are described collectively as the urinary tract because they transport urine out of the body.

The urinary system removes waste products from the bloodstream and also functions in the following ways:

- Storage of urine: Urine is continually produced. The urinary bladder is an expandable sac that can hold up to 1 liter of urine.
- Excretion of urine: The urethra is a tube that transports urine from the urinary bladder so it can be expelled out of the body. This process is called urination or micturition.
- Regulation of blood volume: The kidneys, via certain hormones, control the volume of both the interstitial fluid and blood. Changes in blood volume affect blood pressure. Therefore, the kidneys indirectly affect blood pressure.
- Regulation of erythrocyte production: As the kidneys filter the blood, they indirectly measure its oxygen levels. If this level is reduced, kidney cells secrete a hormone called erythropoietin, which stimulates bone marrow to increase erythrocyte production. With more erythrocytes, the blood can transport more oxygen.

POINT TO REMEMBER

The kidneys remove waste products from the blood. They also assist in the regulation of blood volume, blood pressure, ion levels, and blood pH.

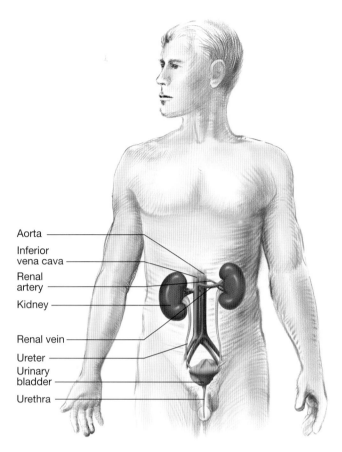

Aorta
Inferior vena cava
Renal artery
Kidney
Renal vein
Ureter
Urinary bladder
Urethra

FIGURE 13–1 The urinary system.

Kidneys

The kidneys are two symmetrical, bean-shaped organs located along the posterior wall of the abdomen. They are situated laterally to the vertebral column (see **Figure 13–2**).

Each kidney has a concave (inwardly curving) border called the hilum, and it is covered by a fibrous capsule. This is the point where nerves, the ureter, and vessels connect to each kidney. The hilum is continuous with a space inside each kidney known as the renal sinus. Each kidney is made up of an outer renal cortex and an inner renal medulla. The medulla is usually darker in color than the cortex. Renal columns extend from the cortex, projecting into the medulla and subdividing it into renal pyramids. The apex (tip) of each renal pyramid is called the renal papilla, which projects toward the renal sinus.

Renal papillae project into funnel-shaped spaces called minor calyces. In each kidney, there are between 8 and 15 minor calyces. These structures merge to form larger spaces known as major calyces. Urine from the renal pyramids collects in the minor calyces and then drains into the major calyces. These merge to form the large, funnel-shaped renal pelvis. Urine collects here and is then transported into the ureter.

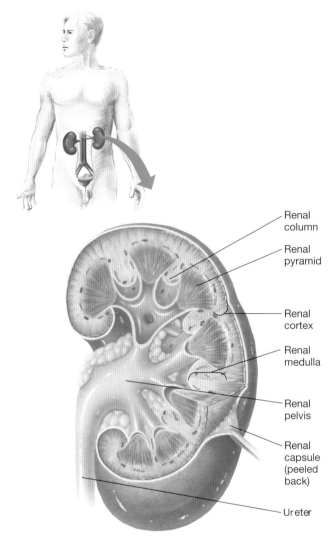

FIGURE 13–2 Gross anatomy of the kidney.

Renal column

Renal pyramid

Renal cortex

Renal medulla

Renal pelvis

Renal capsule (peeled back)

Ureter

Nephrons

POINT TO REMEMBER

Any condition that leads to a massive immune response, including bacterial or viral infections and autoimmune disorders, can cause glomerulonephritis.

The kidney's functional filtration unit is known as the nephron. Each nephron consists of a renal corpuscle, proximal convoluted tubule, nephron loop, and a distal convoluted tubule (see Figure 13–3). The renal corpuscle is composed of a glomerulus and a glomerular capsule. The kidneys contain a combined total of approximately 2.5 million nephrons.

The nephrons form urine through three interrelated processes: filtration, reabsorption, and secretion:

1. Filtration is the process in which water and some dissolved solutes in the blood plasma move out of each glomerulus into the capsular space of each renal corpuscle. This occurs due to pressure differences across the filtration membrane. This water and its dissolved solutes are collectively known as filtrate.

2. Tubular reabsorption occurs when filtrate substances move (by active transport or diffusion) across the convoluted tubule walls and nephron loops to return to the blood (see Figure 13–4). This modified filtrate is called tubular fluid. Usually, all the solutes and most of the water that previously formed the filtrate are reabsorbed by the blood. As this reabsorption occurs, some excess solutes, water, and waste products remain in the tubular fluid.

3. Tubular secretion is the active transport of solutes out of the blood into the tubular fluid.

Juxtaglomerular Apparatus

The juxtaglomerular apparatus is a collection of cells beside each renal glomerulus. It is made up of part of the distal convoluted tubule of the glomerulus, sections of the closest afferent and efferent arterioles, and cells found in between these various structures (see Figure 13–5).

POINT TO REMEMBER

Renal failure refers to greatly diminished or absent renal function caused by the destruction of about 90% of the tissue in the kidney.

These juxtaglomerular cells are actually modified smooth muscle cells of the afferent arteriole near the renal corpuscle's entrance. The macula densa is a group of modified cells in a distal convoluted tubule that touch the juxtaglomerular cells. These cells are located only on the tubule side near the afferent arteriole.

The collective juxtaglomerular apparatus structures regulate blood pressure. The macula densa monitors ion concentration in the tubular fluid. When either blood volume or solute concentration becomes reduced, the tubular fluid reacts similarly. The macula densa senses this and stimulates the juxtaglomerular apparatus to release renin, activating the renin–angiotensin pathway. This results in the production of aldosterone, increasing blood sodium concentrations and blood volume. These changes are important in maintaining the homeostasis of blood volume and blood pressure.

Control of Urine Volume

When the tubular fluid leaves the distal convoluted tubules, it travels through a series of small collecting tubules and empties into collecting ducts. Then, antidiuretic hormone (ADH) is secreted by the posterior pituitary gland. This results in increased water absorption from the tubular fluid in the collecting ducts. Water

POINT TO REMEMBER

A kidney transplant from a genetically similar person may successfully restore renal function.

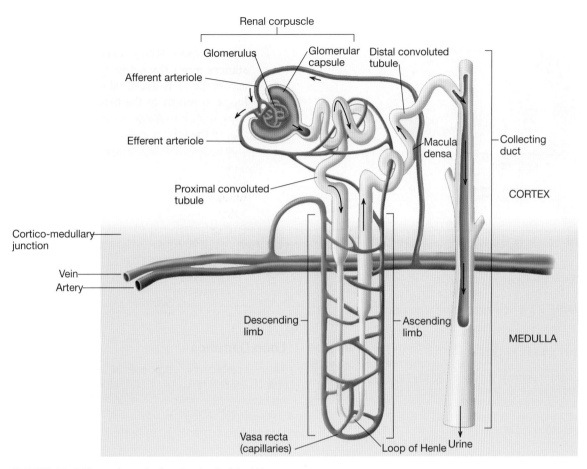

FIGURE 13–3 The nephron; the functional unit of the kidney.

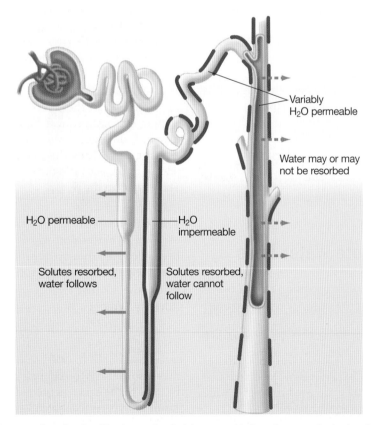

FIGURE 13–4 Tubular resorption of water. The descending limb is permeable to water, so water is absorbed by osmosis. The ascending limb is impermeable to water, so osmosis cannot occur there. The distal convoluted tubule and collecting duct are variably permiable to water, so osmosis in those locations can be regulated.

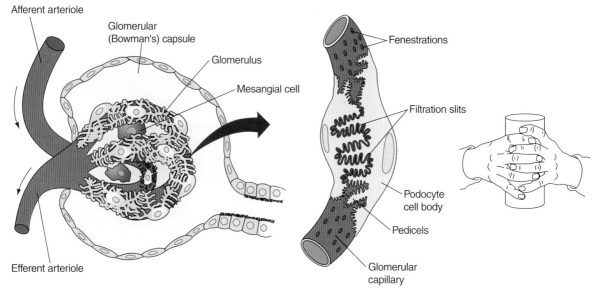

FIGURE 13–5 Structure of the renal corpuscle.

POINT TO REMEMBER

A woman is more prone to a urinary tract infection because the urethra is shorter in length than that of a man. It is close to the anus, allowing bacteria from the gastrointestinal tract to more readily enter the female urethra.

loss from the kidneys is thereby reduced. ADH is secreted in response to either a rise in concentrations of ions in the blood or because of a fall in blood volume (such as when the body is dehydrated and needs to conserve water). When a person is well hydrated, the collecting ducts transport the tubular fluid without modifying it. When a person is dehydrated, water is conserved, and a more concentrated urine is produced (see **Figure 13–6**).

After the tubular fluid leaves the collecting duct, it is then called urine. The remaining kidney structures then simply transport the urine, with the renal pelvis conducting it into each ureter. The **ureters** are long, fibrous, muscular tubes that conduct urine into the **urinary bladder**. This is an expandable, muscular sac that holds the urine. The **urethra** is a fibromuscular tube that begins at the neck of the urinary bladder. It conducts urine outside of the body.

Drugs That Promote Water Loss from the Kidneys

Diuretics promote urine formation and elimination. Most diuretics work by causing the kidneys to eliminate more sodium than they ordinarily would. Sodium passing through the kidneys attracts water from the circulatory system and increases the volume of urine. Diuretics are most often used to treat hypertension and congestive heart failure. In addition, they are used to treat a wide variety of kidney and cardiovascular problems.

Loop Diuretics

Loop diuretics are sometimes called high-ceiling diuretics. They must be used carefully because larger doses can increase urine output to a great degree. This may lead to severely decreased blood volume and even death. The loop diuretics are listed in **Table 13–1**.

Method of Action

Loop diuretics affect the loop of Henle in the kidneys, inhibiting sodium and chloride reabsorption. They act in a similar way to thiazide diuretics, increasing excretion of water, chloride, potassium, and sodium.

Clinical Implications

Loop diuretics are used as the drugs of choice for acute pulmonary edema due to congestive heart failure and for hypercalcemia.

POINT TO REMEMBER

Loop diuretics are effective when taken orally, and they are eliminated by active proximal tubular secretion.

They have a rapid onset of action. Loop diuretics are also used for hypertension when other measures have not been effective. They are the only type of diuretic capable of reducing edema in nephrotic syndrome.

Adverse Effects

Loop diuretics may cause fluid or electrolyte imbalance, hyponatremia, circulatory collapse, hypotension, thromboembolism, and **hepatic encephalopathy**. They may also cause hypokalemia or hypocalcemia and may be toxic to the ears. Furosemide and ethacrynic acid may result in hyperuricemia and gout. Other adverse effects

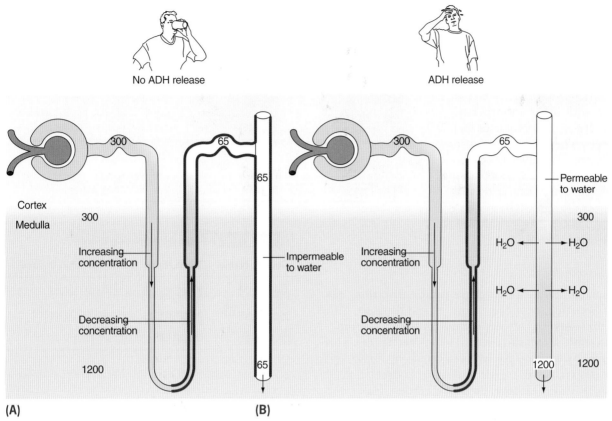

FIGURE 13–6 Mechanisms of urine concentration and dilution. When ADH is not secreted (**A**), the distal convoluted tubule and collecting duct are impermeable to water, resulting in dilute urine. When ADH is secreted (**B**), these structures are permeable to water, allowing water to leave by osmosis, resulting in concentrated urine.

TABLE 13–1 Loop Diuretics		
Generic Name	**Trade Name**	**Average Adult Dosage**
bumetanide	Bumex	PO: 0.5–2 mg/day; IV: 0.5–1 mg over 1–2 min, repeated q2–3h p.r.n. (max: 10 mg/day)
ethacrynic acid	Edecrin	PO: 50–100 mg 1–2 times/day (max: 400 mg/day); IV: 0.5–1 mg/kg
furosemide	Lasix	PO: 20–80 mg/day in 1 or several divided doses (max: 600 mg/day); IM/IV: 20–40 mg in 1 or several divided doses up to 600 mg/day
torsemide	Demadex	PO/IV: 4–20 mg/day

include photosensitivity, hypotension, shock, cardiac arrhythmias, bone-marrow depression, and skin rashes.

Contraindications

Loop diuretics are contraindicated in hypersensitive patients, severe diarrhea, dehydration, electrolyte imbalance, and hypotension. They should be used cautiously in lactating women and infants.

Precautions

Loop diuretics should be used with caution in diabetes mellitus, hepatic cirrhosis, pulmonary edema, gout, and pregnancy. They have many drug interactions and should not be used with thiazide diuretics.

Thiazide and Thiazide-Like Diuretics

Thiazide diuretics are derived from the chemical benzothiadiazine. Thiazide-like drugs are chemically different but have the same method of action as thiazides. They are the most commonly used type of diuretics. Thiazide diuretics include chlorothiazide, cyclothiazide, hydrochlorothiazide, hydroflumethiazide, methyclothiazide, and polythiazide. Thiazide-like diuretics include chlorthalidone and indapamide (see **Table 13–2**).

Method of Action

These diuretics increase urinary excretion of water and sodium. They inhibit sodium reabsorption on the distal convoluted tubules and collecting ducts. They increase bicarbonate, chloride, and potassium ion excretion.

Clinical Implications

Thiazide and thiazide-like diuretics are the most commonly used class of diuretic drugs. These agents are used primarily for hypertension. They may be used with other antihypertensive drugs and potentiate their effects. They are also used for adjunctive therapies in corticosteroid therapy, edema due to congestive heart failure or acute glomerulonephritis, chronic renal failure, estrogen therapy, or hepatic cirrhosis.

Adverse Effects

Thiazide diuretics may cause gastric irritation, nausea, vomiting, cramping, anorexia, and diarrhea. More serious adverse effects include anorexia, jaundice, pancreatitis, aplastic anemia, hypokalemia, hyperuricemia, hyperglycemia, hypercalcemia, hyponatremia, and respiratory distress. Other adverse effects include constipation, headache, dizziness, vertigo, leukopenia, orthostatic hypotension, fever, anaphylactic reactions, and hyperglycemia.

Contraindications

These diuretics are contraindicated in diabetes, gout, impaired liver function, severe renal disease, and in the elderly. They are not recommended to be used by lactating women.

Precautions

POINT TO REMEMBER

The symptoms of hypokalemia include neurological and muscular weakness, cardiac arrhythmias, and respiratory arrest.

Patients with diabetes should monitor their blood glucose levels when taking these diuretics to avoid hyperglycemia.

Potassium-Sparing Diuretics

Potassium-sparing diuretics can produce mild diuretic effects without changing blood potassium levels. They promote sodium and chloride excretion without resulting loss of potassium. Their activity depends on the presence of endogenous or exogenous aldosterone. This is true of spironolactone. There are two groups of potassium-sparing diuretics: the aldosterone antagonists (including spironolactone) and those that work regardless of the presence or absence of aldosterone (such as amiloride and triamterene). **Table 13–3** summarizes potassium-sparing diuretics.

TABLE 13–2 Thiazide and Thiazide-Like Diuretics

Generic Name	Trade Name	Average Adult Dosage
Thiazide diuretics		
• chlorothiazide	• Diuril, Duragen	• PO: 250–500 mg 1–2 times/day
• cyclothiazide	• Anhydron	• PO: 2 mg/day
• hydrochlorothiazide	• HydroDIURIL, Esidrix	• PO: 12.5–100 mg/day
• hydroflumethiazide	• Diucardin, Saluron	• PO: 25–100 mg 1–2 times/day
• methyclothiazide	• Aquatensen, Enduron	• PO: 2.5–10 mg/day
• polythiazide	• Renese	• PO: 1–4 mg/day
Thiazide-like diuretics		
• chlorthalidone	• Hygroton	• PO: 50–100 mg/day
• indapamide	• Lozol	• PO: 2.5–5 mg/day

TABLE 13–3 Potassium-Sparing Diuretics

Generic Name	Trade Name	Average Adult Dosage
amiloride	Midamor	PO: 5–20 mg/day
spironolactone	Aldactone	PO: Up to 400 mg/day
triamterene	Dyrenium	PO: Up to 300 mg/day

Method of Action

Potassium-sparing diuretics prevent sodium reabsorption in the distal tubule and collecting ducts, either by competing with aldosterone for intracellular cytoplasmic receptor sites or by directly translocating into the target cell nuclei. The serum potassium is elevated as a result of this action.

Clinical Implications

Potassium-sparing diuretics are used for edema associated with congestive heart failure, hepatic cirrhosis with ascites, renal failure, and nephrotic syndrome. They are used mainly in combination with other drugs to manage hypertension and correct hypokalemic conditions. Spironolactone is also used for primary hyperaldosteronism.

Adverse Effects

These diuretics may cause life-threatening hyperkalemia (high potassium levels in the blood). Common adverse effects include acute renal failure, kidney stones, lethargy, headache, mental confusion, and nausea. Spironolactone may cause gynecomastia in men and menstrual irregularities in women.

Contraindications

Potassium-sparing diuretics are contraindicated in acute renal insufficiency, anuria, hyperkalemia, and impaired renal function.

TABLE 13–4 Osmotic Diuretics

Generic Name	Trade Name	Average Adult Dosage
glycerin	Osmoglyn	PO: 1–2 g/kg
isosorbide	Ismotic	PO: 1–3 mg/kg b.i.d.–q.i.d.
mannitol	Osmitrol	IV: 50–100 g as 10–20% solution over 2–6 hours (used for edema or ascites)
urea	Ureaphil	IV: 1–1.5 g/kg/day

TABLE 13–5 Carbonic Anhydrase Inhibitors

Generic Name	Trade Name	Average Adult Dosage
acetazolamide	Diamox Sequels	PO: 250 mg/day 1–4 times/day; 500 mg sustained release b.i.d.
	Diamox Parenteral	IV/IM: 500 mg, may repeat in 2–4 hours
dichlorphenamide	Daranide, Oratrol	PO: 100–200 mg followed by 100 mg q12h until desired response is obtained
methazolamide	Neptazane	PO: 50–100 mg b.i.d.–t.i.d.

Precautions

Potassium-sparing diuretics should be used with caution in patients with hepatic cirrhosis and during pregnancy or lactation. Potassium supplements should be avoided.

Osmotic Diuretics

Osmotic diuretics increase urine formation by exceeding the reabsorption capacity of the tubules. This type includes osmotic electrolytes (potassium and sodium salts), osmotic nonelectrolytes (glycerin, mannitol, and urea), and acid-forming salts, such as ammonium chloride (see **Table 13–4**).

Method of Action

> **POINT TO REMEMBER**
>
> Osmotic diuretics osmotically hold water in the tubules and increase urine flow.

Osmotic diuretics affect various areas of the nephrons, decreasing solute content. This results in less water reabsorption from the descending loop of Henle and collecting duct. Therefore, less sodium chloride is reabsorbed in the proximal tubule and ascending loop of Henle.

Clinical Implications

Osmotic diuretics are very effective in treating cerebral edema. They are used mostly for this condition.

Adverse Effects

Osmotic diuretics may cause headache, convulsions, tremor, dizziness, blurred vision, and dry mouth. More serious adverse effects may include hypertension or hypotension, thrombophlebitis, and allergic reactions. Other adverse effects include nausea, vomiting, and chills or fever.

Contraindications

Osmotic diuretics are contraindicated in anuria, marked edema or pulmonary congestion, organic CNS disease, and severe dehydration or congestive heart failure. They are also contraindicated in intracranial bleeding, shock, history of allergy, and during pregnancy or lactation.

Precautions

Glycerin should be used with caution in cardiac disease, hepatic disease, diabetes mellitus, mild renal impairment, thyroid disease, dehydrated patients, or older adults. Mannitol should be used cautiously in older adults and those with electrolyte imbalance. Ammonium chloride should be used with caution in cardiac edema or insufficiency, pulmonary insufficiency, and during pregnancy or lactation.

Carbonic Anhydrase Inhibitors

Carbonic anhydrase inhibitors are often used for epilepsy, glaucoma, and to lessen the effects of higher altitudes. Their action in the kidneys mainly affects the proximal tubules. The carbonic anhydrase inhibitors are listed in **Table 13–5**.

Method of Action

Carbonic anhydrase inhibitors stop the conversion of carbon dioxide into bicarbonate and carbonic acid ions. This reaction occurs in the proximal tubules of the kidneys and in other parts of the body, affecting acid-base balance.

Clinical Implications

Carbonic anhydrase inhibitors are used for seizures (absence, focal, and generalized tonic-clonic), to reduce intraocular pressure in glaucoma, and for acute high-altitude sickness.

Adverse Effects

Carbonic anhydrase inhibitors may cause nausea, vomiting, weight loss, dry mouth and thirst, diarrhea, fatigue, dizziness, drowsiness, and exacerbation of gout. More serious adverse effects may include anorexia, bone-marrow depression, hyperglycemia, and hepatic dysfunction.

Contraindications

Carbonic anhydrase inhibitors are contraindicated in hypersensitive patients, marked renal or hepatic dysfunction, adrenocortical insufficiencies, hyponatremia, and hypokalemia. They are also contraindicated in hypochloremic acidosis and have not been established as safe to use during pregnancy or lactation.

Precautions

Carbonic anhydrase inhibitors should be used with caution in diabetes mellitus, gout, history of hypercalciuria, obstructive pulmonary disease, and respiratory acidosis. They may interact with many other drugs, including digitalis.

Patient Education

The respiratory therapist should emphasize to patients on long-term loop or thiazide diuretic therapy that they should have a diet rich in potassium. This includes apricots, wheat bran, raisins, potato chips, figs, and bananas. Diuretics should be taken in the morning instead of in the evening or at bedtime.

SUMMARY

The urinary system is composed of the kidneys and the urinary tract (paired ureters, a urinary bladder, and a urethra). The urinary system filters the blood, transports urine, stores urine, excretes urine, helps to maintain blood volume, and regulates erythrocyte production. The kidneys are located along the abdomen's posterior wall. Urine deposited within the minor calyx flows into the major calyx and then into the renal pelvis. The nephron is the structural and functional unit of the kidneys. Nephrons are composed of a renal corpuscle and a renal tubule. The juxtaglomerular apparatus releases renin to regulate blood pressure. Urine volume is controlled, in large part, by antidiuretic hormone (ADH), which is secreted in response to either a rise in concentrations of ions in the blood or because of a fall in blood volume. Diuretics promote urine formation and elimination. They include loop diuretics, thiazide and thiazide-like diuretics, potassium-sparing diuretics, and osmotic diuretics. Carbonic anhydrase inhibitors are also used for various conditions related to the kidneys.

LEARNING GOALS

These learning goals correspond to the objectives at the beginning of the chapter, providing a clear summary of the chapter's most important points.

1. The urinary system is composed of the kidneys, ureters, urinary bladder, and urethra. The kidneys filter waste products from the bloodstream, converting this filtrate into urine. The urinary tract transports urine out of the body.
2. The nephrons are the functional filtration units of the kidneys. They consist of a renal corpuscle, proximal convoluted tubule, nephron loop, and a distal convoluted tubule. There are about 2.5 million nephrons in the two kidneys. The nephrons function in filtration, reabsorption, and secretion.
3. ADH is secreted by the posterior pituitary gland. It increases water absorption from the tubular fluid in the collecting ducts. This reduces water loss from the kidneys. ADH is secreted either in response to a rise in the concentrations of ions in the blood or a fall in blood volume.
4. Diuretics are indicated for many different conditions, including hypertension, congestive heart failure, acute pulmonary edema, hypercalcemia, hepatic cirrhosis, nephrotic syndrome, cerebral edema, and other conditions.
5. The major types of diuretics include loop diuretics, thiazide and thiazide-like diuretics, potassium-sparing diuretics, osmotic diuretics, and carbonic anhydrase inhibitors.
6. Thiazide diuretics work by increasing urinary excretion of water and sodium. They inhibit sodium reabsorption and increase the excretion of bicarbonate, chloride, and potassium ions.
7. The major adverse effect of potassium-sparing diuretics is life-threatening hyperkalemia, with common adverse effects including acute renal failure, kidney stones, lethargy, headache, mental confusion, and nausea.
8. The contraindications of thiazide diuretics include diabetes, gout, impaired liver function, and severe renal disease. They are also not recommended to be used by lactating women or elderly patients.
9. Osmotic diuretics are very effective in treating cerebral edema and are used mostly for this condition.
10. Loop diuretics are sometimes called high-ceiling diuretics, and they must be used carefully

because larger doses can increase urine output to a great degree. This may lead to severely decreased blood volume and even death.

CRITICAL THINKING QUESTIONS

A college student drank a dozen bottles of beer at a party. During the evening, he had to urinate many times. The next morning, he had a headache, was dizzy, and was very dehydrated.

1. Explain the method of action of this condition.
2. Describe what will happen if this student drinks a lot of pure water.

WEB SITES

http://kidney.niddk.nih.gov/Kudiseases/pubs/
    yourkidneys/
http://www.drugs.com/cons/carbonic-anhydrase-
    inhibitors.html
http://www.drugs.com/cons/diuretics-loop.html
http://www.ivy-rose.co.uk/HumanBody/Urinary/
    Urinary_System_Nephron_Diagram.php
http://www.mayoclinic.com/health/diuretics/HI00030
http://www.merck.com/mmhe/sec12/ch158/ch158a
    .html
http://www.nsbri.org/HumanPhysSpace/focus4/
    ep-urinecontrol.html
http://www.youtube.com/watch?v=0q2mQEkUxDc

REVIEW QUESTIONS

Multiple Choice

Select the best response to each question.

1. The apex of a renal pyramid is called the renal
   A. calyx
   B. capsule
   C. papilla
   D. cortex
2. Urine in a major calyx of the kidney next travels to the
   A. minor calyx
   B. ureter
   C. urinary bladder
   D. renal pelvis
3. Which of the following organs is responsible for filtering the blood?
   A. ureter
   B. kidney
   C. urethra
   D. urinary bladder
4. Which of the following diuretics are the drugs of choice for acute pulmonary edema due to congestive heart failure and for hypercalcemia?
   A. osmotic diuretics
   B. loop diuretics
   C. thiazide diuretics
   D. potassium-sparing diuretics
5. Urine formation begins with which of the following processes?
   A. urinary excretion
   B. glomerular filtration
   C. tubular reabsorption
   D. tubular secretion
6. Which of the following is a major adverse effect of potassium-sparing diuretics?
   A. hyperkalemia
   B. hypercalcemia
   C. hypocalcemia
   D. hypokalemia
7. Antidiuretic hormone is also called
   A. erythropoietin
   B. vasopressin
   C. aldosterone
   D. renin
8. Which of the following are the most commonly used type of diuretics?
   A. osmotic diuretics
   B. loop diuretics
   C. carbonic anhydrase inhibitors
   D. thiazide and thiazide-like diuretics
9. Spironolactone is classified as
   A. a carbonic anhydrase inhibitor
   B. a potassium-sparing diuretic
   C. a thiazide or thiazide-like diuretic
   D. an osmotic diuretic
10. Osmotic diuretics are very effective in treating
    A. cerebral edema
    B. pulmonary congestion
    C. intracranial bleeding
    D. glaucoma
11. Which of the following organs secretes erythropoietin?
    A. lung
    B. bone
    C. kidney
    D. brain
12. Carbonic anhydrase inhibitors are used for
    A. weight loss and hyperglycemia
    B. glaucoma and seizures
    C. bone-marrow depression and anorexia
    D. hepatic dysfunction and gout

13. Which of the following drugs is classified as a loop diuretic?
    A. indapamide (Lozol)
    B. chlorthalidone (Hygroton)
    C. amiloride (Midamor)
    D. furosemide (Lasix)

14. Which of the following is the generic name of Aldactone?
    A. spironolactone
    B. triamterene
    C. amiloride
    D. bumetanide

15. Which of the following statements is false about the method of action of thiazide diuretics?
    A. They increase urinary excretion of water and sodium.
    B. They inhibit sodium reabsorption on the distal convoluted tubules and collecting ducts.
    C. They decrease bicarbonate and potassium ion excretion.
    D. They increase bicarbonate, chloride, and potassium ion excretion.

CASE STUDY

A 57-year-old female was diagnosed with congestive heart failure and cirrhosis of the liver. She had been on loop diuretics for several months and was particularly sensitive to potassium loss. Her neurological symptoms included drowsiness, irritability, confusion, and loss of sensation. She also had muscular weakness, cardiac arrhythmias, and tetany. Shortly after her diagnoses, this patient died of respiratory arrest.

1. If the patient had hypokalemia, could it have been related to her diuretic therapy?
2. List which diuretics can cause hypokalemia.
3. How can hypokalemia be prevented?

Medications for Coagulation Disorders

OBJECTIVES

Upon completion of this chapter, the reader should be able to the following:

1. Explain the important steps of hemostasis.
2. Identify the main drugs affecting coagulation.
3. Differentiate between the anticoagulants heparin and warfarin.
4. Explain antiplatelet drugs and their methods of action.
5. Differentiate clotting factors from hemostatic agents.
6. Identify the main adverse effects of heparin.
7. Explain the clinical implications of low-molecular-weight heparins.
8. Describe the methods of action of thrombolytic medications.
9. List examples of hemostatic agents.
10. List five examples of common low-molecular-weight heparins.

KEY TERMS

Antidote	Serotonin
Coagulation	Thrombocytopenia
Endothelial	Thrombus
Hematomas	Tourniquets
Hemophilia	Urticaria
Hemostasis	
Heparin	
Microfibrillar collagen	
Platelet plug	

INTRODUCTION

Hemostasis protects the body from injury by controlling the blood clotting process. The human body, without hemostasis, could experience shock leading to death from loss of blood. Hemostasis controls the level of clotting needed to plug an injury without causing clots to become too large. Anticoagulants are drugs administered to keep clotting from becoming too excessive in conditions such as cerebrovascular accident (CVA) or stroke, myocardial infarction (MI), diseases of the heart valves, conditions involving the use of catheters, and venous thrombus. Thromboembolic disorders are caused by thrombi and emboli, thrombocytopenia, and bleeding disorders such as hemophilia.

Hemostasis

When a blood vessel is injured, many physiological mechanisms are activated that promote **hemostasis** (the cessation of bleeding). Breakage of the **endothelial** lining of a vessel exposes collagen proteins to the blood. This begins three separate yet overlapping hemostatic mechanisms:

1. Vasoconstriction: This decreases blood loss until clotting can occur. It is caused by the release of the neurotransmitter **serotonin** by the platelets.
2. The formation of a platelet plug: When a blood vessel is damaged, the platelets are activated by its inner lining, becoming sticky and adhering to each other as well as the injured vessel to form a **platelet plug**. An inactive glycoprotein called prothrombin is converted into the active enzyme thrombin. Thrombin then converts a soluble protein known as fibrinogen into fibrin. **Figure 14–1** shows the steps in platelet plug formation.
3. Blood clotting: Blood clotting is the production of a netlike or weblike structure of fibrin proteins that penetrates and surrounds the platelet plug, caused by activated blood clotting factors, sealing off the injured area. More serious injuries to

blood vessels are handled by the formation of blood clots. The **process** of blood clotting is known as **coagulation**. The mechanism of clotting is shown in **Figure 14–2**.

> **POINT TO REMEMBER**
>
> Clot formation requires a sequence or cascade of events.

Anticoagulants

Anticoagulant agents prolong bleeding time and help to prevent potentially harmful clots from forming in blood vessels. Although they do not actually thin the blood, they are sometimes referred to as blood thinners. Anticoagulants do not dissolve clots that already exist in a blood vessel. They can prevent clots from enlarging, however. Anticoagulants work by preventing prothrombin from being converted into thrombin, therefore stopping the conversion of fibrinogen into fibrin. They fall into two main groups: orally administered and parenterally administered anticoagulants. The primary anticoagulants include warfarin (oral), fondaparinux (subcutaneous), and heparin (intravenous or subcutaneous). **Table 14–1** lists the primary anticoagulants.

> **POINT TO REMEMBER**
>
> The circulating clotting factors are produced primarily in the liver.

> **POINT TO REMEMBER**
>
> Vitamin K is required for the synthesis of most clotting factors, and calcium ions are essential for many steps in the clotting process.

Heparin

Heparin is a mucopolysaccharide that has anticoagulant effects. The original type, known as unfractionated (standard) heparin, is extracted from pigs. Heparin sodium is produced by and potentially released by mast cells located in the liver, lung, intestines, and other parts of the body. Heparin is a very large, water-soluble molecule. It must be given intravenously or subcutaneously.

> **POINT TO REMEMBER**
>
> High endogenous heparin concentrations occur in the mast cells in the lungs.

> **POINT TO REMEMBER**
>
> The distribution of heparin is limited to the vascular space, making it useful for anticoagulation during pregnancy.

Method of Action

Heparin works by increasing the length of clotting time and preventing thrombi from forming or growing larger. This is accomplished by the blockage of the conversion

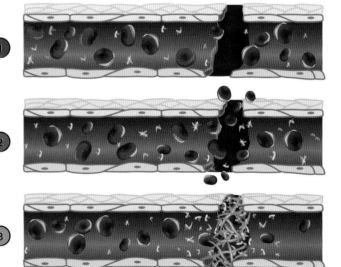

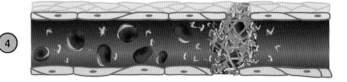

1. Vessel wall break
2. Bleeding starts
3. Thrombocytes stick together to seal the area of the breakage
4. Thrombocytes form a platelet plug to stop bleeding

FIGURE 14–1 The formation of a platelet plug.

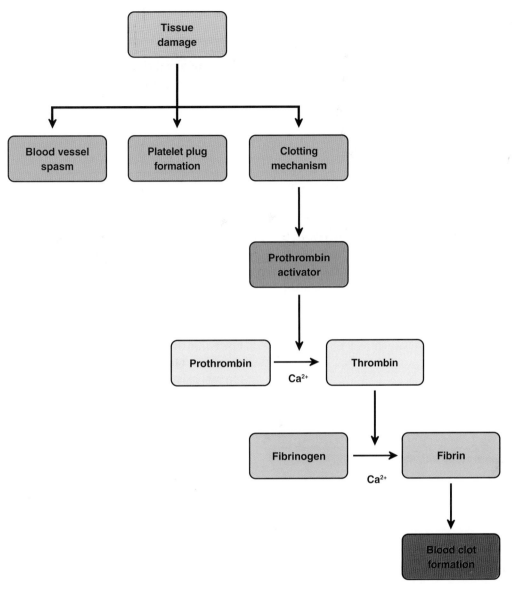

FIGURE 14–2 Mechanisms of clotting.

TABLE 14–1 Primary Anticoagulants		
Generic Name	**Trade Name**	**Average Adult Dosage**
fondaparinux	Arixtra	SC: 2.5 mg/day for 7 days
heparin	Hep-Lock	IV infusion: 5000–40,000/day; SC: 15,000–20,000 units b.i.d.
warfarin	Coumadin	PO: 2–15 mg/day

of prothrombin to thrombin and fibrinogen to fibrin, disabling the clotting process.

Clinical Implications

Heparin is used for specific cardiovascular and lung disorders, and during open-heart surgery, coronary artery bypass graft surgery, and dialysis. Heparin dosage is determined on an individual basis. Because it is not absorbed via oral administration, heparin is given either by intravenous or subcutaneous routes. Intramuscular administration is discouraged because the absorption is erratic and may cause large hematomas.

Adverse Effects

Heparin's main adverse effect is the potential for bleeding. The most common bleeding sites are the GI tract, urinary

TABLE 14–2 Low-Molecular-Weight Heparins (LMWHs)

Generic Name	Trade Name	Average Adult Dosage
ardeparin	Normiflo	SC: 50 units/kg b.i.d. for 14 days
dalteparin	Fragmin	SC: 2500–5000 units/day for 5–10 days
danaparoid	Orgaran	SC: 750 units b.i.d. for 7–10 days
enoxaparin	Lovenox	SC: 30 mg b.i.d. for 7–10 days
tinzaparin	Innohep	SC: 175 units/kg/day for at least 6 days

POINT TO REMEMBER

A mild heparin overdose can be treated by discontinuing administration of heparin, and protamine is the antidote for heparin to treat a more serious heparin overdose.

tract, and soft tissues. Other adverse effects may include subdural hematoma, acute hemorrhagic pancreatitis, ecchymosis (bleeding into the skin), and hemarthrosis (bleeding into a joint). Less common adverse effects include fever, alopecia, hypersensitivity reactions, ostealgia (bone pain), and osteoporosis. Protamine sulfate is the antidote for heparin overdosage.

Contraindications

Heparin is contraindicated if there is serious or intracranial bleeding, hemophilia, severe liver or kidney disease, severe thrombocytopenia, or malignant hypertension.

Precautions

Heparin should be used with caution when taking aspirin or other OTC medications; if changes in the color of urine, vomitus, or stools occur; if any other signs of bleeding occur; if bruises appear; if epistaxis or bloody sputum, pain in the chest, abdomen, back, or pelvis occurs; if menstruation increases; or if there is persistent headache, dizziness, or faintness.

Low-Molecular-Weight Heparins (LMWHs)

These newer types of heparin are derived from unfractionated heparin and are similar in action. LMWHs are more readily absorbed after subcutaneous injection into the bloodstream than standard heparin and have longer-lasting effects. They have a more predictable dose response than standard heparin. **Table 14–2** summarizes the LMWHs.

Method of Action

The methods of action of LMWHs are similar to that of standard heparin.

Clinical Implications

LMWHs are used for preventing and treating venous thromboembolism, including deep vein thrombosis

(DVT), acute coronary disease, and pulmonary embolism. They are also used for preventing venous thrombosis in hip replacement patients. LMWHs are used according to body weight and do not require laboratory monitoring. LMWHs are administered subcutaneously and generally have less potential for patient harm than does standard heparin.

Adverse Effects

Abnormal bleeding is common during heparin therapy. LMWHs may cause nausea, vomiting, allergic reactions (rash, urticaria), and pain at the injection site. Overdose of LMWHs may be treated with protamine. Protamine sulfate has an onset time of 5 minutes and is also a blocker of the LMWHs.

Contraindications

LMWHs are contraindicated in children. In adults, they should not be used with allergy to heparin (or pork), active bleeding, thrombocytopenia, and unstable angina. They should not be used in patients with renal failure.

Precautions

LMWHs have the same precautions as standard heparin.

Warfarin

Warfarin is the oral anticoagulant of choice because of its potency and reliable bioavailability. It is a fat-soluble derivative of coumarin and is similar to vitamin K. Coumarin-derived drugs, such as warfarin, are preferred over those derived from the drug indandione because they have less toxicity.

Method of Action

Warfarin interferes with the liver's synthesis of vitamin K-dependent clotting factors. This prolongs clotting time. Warfarin acts by binding to plasma proteins, which can cross the placenta during pregnancy. The onset of action is delayed by 8–12 hours because stores of the clotting factors must be depleted. The maximum anticoagulant effect of warfarin occurs after 1 week of administration.

TABLE 14-3 Antiplatelet Medications

Generic Name	Trade Name	Average Adult Dosage
abciximab	ReoPro	IV: 0.25 mg/kg initially over 5 minutes, then 10 mcg/min for 12 hours
aspirin	Ecotrin, etc.	PO: 80 mg/day to 650 mg b.i.d.
cilostazol	Pletal	PO: 100 mg b.i.d.
clopidogrel	Plavix	PO: 75 mg/day
dipyridamole	Persantine	PO: 75–100 mg q.i.d.
eptifibatide	Integrilin	IV: 180 mcg/kg initial bolus over 1–2 minutes, then 2 mcg/kg/min for 24–72 hours
pentoxifylline	Trental	PO: 400 mg t.i.d.
ticlopidine	Ticlid	PO: 250 mg b.i.d.
tirofiban	Aggrastat	IV: 0.4 mcg/kg/min for 30 minutes, then 0.1 mcg/kg/min for 12–24 hours

Clinical Implications

POINT TO REMEMBER

Because warfarin is effective when given orally, it is more useful than heparin for outpatients.

Warfarin is used when long-term anticoagulant therapy is needed. It is administered in conventional or minidoses as needed and usually lasts from 2 to 5 days.

Adverse Effects

POINT TO REMEMBER

Because warfarin readily crosses the placenta and affects bone formation in the developing fetus, teratogenicity must be kept in mind.

Warfarin's major adverse effect is hemorrhage, especially at ulcer or tumor sites. Prolonged used of coumarin-derived drugs is usually free of adverse effects, although bleeding may occur at various sites throughout the body. Close monitoring of the degree of anticoagulation is required. Treatment with warfarin should be done over as short a time period as possible. Rare adverse effects include diarrhea, alopecia, itching, dermatitis, and skin necrosis. Intracranial hemorrhage is the most serious adverse effect of warfarin use and often results in permanent disability or death.

Contraindications

Absolute contraindications to warfarin include active bleeding, hemorrhagic tendencies, history of warfarin-induced skin necrosis, and pregnancy.

Precautions

Warfarin should be used with great caution in patients with a history of GI bleeding, alcoholic liver disease, recent neurosurgery, severe renal impairment, or inability to keep follow-up appointments for monitoring. Warfarin should be taken at the same time each day. Females should use contraceptives to prevent pregnancy during warfarin administration and should not breastfeed due to potential toxicity via the breast milk.

POINT TO REMEMBER

Nicotine, digoxin, tetracycline, or antihistamines may inhibit anticoagulation.

Antiplatelet Medications

Antiplatelet medications are used to prevent thrombosis. They counteract many of the steps of platelet activation and adhesion. Examples of antiplatelet medications such as aspirin, clopidogrel, eptifibatide, and ticlopidine are shown in **Table 14-3**.

Method of Action

Antiplatelet medications reduce the likelihood that the platelets will aggregate and form potentially harmful blood clots.

Clinical Implications

Antiplatelet medications are used prophylactically for arterial thrombosis and to manage MI and stroke. These drugs are commonly used in patients who have

TABLE 14-4 Thrombolytic Medications

Generic Name	Trade Name	Average Adult Dosage
alteplase recombinant	Activase	IV: Start with 60 mg, then infuse 20 mg/hour over next 2 hours
anistreplase	Eminase	IV: 30 units over 2–5 minutes
reteplase recombinant	Retavase	IV: 10 units over 2 minutes; repeat dose in 30 minutes
streptokinase	Streptase, Kabikinase	IV: 250,000–1.5 million units over a short period
tenecteplase	TNKase	IV: Up to 50 mg bolus over 5 seconds based on patient weight
urokinase	Abbokinase	IV: 4400–6000 units over several minutes to 12 hours

acute coronary syndromes or who have received stents. They are administered as adjuncts to thrombolytic therapy.

Adverse Effects

The major adverse effect of antiplatelet drugs is bleeding. These drugs may cause epigastric pain, heartburn, diarrhea, and nausea. Abciximab may also cause pain at the injection site, dizziness, and dyspepsia.

Contraindications

Antiplatelet medications are contraindicated in history of GI ulcers, asthma, allergies, hypertension, and nasal polyps.

Precautions

Patients should tell their physicians about any other medications they are taking before starting antiplatelet therapy. This includes herbal remedies and nutritional supplements. Patients should be instructed to report any diarrhea, nausea, rash, infection, sore throat, signs of bleeding, dark urine, yellow skin, or clay-colored stools. They should keep all appointments for follow-up blood tests.

Thrombolytic Medications

Thrombolytic medications (thrombolytics) are used for excessive bleeding as a result of surgery. Only six thrombolytics are currently available, as listed in **Table 14-4**.

Method of Action

Thrombolytic medications facilitate the conversion of plasminogen to plasmin. This conversion hydrolyzes fibrin to dissolve already-formed thrombi or blood clots. Newer types, such as tenecteplase, bind to fibrin and activate its breakdown more than breaking down fibrinogen.

Clinical Implications

Thrombolytic medications are used to treat deep vein thrombosis (DVT), arterial thromboembolism, and severe pulmonary embolism. They are very important for use after MI or acute ischemic stroke.

Adverse Effects

Thrombolytic medications usually cause bleeding at the site of injury, which is caused by the breakdown of fibrin or fibrinogen. Therapy must be stopped if life-threatening intracranial bleeding occurs.

Contraindications

Thrombolytic medications are contraindicated in active bleeding, intracranial trauma, cancer, vascular disease, and during pregnancy or lactation.

Precautions

Patients should be instructed to avoid taking thrombolytic medications with anticoagulants and aspirin. They should also avoid certain herbs for the same reason, including ginger and gingko. Patients should be instructed to immediately report signs of bleeding and changes in consciousness to their physician.

Hemostatics

Hemostatics are substances, devices, or procedures that arrest blood flow. Procedures that are hemostatic include direct pressure, surgical clamps, and tourniquets. Other procedures include cold compresses, such as an ice bag, and irrigation of the stomach with an iced solution to slow gastric bleeding. During surgical procedures, hemostatic measures include gelatin sponges, thrombin solutions, and microfibrillar collagen. Phytonadione (vitamin K_1) is used to prevent and treat hemorrhagic disease in newborns and to treat prothrombin deficiency that can be induced by anticoagulants and other drugs.

Patient Education

Respiratory therapists should instruct patients about the procedures involved in anticoagulant therapy and why they are necessary prior to beginning thrombolytic therapy. Patients should be advised of an increased risk of bleeding. Their activity should be restricted, and there must be frequent monitoring of the blood during this time.

SUMMARY

Hemostasis is a complex process involving multiple steps and many enzymes and clotting factors. The final product of hemostasis is a fibrin clot that stops blood loss. Diseases of hemostasis include thromboembolic disorders caused by thrombi and emboli, thrombocytopenia, and bleeding disorders, such as hemophilia. The normal coagulation process can be modified by a number of different mechanisms, including specific clotting factors, dissolving fibrin, and inhibiting platelet function.

Anticoagulants are used to prevent thrombi from forming or enlarging. The primary drugs in this category are heparin (parenteral) and warfarin (oral), although low-molecular-weight heparins and thrombin inhibitors are also available. Thrombolytics are used to dissolve existing intravascular clots in patients with myocardial infarctions or stroke.

LEARNING GOALS

These learning goals correspond to the objectives at the beginning of the chapter, providing a clear summary of the chapter's most important points.

1. Hemostasis occurs in the following important steps:
    A. Vasoconstriction: Vasoconstriction is caused by the release of serotonin.
    B. Formation of platelet plug: The platelets become sticky.
    C. Blood clotting (coagulation): A netlike structure of fibrin seals the injured area.
2. The main drugs that affect coagulation are the following anticoagulants: warfarin (oral), pentoxifylline (oral), and heparin (IV or SC).
3. The main differences between heparin and warfarin are as follows:
    -   Heparin is a protein with anticoagulant effects. It was originally extracted from pigs, although it is produced by the human body as well. Heparin increases the length of clotting time and prevents thrombi from forming or growing larger.
    -   Warfarin is more potent and has more reliable bioavailability. It is derived from coumarin and is similar to vitamin K. Warfarin interferes with the liver's synthesis of vitamin K-dependent clotting factors to prolong clotting time.
4. Antiplatelet drugs prevent thrombosis, counteracting many steps of platelet activation and adhesion. They reduce the likelihood of platelets to aggregate and form potentially harmful blood clots.
5. Clotting factors are activated substances in the blood that produce a netlike web of fibrin proteins to surround platelet plugs and seal off injured areas. They are natural substances that the body produces for this purpose. Hemostatics are substances, devices, or procedures that arrest blood flow and are not produced within the body. However, one hemostatic substance is vitamin K_1. Although it is produced in the body, it may be introduced into the body from an outside source to prevent and treat hemorrhagic disease in newborns or to treat prothrombin deficiency.
6. The main adverse effects of heparin include the potential for bleeding, subdural hematoma, acute hemorrhagic pancreatitis, ecchymosis, and hemarthrosis.
7. Low-molecular-weight heparins (LMWHs) are indicated for venous thromboembolism, including deep vein thrombosis (DVT), acute coronary disease, and pulmonary embolism.
8. Thrombolytic medications facilitate the conversion of plasminogen to plasmin to dissolve already-formed thrombi or blood clots.
9. Hemostatic agents include substances, devices, and procedures that arrest blood flow:
    -   Hemostatic substances: thrombin solutions, microfibrillar collagen, phytonadione (vitamin K_1)
    -   Hemostatic devices and procedures: direct pressure, surgical clamps, tourniquets, cold compresses, irrigation of the stomach with an iced solution, gelatin sponges
10. Five examples of common low-molecular-weight heparins include ardeparin (Normiflo), dalteparin (Fragmin), danaparoid (Orgaran), enoxaparin (Lovenox), and tinzaparin (Innohep).

CRITICAL THINKING QUESTIONS

1. Why doesn't blood normally clot in the blood vessels?
2. List three ways that normal blood clotting could be impaired and three ways that inappropriate blood clotting could develop.

WEB SITES

http://www.aafp.org/afp/990315ap/1607.html
http://www.americanheart.org/presenter
.jhtml?identifier=4443
http://www.clotcare.com/clotcare/index.aspx
http://www.hemophiliamoms.com/

http://www.hrsonline.org/PatientInfo/Treatments/
Medications/ThromTher/

http://www.mhhe.com/biosci/esp/2002_general/Esp/
folder_structure/tr/m1/s7/trm1s7_3.htm

http://www.rxlist.com/heparin-drug.htm

http://www.webmd.com/heart-disease/
antiplatelet-drugs

REVIEW QUESTIONS

Multiple Choice

Select the best response to each question.

1. The principal toxic effect of heparin is
   A. hemorrhage
   B. hair loss
   C. bronchospasm
   D. fever

2. Tenecteplase (TNKase) is used primarily to reduce mortality associated with which of the following clinical problems?
   A. hemorrhage
   B. pulmonary edema
   C. myocardial infarction
   D. stroke

3. The action of heparin is terminated by
   A. insulin
   B. coumarin
   C. sulfonamides
   D. protamine sulfate

4. Which of the following is *not* a low-molecular-weight heparin?
   A. tinzaparin
   B. dalteparin
   C. warfarin
   D. enoxaparin

5. Streptokinase is used to
   A. treat digestive disorders
   B. dissolve blood clots
   C. promote carbohydrate degradation
   D. replace pepsin

6. Standard heparin is also called
   A. eptifibatide
   B. ardeparin
   C. unfractionated heparin
   D. low-molecular-weight heparin

7. Which of the following is an absolute contraindication for heparin therapy?
   A. infancy
   B. prostate cancer
   C. breastfeeding
   D. intracranial bleeding

8. The generic name of Fragmin is
   A. dalteparin
   B. danaparoid
   C. enoxaparin
   D. ardeparin

9. Stoppage of blood flow is referred to as
   A. hemolysis
   B. hemopoiesis
   C. hemostasis
   D. hemosiderosis

10. Which of the following anticoagulants is given orally?
    A. streptokinase
    B. urokinase
    C. heparin
    D. Coumadin

11. An example of an antiplatelet drug is
    A. warfarin
    B. heparin
    C. abciximab
    D. Abbokinase

12. Which of the following anticoagulants is contraindicated during pregnancy?
    A. enoxaparin
    B. ardeparin
    C. warfarin
    D. heparin

13. The generic name of Plavix is
    A. clopidogrel
    B. abciximab
    C. ticlopidine
    D. tirofiban

14. Which of the following agents is used in the prevention and treatment of bleeding in newborns?
    A. enoxaparin
    B. aspirin
    C. vitamin A
    D. vitamin K_1

15. Which of the following chemical substances may be released by the platelets to cause vascular spasms to stop bleeding?
    A. renin
    B. serotonin
    C. vitamin K_1
    D. heparin

CASE STUDY

Mrs. Gregg was admitted to the hospital with chest pain and suspected pulmonary embolus. She was immediately placed on heparin for 48 hours, and then her drug therapy was switched to warfarin. She was allowed to leave the hospital with instructions to have laboratory blood testing every other day for the next 2 weeks.

1. Why did the physician first place Mrs. Gregg on heparin therapy instead of warfarin?
2. What laboratory tests will likely be performed during the 2 weeks after her discharge?

Treatment of Respiratory Disorders

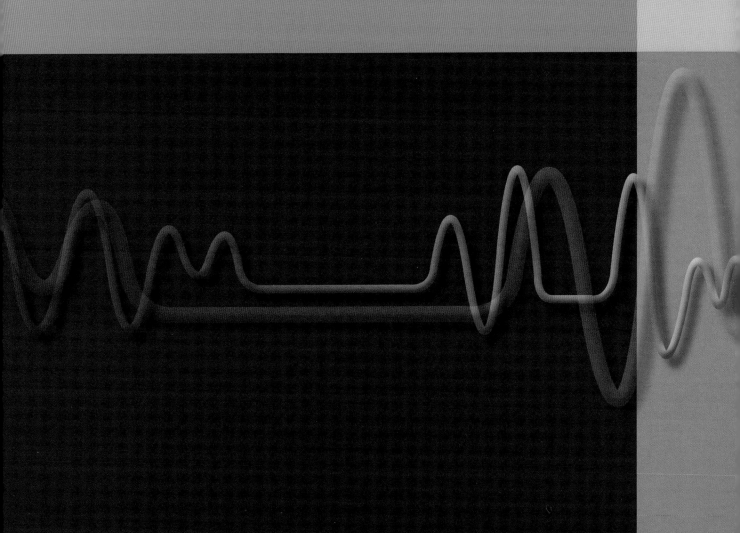

Antiasthma Medications

OBJECTIVES

Upon completion of this chapter, the reader should be able to do the following:

1. Describe the various types of asthma.
2. Explain and contrast the agents used for acute and chronic asthma.
3. Classify drugs indicated in asthma therapy.
4. Describe the advantages of combination controller therapy.
5. Explain and contrast leukotriene modifiers and mast cell stabilizers in treating asthma.
6. Identify the common adverse effects of xanthine derivatives.
7. Discuss adverse effects of anticholinergics.
8. Explain the contraindications of beta$_2$-adrenergic agonists.
9. Describe the clinical implications of glucocorticoids as anti-inflammatory agents.
10. Discuss the method of action of beta$_2$-adrenergic agonists.

KEY TERMS

Allergens	Leukotriene
Anticholinergics	Macrophages
Bronchodilators	Mast cell stabilizers
Histamine	Mast cells
Immunoglobulin E (IgE) antibodies	Muscarinic receptors
Leukocytes	Sympathomimetic

INTRODUCTION

The National Asthma Education and Prevention Program (NAEPP) defines asthma as "a chronic inflammatory disorder of the airways in which many cells and cellular elements play a role." Patients with asthma experience inflammation and resulting breathlessness, chest tightness, coughing, and wheezing. These symptoms are usually associated with obstructed airflow that may be reversed spontaneously or with treatment. Airway inflammation also causes increased bronchial responsiveness to different types of stimuli.

Asthma is classified as an intermittent, obstructive, reversible lung disease. It is a growing health problem in the United States. Approximately 20 million people are affected by asthma. In the past 25 years, the number of children with asthma has grown immensely. It is now the leading serious chronic illness in children. Nearly 75% of children with asthma continue to have chronic problems in adulthood. This condition kills more than 500,000 US patients every year. Asthma is more common in males younger than age 18 years. However, in adults, asthma is more common in females. Prescribers must choose specific medications to manage each type of asthma effectively. These agents will be discussed in detail in later chapters. The classifications of asthma are listed in Table 15–1.

Risk Factors Causing Asthma

Asthma is caused by various environmental and genetic factors, including animal dander, mites, cockroaches, pollen from trees, mold (indoor and outdoor), dust, chemicals and drugs, hormonal changes, emotional upsets, airborne pollutants, cigarette smoke, gastroesophageal reflux, and respiratory tract infections. Bronchial asthma that begins in childhood or adolescence is usually genetically linked. Patients with this type of asthma usually have other allergic conditions, such as eczema, hay fever, and hives.

Bronchial asthma that results from exercise occurs in 40 to 90% of patients. This condition most often affects patients who exercise in a cold environment rather than in a warmer environment. The wearing of a mask during exercise may sufficiently warm air to the lungs and prevent this type of asthma.

POINT TO REMEMBER

In asthma, histamine attaches to receptor sites in larger bronchi, causing swelling of the smooth muscles.

Irritants that may induce asthma include tobacco, strong odors, irritating gases, fumes, dusts, and other chemicals. Irritant gases include nitrogen dioxide, ozone, and sulfur dioxide. In the workplace, common causes of asthma include epoxy resins, plastics, toluene, cotton dust, platinum dust, wood dust, and chemicals such as formaldehyde. Some asthma patients have their symptoms worsened by aspirin, NSAIDs, nonselective beta-blockers, certain ophthalmic preparations, and sulfites that are used as food preservatives.

Changes in hormone levels can induce asthma symptoms. For example, nearly 40% of women with asthma report increased symptoms during their premenstrual period. Also, the reflux of gastric secretions may act as a trigger for bronchospasm and related asthma. Nocturnal asthma can be caused by reflux during sleep.

POINT TO REMEMBER

Leukotrienes attach to receptor sites in the smaller bronchi and cause swelling of smooth muscle in these sites.

Treating Acute and Chronic Asthma

Antiasthma medications can be divided into those used for symptom relief (beta$_2$-adrenergic agonists, theophylline, and anticholinergics) and those used for long-term control (corticosteroids, cromolyn, and leukotriene modifiers). Beta-adrenergic (**sympathomimetic**) agonists are preferred for treating acute bronchoconstriction associated with asthma. They may activate only one type of receptor or both beta$_1$- and beta$_2$-receptors. The agonists that specifically activate beta$_2$-receptors have become the preferred agonists over the nonselective types because of fewer cardiac-related adverse effects. Beta-adrenergic agonists are commonly called **bronchodilators**. They relax bronchial smooth muscle to widen airways and make breathing easier. They have no anti-inflammatory properties.

Therefore, for chronic asthma, other types of drugs are required to control related inflammation. Bronchodilators are classified according to their duration of

TABLE 15–1 Classifications of Asthma

Classification	Description
Mild intermittent	• Symptoms less than twice a week: coughing, wheezing, chest tightness, difficulty breathing • Symptoms less than twice a month: nighttime symptoms
Mild persistent	• Symptoms more than three to six times a week: coughing, wheezing, chest tightness, difficulty breathing • Symptoms three to four times a month: nighttime symptoms
Moderate persistent	• Daily symptoms: coughing, wheezing, chest tightness, difficulty breathing • Symptoms five or more times a month: nighttime symptoms
Severe persistent	• Continual symptoms: coughing, wheezing, chest tightness, difficulty breathing • Frequent symptoms: nighttime symptoms

action: ultrashort acting, short acting, intermediate acting, and long acting. The effects of the various types of bronchodilators range from 2 to 12 hours. Acute asthmatic attacks are treated with either ultrashort-, short-, or intermediate-acting bronchodilators. Persistent chronic asthma is often treated with long-acting bronchodilators used in combination with inhaled glucocorticoids. Many beta-adrenergic agonists cause fewer adverse effects when administered via inhalation rather than oral tablets. Chronic use of these agents may cause tolerance to occur, meaning that doses need to be increased for an appropriate effect.

Anticholinergics are often used to treat chronic asthma. They act by blocking parasympathetic nervous system effects to cause bronchodilation. They have a slower onset of action than most beta-agonists, with more prolonged effects. Though they may cause many different adverse effects when administered systemically, they offer very few adverse effects when inhaled. These agents will be discussed in further detail later.

Antiallergic Agents (Bronchodilators)

Inhaled allergens cause an early-phase allergic reaction. Histamine, along with other mediators released from mast cells and basophils, plays a role in mediating allergies. It acts on histamine receptors to cause contraction of smooth muscles of the airway, increased vasopermeability and vasodilation, enhanced mucus production, pruritus, and cutaneous vasodilation.

The early-phase allergic reaction is characterized by cells becoming activated that contain allergen-specific immunoglobulin E (IgE) antibodies. Airway mast cells and macrophages are rapidly activated. Mast cells release proinflammatory mediators, such as histamine. Contraction of airway smooth muscle, mucus secretion, excretion of airway plasma, and vasodilation is caused by the release of histamine. These events induce a thickened airway wall, narrowed airway lumen, and reduced mucus clearance (see Figure 2–3). Antiallergic agents include beta-adrenergic agonists, anticholinergics, and xanthine derivatives.

Beta-Adrenergic Agonists

Short-acting beta$_2$-agonists are the most effective bronchodilators available today. When they are administered in aerosol form, they enhance bronchoselectivity, providing a more rapid response and greater protection against bronchospasm (which may be caused by allergens or exercise). The aerosol method of administering these agonists is safer and more effective than when they are administered in any other manner. Three devices commonly used to deliver respiratory drugs are shown in Figure 15–1.

The most commonly used beta$_2$-adrenergic agonists are listed in Table 15–2.

Method of Action

Beta$_2$-adrenergic agonists produce bronchodilation by relaxing the bronchial tree's smooth muscles. They affect the nervous system, targeting the nerves that supply the muscles around the airways. This decreases airway resistance, encourages mucus drainage, and increases vital capacity.

Clinical Implications

Beta-adrenergic agents are the most commonly prescribed bronchodilators. They are the drugs of choice in the treatment of acute bronchoconstriction.

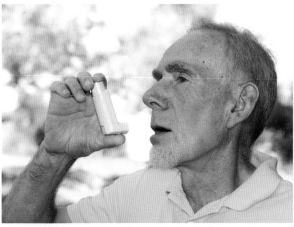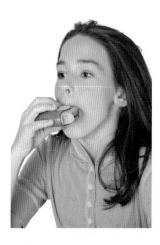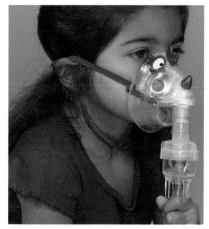

FIGURE 15–1 Devices used to deliver respiratory drugs.

TABLE 15–2 Beta$_2$-adrenergic Agonists

Generic Name	Trade Name	Average Adult Dosage
albuterol	Proventil, Ventolin	PO: 2–4 mg t.i.d.; inhalation: 1–2 inhalations q4–6h; 2 inhalations before exercise
arformoterol	Brovana	Inhalation (nebulizer): one 15-mg inhalation every morning and evening
formoterol	Foradil, Perforomist	Inhalation (Aerolizer inhaler): one 12-mg capsule q12h
levalbuterol	Xopenex	Inhalation (nebulizer): 0.63 mg t.i.d. q6–8h, may increase to 1.25 mg t.i.d. p.r.n.
pirbuterol	Maxair	Inhalation: 2 inhalations (0.4 mg) q6h (max: 12 inhalations/day)
salmeterol	Serevent	Inhalation (various): 2 inhalations of aerosol (42 mcg) or 1 powder Diskus (50 mcg) b.i.d., 12 hours apart

TABLE 15–3 Anticholinergics

Generic Name	Trade Name	Average Adult Dosage
albuterol with ipratropium	DuoNeb	Inhalation (nebulizer): one 3-mL vial administered 4 times/day (max: 6 inhalations/day)
ipratropium bromide	Atrovent, Combivent	Inhalation (MDI): 2 inhalations q.i.d. (max: 12 inhalations/day)
tiotropium	Spiriva	Inhalation (HandiHaler device): 1 capsule inhaled/day

Beta$_2$-adrenergic agonists are used for other reversible airway diseases that are obstructive and bronchospasm that is exercise induced. They are often inhaled using a nebulizer that disperses a fine-particle mist of medication. Therefore, they produce rapid bronchodilation by relaxing bronchiolar smooth muscle.

Adverse Effects

When given orally, the adverse effects of beta$_2$-adrenergic agonists include headache, dizziness, palpitations, restlessness, insomnia, nausea, vomiting, anorexia, and tachycardia. Inhaled beta-adrenergic agents produce little systemic toxicity because only small amounts of the drugs are absorbed.

Contraindications

Beta$_2$-adrenergic agonists are contraindicated in hypersensitive patients, narrow-angle glaucoma, and shock. They are not proven to be safe for use during pregnancy and lactation.

Precautions

Beta$_2$-adrenergic agonists should be used cautiously in older adults, debilitated patients, hypertension, diabetes mellitus, hyperthyroidism, Parkinson disease, prostatic hypertrophy, psychoneurosis, and tuberculosis.

Anticholinergics

Anticholinergic agents are competitive inhibitors of muscarinic receptors. They produce bronchodilation *only* in cholinergic-mediated bronchoconstriction.

Anticholinergics are not as potent as beta$_2$-agonists but have a synergistic relationship with them. See **Table 15–3** for commonly used anticholinergics.

Method of Action

Anticholinergics work by inhibiting the muscarine receptors located in the brain's basal ganglia. This lessens chemical imbalances by blocking acetylcholinic effects. Anticholinergics cause the acetylcholine receptors in muscles to become blocked, reducing the amount of acetylcholine they contain and causing muscular relaxation.

POINT TO REMEMBER

In 2005, a new anticholinergic called tiotropium was approved, which has a long duration of action that allows for once-daily dosing.

Clinical Implications

Anticholinergics are used by inhalation, in various methods, for asthmatic conditions. Interestingly, anticholinergics that are centrally acting are used effectively in treating Parkinson disease. The most widely used drug in this class is ipratropium, which is taken via inhalation to rapidly relieve bronchospasm. Inhaled anticholinergics are more effective when used with other bronchodilators.

Adverse Effects

Anticholinergics may cause anxiety, agitation, confusion, decreased sweating and heat release, drowsiness, dry mouth, urine retention, paresthesias, sinus tachycardia,

TABLE 15–4 Xanthine Derivatives

Generic Name	Trade Name	Average Adult Dosage
aminophylline	Phyllocontin, Truphylline	IV: loading dose 6 mg/kg over 30 minutes; maintenance dose 0.25–0.75 mg/kg/hour; PO: 0.5 mg/kg/hour q.i.d.
dyphylline	Dilor, Lufyllin, etc.	PO: 200–800 mg q6h up to 15 mg/kg q.i.d.
oxtriphylline	Choledyl	PO: 200–800 mg q6h up to 15 mg/kg
theophylline	Somophyllin, Theo-Dur, etc.	PO (loading dose): 5 mg/kg; PO (sustained release maintenance dose): 0.5 mg q8–12h

and urticaria. Some patients may experience an allergic reaction to certain metered dose inhaler formulations of Atrovent.

Contraindications

Anticholinergics are contraindicated for use along with other antimuscarinic agents. They have not been established as safe to use in pregnant women.

Precautions

Patients should be instructed to avoid consuming alcohol while taking anticholinergics. They should eat a high-fiber diet to avoid constipation. They should also avoid driving or operating heavy machinery due to potential drowsiness.

Xanthine Derivatives

The methylxanthines appear to produce bronchodilation but are ineffective via aerosol. They must be administered orally or intravenously for their systemic effects to occur. The preferred xanthine derivative for oral use is sustained-release theophylline. **Table 15–4** lists the xanthine derivatives.

Method of Action

Xanthine derivatives work by relaxing smooth muscle in the bronchi and pulmonary vessels. They stimulate the respiratory center of the medulla oblongata to increase the lungs' vital capacity.

Clinical Implications

Xanthine derivatives are used for the prophylaxis and relief of bronchial asthma, bronchospasm associated with chronic bronchitis, and emphysema.

Adverse Effects

Xanthine derivatives may cause palpitations, flushing, hypotension, insomnia, nervousness, nausea, vomiting, tachycardia, diarrhea, and tachypnea. Their most serious adverse effect is potential respiratory arrest.

Contraindications

Xanthine derivatives are contraindicated in hypersensitive patients, coronary artery disease, history of angina pectoris, and severe hepatic or renal impairment. They have not been proven safe for pregnant or lactating women.

Precautions

Xanthine derivatives should be used with caution in children and the elderly and in patients with hypertension, hyperthyroidism, peptic ulcer, glaucoma, diabetes mellitus, and prostatic hypertrophy. Patients should be instructed to take these medications at the same time every day. They should avoid eating charbroiled food, limit caffeine intake, and avoid cigarette smoking while taking xanthine derivatives.

Anti-Inflammatory Agents

Anti-inflammatory agents reduce inflammation. The most common anti-inflammatory agents used for asthma include inhaled glucocorticoids, leukotriene modifiers, and mast cell stabilizers. Anti-inflammatory agents are listed in **Table 15–5**.

Glucocorticoids

Glucocorticoids are adrenocortical steroid hormones. They are the most potent natural anti-inflammatory substances known. They are used for asthma, allergic reactions, and arthritis, among other conditions. Glucocorticoids are commonly administered by inhalation for asthmatic conditions; they are listed in Table 15–5.

Method of Action

The actions of glucocorticoids are not precisely understood, but these agents appear to diminish activation of inflammatory cells. This increases production of anti-inflammatory mediators, reducing mucus production and edema. Their action also decreases airway obstruction.

TABLE 15–5 Anti-Inflammatory Agents

Generic Name	Trade Name	Average Adult Dosage
Inhaled glucocorticoids		
• beclomethasone	Beclovent, Vanceril, etc.	MDI: 1–2 inhalations t.i.d.–q.i.d. (max: 20 inhalations/day)
• budesonide	Pulmicort Turbuhaler	DPI: 1–2 inhalations (200 mcg/inhalation) q.i.d. (max: 800 mcg/day)
• flunisolide	AeroBid	MDI: 2–3 inhalations b.i.d.–t.i.d. (12 inhalations/day)
• fluticasone	Flonase, Flovent	MDI: 44 mcg (2 inhalations) b.i.d. (max: 10 inhalations/day)
• triamcinolone	Azmacort	MDI: 2 inhalations t.i.d.–q.i.d. (max: 16 inhalations/day)
Leukotriene modifiers		
• montelukast	Singulair	PO: 10 mg/day in the evening
• zafirlukast	Accolate	PO: 20 mg b.i.d. 1 hour before or 2 hours after meals
• zileuton	Zyflo	PO: 600 mg q.i.d.
Mast cell stabilizers		
• cromolyn sodium	Intal	MDI or nebulizer: 1 inhalation q.i.d.
• nedocromil sodium	Tilade	MDI: 2 inhalations q.i.d.

Clinical Implications

Glucocorticoids are used for nasal congestion and other respiratory conditions, as well as allergic conditions such as asthma and rhinitis. Inhaled glucocorticoids are the drugs of choice for asthma prophylaxis.

Adverse Effects

The inhaled glucocorticoids, even when used on a long-term basis, produce few side effects compared to oral glucocorticoids. Therefore, oral glucocorticoids may cause headache, irritated mucous membranes, epistaxis, nausea, vomiting, asthmalike symptoms, coughing, and pharyngitis. Less common adverse effects include bloody nasal mucous, abdominal pain, diarrhea, fever, flulike symptoms, body aches, dizziness, bronchitis, and increased nasal secretions.

Contraindications

Glucocorticoids are contraindicated in hypersensitive patients, when symptoms of hypercortism are present, and in children younger than age 4 years. They should not be used with ritonavir, ketoconazole, other cytochrome P-450 inhibitors, and other similar inhaled medications.

Precautions

Glucocorticoids must be used with caution in patients with immune system infections, herpes simplex, tuberculosis, nasal surgery or trauma, ulcers, and during pregnancy or lactation. Patients should avoid exposure to chickenpox or measles while taking these agents.

Leukotriene Modifiers

Leukotriene is a term for a class of biologically active compounds that occur naturally in leukocytes. They produce allergic and inflammatory reactions similar to those of histamine. They are thought to play a role in the development of allergies and asthma. Leukotriene modifiers are receptor antagonists that reduce inflammation and bronchoconstriction. The leukotriene modifiers are listed in Table 15–5.

POINT TO REMEMBER

Leukotriene modifiers and mast cell stabilizers are alternative anti-inflammatory drugs for the prophylaxis of asthma.

Method of Action

Leukotriene modifiers affect the synthesis of, and the body's response to, leukotrienes. This blocks the inflammatory response and controls asthma attacks.

Clinical Implications

Leukotriene modifiers are used for prophylaxis and treatment of allergic rhinitis or chronic asthma.

Adverse Effects

Leukotriene modifiers may cause arrhythmias, dizziness, anxiety, headache, euphoria, and light-headedness. Other common adverse effects are diarrhea, dry mouth, abdominal discomfort, and nausea.

Contraindications

Leukotriene modifiers are contraindicated in hypersensitive patients, bronchoconstriction due to asthma or NSAIDs, severe asthma attacks, and status asthmaticus. They should not be used by lactating women.

Precautions

Leukotriene modifiers should be used with caution during pregnancy, in severe liver disease, and in children younger than 1 year of age. They should not be used to reverse an acute asthmatic attack.

Mast Cell Stabilizers

Mast cells are large cells found in connective tissue. They contain a wide variety of biochemicals, including histamine. Mast cells are involved in inflammation secondary to injuries and infections. They are sometimes implicated in allergic reactions. **Mast cell stabilizers** have beneficial effects that appear to result from the stabilization of mast cell membranes. They are effective only when administered by inhalation via metered dose inhalers (MDIs). Cromolyn is also available as a nebulizer solution. Mast cell stabilizers are listed in Table 15–5.

Method of Action

Mast cell stabilizers inhibit the release of bronchoconstrictors, such as histamine, from pulmonary mast cells. This suppresses the allergic response.

Clinical Implications

Mast cell stabilizers are used for various respiratory conditions. The mast cell stabilizer known as cromolyn sodium is primarily used for prophylaxis of bronchial asthma and allergic rhinitis, as well as to prevent exercise-related bronchospasm and acute bronchospasm from pollutants or antigens. Nedocromil sodium is used for the maintenance of mild to moderate asthma.

Adverse Effects

Mast cell stabilizers commonly cause nausea, vomiting, dry mouth, coughing, hoarseness, slightly bitter aftertaste, throat irritation, dizziness, headache, rash, and urticaria.

Contraindications

Mast cell stabilizers are contraindicated in coronary artery disease, history of arrhythmias, acute asthma, dyspnea, and status asthmaticus. They should not be used during pregnancy or in children younger than age 6 years.

Precautions

Cromolyn sodium should be used cautiously in renal or hepatic dysfunction. Patients should be instructed to gargle with water, drink water, or use a throat lozenge after taking each dose of a mast cell stabilizer. Lactating women should not use these agents.

Combination Controller Therapy

Combination controller therapy involves the addition of a second long-term control medication to inhaled corticosteroid therapy. This is a recommended treatment option for moderate to severe persistent asthma. Single-inhaler combination products containing a combination of a corticosteroid and a long-acting beta$_2$-adrenergic agonist are available. These include fluticasone and salmeterol (Advair) and budesonide and formoterol (Symbicort). Symbicort is the more recent combination of the two and has been shown to be very effective for the treatment of chronic asthma. Combination therapy is more effective than higher-dose inhaled corticosteroids alone for reducing asthma symptoms in patients with persistent asthma.

Patient Education

Respiratory therapists should instruct patients to use medications as directed, even if no symptoms persist. They must report any difficulty in breathing, as well as symptoms of deteriorating respiratory status. These include increased dyspnea (shortness of breath), breathlessness with speech, or orthopnea (difficulty breathing when lying down). Proper use of metered dose inhalers should be discussed. Patients should use their medications strictly as prescribed and should never double their dose.

SUMMARY

Asthma is a chronic disease that causes inflammation and irritation of the airways, resulting in difficulty breathing. There are several types of asthma: acute (asthma attack), mild intermittent, mild persistent, moderate persistent, and severe persistent. Many risk factors can cause asthma, including genetics (family history), air pollution, exposure to certain allergens, smoking, and childhood infections. Asthma triggers can precipitate an asthma attack.

Drugs used for the treatment and management of asthma are classified as short-acting beta$_2$-adrenergic agonists, and they provide short-term relief of acute symptoms. Drugs intended for long-term use are taken daily to prevent asthma symptoms and are referred to as controllers. Long-acting beta$_2$-adrenergic agonists, leukotriene modifiers, xanthine derivatives, inhaled corticosteroids, and mast cell stabilizers are used for prophylaxis of asthma.

LEARNING GOALS

These learning goals correspond to the objectives at the beginning of the chapter, providing a clear summary of the chapter's most important points.

1. The various types of asthma are as follows:
   - Mild intermittent: symptoms less than twice a week; less than twice a month involves nighttime symptoms
   - Mild persistent: symptoms more than three to six times a week; three to four times a month involves nighttime symptoms
   - Moderate persistent: daily symptoms; five or more times a month involves nighttime symptoms
   - Severe persistent: continual symptoms; frequent nighttime symptoms

2. Asthma medications designed for symptom relief include beta$_2$-adrenergic agonists, theophylline, and anticholinergics. Asthma medications designed for long-term control include corticosteroids, cromolyn, and leukotriene modifiers. Acute attacks and persistent chronic asthma are treated as follows:

- Acute bronchoconstriction is treated with beta-adrenergic (sympathomimetic) agonists. Acute asthma attacks are treated with either ultrashort-, short-, or intermediate-acting bronchodilators.

- Persistent chronic asthma is often treated with long-acting bronchodilators used in combination with inhaled glucocorticoids. Anticholinergics are also often used to treat chronic asthma.

3. There are basically two categories of agents used to treat asthma:

- Antiallergic agents (bronchodilators): beta-adrenergic agonists, anticholinergics, and xanthine derivatives

- Anti-inflammatory agents: glucocorticoids, leukotriene modifiers, and mast cell stabilizers

4. Combination controller therapy is more effective than higher-dose inhaled corticosteroids alone for reducing symptoms of persistent asthma. It involves the addition of a second long-term control medication to inhaled corticosteroid therapy.

5. Leukotriene modifiers occur naturally in leukocytes, producing allergic and inflammatory reactions similar to those of histamine. They block the inflammatory response and control asthma attacks, and they are indicated for allergic rhinitis or chronic asthma. Mast cells are found in connective tissue and are involved in inflammation secondary to injuries and infections. Their beneficial effects appear to result from stabilization of mast cell membranes. They are effective only by inhalation, whereby they inhibit the release of bronchoconstrictors to suppress the allergic response. They are indicated for bronchial asthma, allergic rhinitis, exercise-related bronchospasm, acute bronchospasm, and for maintenance of mild to moderate asthma.

6. The common adverse effects of xanthine derivatives include palpitations, flushing, hypotension, insomnia, nervousness, nausea, vomiting, tachycardia, diarrhea, and tachypnea. Their most serious adverse effect is potential respiratory arrest.

7. The adverse effects of anticholinergics include anxiety, agitation, confusion, decreased sweating and heat release, drowsiness, dry mouth, urine retention, paresthesias, sinus tachycardia, and urticaria.

8. Beta$_2$-adrenergic agonists are contraindicated in hypersensitive patients, narrow-angle glaucoma, and shock. They are also not proven to be safe during pregnancy and lactation.

9. The clinical implications of glucocorticoids include nasal congestion and other respiratory conditions, as well as allergic conditions such as asthma and rhinitis.

10. The method of action of beta$_2$-adrenergic agonists is the production of bronchodilation by relaxing the bronchial tree's smooth muscles, decreasing airway resistance, encouraging mucus drainage, and increasing vital capacity.

CRITICAL THINKING QUESTIONS

1. Which antiasthmatics are effective only when administered by inhalation via metered dose inhalers?
2. Discuss the best treatment for acute asthma in children.

WEB SITES

http://asthma.about.com/od/medicationguid1/p/leukotrienes.htm
http://www.aafa.org/
http://www.healthline.com/galecontent/anticholinergics
http://www.medicinenet.com/xanthine_derivatives-oral/article.htm
http://www.medscape.com/viewarticle/584485?src=rss
http://www.pamf.org/asthma/medications/inhaled/mastcell.html
http://www.vivo.colostate.edu/hbooks/pathphys/endocrine/adrenal/gluco.html
http://www.webmd.com/asthma/guide/asthma_inhalers_bronchodilators

REVIEW QUESTIONS

Multiple Choice

Select the best response to each question.

1. Cromolyn sodium acts by
   A. releasing histamine
   B. destroying histamine
   C. metabolizing histamine
   D. preventing the release of histamine
2. Signs and symptoms of theophylline toxicity include
   A. insomnia
   B. seizures
   C. nausea and vomiting
   D. all of the above

3. Albuterol is usually administered by which of the following routes?
   A. oral
   B. nasal
   C. intravenous
   D. intramuscular

4. The adverse effects of beta-adrenergic agonists include all of the following except
   A. dizziness and headache
   B. nausea and vomiting
   C. bradycardia and bronchospasm
   D. palpitations and restlessness

5. Which of the following statements is false about anticholinergics?
   A. Anticholinergics are competitive inhibitors of muscarinic receptors.
   B. Anticholinergics are more potent than beta$_2$-adrenergic agonists.
   C. Anticholinergics produce bronchodilation.
   D. Atrovent and Spiriva are examples of anticholinergics.

6. Phyllocontin is the trade name of
   A. dyphylline
   B. oxtriphylline
   C. aminophylline
   D. theophylline

7. Xanthine derivatives stimulate the respiratory center of the
   A. medulla oblongata
   B. spinal cord
   C. thalamus
   D. cerebellum

8. Which of the following is an example of combination controller therapy for moderate to severe persistent asthma?
   A. Beclovent
   B. Spiriva
   C. Somophyllin
   D. Symbicort

9. Leukotriene modifiers are used for prophylaxis and treatment of
   A. chronic asthma
   B. contact dermatitis
   C. arrhythmia
   D. coughing

10. The generic name of Singulair is
    A. zafirlukast
    B. montelukast
    C. zileuton
    D. cromolyn sodium

11. The most serious adverse effect of xanthine derivatives is
    A. tachypnea
    B. insomnia
    C. palpitation
    D. respiratory arrest

12. Which of the following antibodies (immunoglobulins) are activated by inhaled allergens?
    A. IgA
    B. IgE
    C. IgD
    D. IgG

13. The trade name of metaproterenol is
    A. Isuprel
    B. Proventil
    C. Alupent
    D. Ventolin

14. Beta$_2$-adrenergic agonists are contraindicated in all of the following except
    A. hypertension
    B. asthma
    C. glaucoma
    D. shock

15. All of the following agents reduce inflammation except
    A. mast cell stabilizers
    B. leukotriene modifiers
    C. xanthine derivatives
    D. glucocorticoids

CASE STUDY

Mrs. Arnold took her 6-year-old daughter to the emergency department with signs and symptoms of an asthma attack. The girl had dyspnea, wheezing, and a bluish discoloration of the face. Her pediatrician confirmed that it was indeed an asthma attack.

1. Which medications would be best for this child?
2. If the patient were discharged, what medications should be prescribed for her to use at home?

Drug Therapy for Smoking Cessation

OBJECTIVES

Upon completion of this chapter, the reader should be able to do the following:

1. Explain the effects of cigarette smoking on the respiratory system.
2. Describe the effects of nicotine on the cardiovascular system.
3. Discuss the physiology of nicotine addiction.
4. Explain nicotine withdrawal.
5. Describe behavioral intervention.
6. Discuss pharmacologic intervention.
7. Explain nicotine replacement therapy.
8. Describe the adverse effects of nicotine nasal spray.
9. Explain the benefits of bupropion for smoking cessation.
10. Describe a brief intervention using the five A's and five R's to effectively counsel patients regarding smoking cessation.

KEY TERMS

Abruptio placentae	Nicotine
Carcinogens	Peptic ulcer
Cotinine	Placenta previa
Gastritis	Stillbirth

INTRODUCTION

Smoking is a modern-day epidemic that causes substantial health burdens and costs. Worldwide estimates suggest that smoking prevalence has increased to approximately 1.1 billion people (one of every three adults). Recent statistics from the Centers for Disease Control and Prevention (CDC) state that more than 443,000 people die in the United States every year due to smoking-related illnesses. Smokers become addicted to tobacco, and quitting smoking or using other types of tobacco products is very difficult. Nearly half of all smokers will die of problems related to smoking. Tobacco smoking affects all body systems—primarily respiration, circulation, and brain activities.

Research shows that a person who quits smoking decreases the risk of lung cancer. The short-term effects of quitting smoking include anxiety, irritability, and weight gain. Today there are a wide variety of products available to help smokers and other tobacco users quit their habit.

In 2004, the US surgeon general published a report that detailed the health consequences of smoking. The report identified these four major conclusions: (1) smoking harms nearly every organ in the body, (2) quitting smoking has immediate and long-term benefits, (3) smoking cigarettes with reduced levels of tar and nicotine does not minimize risks, and (4) the list of diseases caused by smoking has been expanded. These diseases now include abdominal aortic aneurysm, acute myeloid leukemia, cataract, pneumonia, gum disease, and cancers of the cervix, kidneys, bladder, pancreas, and stomach.

Dangers of Cigarette Smoking

Cigarette smoking harms nearly every major organ of the body. Smoking-related diseases include various types of cancers, heart diseases, stroke, hypertension, and chronic lung diseases (such as chronic obstructive pulmonary disease, chronic bronchitis, and asthma).

Epidemiology and Effects of Cigarette Smoking

Many cancers and chronic diseases are associated with a history of smoking. Cancers predominantly associated with smoking include cancers of the mouth, pharynx, larynx, esophagus, lungs, heart, kidneys, urinary bladder, and pancreas. Other related cancers affect the prostate, ovaries, and uterus. Further evidence has shown that cigarette smoking influences cardiovascular disorders, such as heart attack, angina pectoris, hypertension, and stroke.

In the United States, the direct medical costs of smoking exceed $75 billion per year. Adding this total to the costs of lost productivity and related neonatal medical care brings the total to more than $157 billion per year.

Respiratory System

Cigarette smoking increases the risk of lung cancer by more than 10 times compared to the risk of lung cancer in nonsmokers during late middle age. The risk of lung cancer from cigarette smoking is directly related to the duration of smoking as well as the number of cigarettes smoked per day. Individuals with chronic bronchitis or chronic obstructive pulmonary disease (COPD) usually have a history of cigarette smoking.

> **POINT TO REMEMBER**
>
> Tobacco smoke contains about 4000 chemical agents, including more than 60 **carcinogens** that are responsible for 80 to 90% of lung cancers.

COPD is primarily caused by cigarette smoke. Smoking cessation is the most effective means of stopping the progression of COPD.

Although the lung cancer risk from pipe or cigar smoking is similar to that of cigarette smoking, there is some evidence suggesting that the effects of these types of smoking may be less severe. Because smoke from cigars and pipes is more alkaline, **nicotine** absorption in the lungs is decreased. The smoke from cigars and pipes is more irritating to the lungs, causing the smoker to inhale less deeply than with cigarettes.

Another important fact concerns the inhalation of secondhand smoke,

> **POINT TO REMEMBER**
>
> Exposure to parental smoking has been reported to increase the severity of asthma in children.

also called passive smoking. When nonsmokers inhale secondhand smoke, their risk of lung cancer (and other cancers) is increased. Inhaled irritants, such as tobacco smoke, are thought to induce bronchospasm influenced by irritant receptors in the brain.

Cardiovascular System

Cessation of cigarette smoking decreases the risk of coronary disease because smoking appears to increase vasoconstriction and heart rate. This increases the workload on the heart. Smoking also increases platelet adhesion and the risk of thrombus formation. It increases serum lipid levels as well. Carbon monoxide, which is a product of cigarette smoking, displaces oxygen from hemoglobin. Women who smoke while taking oral contraceptives have a much higher risk of developing cardiovascular disease than other women.

Nervous System

During smoking, nicotine is absorbed quickly into the bloodstream. It travels to the brain in a matter of seconds. Nicotine causes addiction to cigarettes that is similar to the addiction produced by using heroin or cocaine. Recent studies show that nicotine promotes the activity of dopaminergic neurons in the brain (see Chapter 22). This explains the similarity of nicotine addiction to other drug addictions. The effects of nicotine on the central and peripheral nervous systems include both stimulation and depression, including peripheral vasoconstriction, which increases blood pressure.

Digestive System

Esophageal cancer occurs predominantly in people with a history of alcohol and tobacco use. Although the cause of pancreatic cancer is unknown, smoking appears to be a major risk factor. The incidence of pancreatic cancer is twice as high among smokers than nonsmokers. Another effect of nicotine is that it reduces appetite. It increases the production of hydrochloric acid in the stomach, which can result in **gastritis** or **peptic ulcer**.

Urinary System

Although the exact cause of kidney cancer remains unknown, several factors seem to predispose a person to kidney cancer. Smokers increase their risk of developing kidney cancer by 40%. Bladder cancer is the most frequent form of urinary tract cancer in the United States. Although the cause of bladder cancer is not well understood, cigarette smoking is an established risk factor. Carcinogens excreted in the urine are stored in the bladder. Bladder

> **POINT TO REMEMBER**
>
> Cigarette smoking is associated with 50 to 80% of bladder cancers in men.

cancer is three times more common in men than women. Additional risk factors for bladder cancer are outside the scope of this chapter.

Reproductive System

When women become pregnant and continue to smoke cigarettes, their babies will usually be born with a lower than normal birth weight, are often born prematurely, and may experience intrauterine growth retardation. The baby will also display signs of increased irritability. Cigarette smoking during pregnancy can cause stillbirth as well as sudden infant death syndrome (SIDS). There is also a higher risk of placenta previa and abruptio placentae.

Nicotine Addiction

Worldwide, approximately 1 billion people smoke cigarettes. Eighty percent of these people reside in low- to middle-income countries. Nicotine is highly addictive and is directly linked to chronic lung disease, cardiovascular disease, stroke, cancer, addiction, and adverse pregnancy outcomes. Nicotine is widely distributed throughout the body and increases heart rate, blood pressure, respiratory rate, and mental alertness. When cigarettes are smoked, the effect of nicotine on the brain takes as little as 10 to 19 seconds. This rapid effect reinforces the behavioral need to smoke. Smoking causes nicotine to be absorbed much more quickly than when it is used in products such as chewing tobacco because the gastrointestinal tract breaks down the drug's concentrations.

However, nicotine is removed quickly from the body. Because nicotinic receptors in the brain signal a rapid decline in nicotine levels as the body processes the drug, each additional period of smoking provides a pleasurable sensation. Over time, the body will require increased amounts of nicotine to maintain the stimulation that the drug provides.

Approximately 80% of nicotine in the body is broken down into cotinine in the liver and lungs for excretion in the urine. Nicotinic acetylcholine receptors throughout the brain are involved in nicotine addiction. The neurochemical effects of nicotine cause the release of acetylcholine, dopamine, and norepinephrine. Withdrawal symptoms from stopping smoking can occur in as little as 24 hours. Symptoms of nicotine withdrawal include depression, difficulty concentrating, drowsiness, headache, hostility, frustration, insomnia, anxiety, craving for tobacco, decreased blood pressure and heart rate, gastrointestinal problems, and weight gain.

Smoking Cessation

Although nicotine is very addictive, there are now effective drugs and various types of interventions to assist people in overcoming their addictions. Evidence shows that smoking cessation can be encouraged via counseling, nicotine replacement, and the use of the drugs bupropion and varenicline. Less well-documented methods of therapy include interventions involving hypnosis, acupuncture, exercise, and anxiolytics.

Benefits of Smoking Cessation

The surgeon general's office has published many papers on the decreased risk of death due to smoking after a person quits, and these risks decrease continually with each year that passes. Since 2002, the number of former smokers in the United States is greater than the number of current smokers. Quitting smoking at various ages has been shown to result in the following average number of years of life that are gained:

- Quitting at age 30: 10 years of life gained
- Quitting at age 40: 9 years of life gained
- Quitting at age 50: 6 years of life gained
- Quitting at age 60: 3 years of life gained

People who continue smoking usually lose an average of 10 years of their normal life expectancy. Nonsmokers save large amounts of money due to the high cost of tobacco products. Withdrawal symptoms from smoking are usually serious only during the first month after quitting, and they subside quite quickly thereafter. Getting through the first month has never been easier due to the variety of products and therapies now available.

Nicotine Replacement Therapy

Nicotine replacement therapy (NRT) commonly involves the use of nicotine gums, patches, nasal sprays, and inhalers. The FDA first approved a nicotine gum in 1984, and it was the original NRT product available in the United States. In 1996, its prescription-only status was removed, and the product was then sold over the counter (OTC). Nicotine patches became available in 1991 and became OTC products in 1996. Nicotine nasal sprays and inhalers were approved in 1996 and 1997, respectively, and are available by prescription only. Nicotine lozenges were approved for OTC sales in 2002. NRT agents include all varieties of the generic drug nicotine polacrilex. NRT offsets the craving for nicotine. The success rates for each type of nicotine replacement therapy are listed in **Table 16–1**.

Table 16–2 lists drugs used as nicotine replacement agents.

Nicotine Gum

Nicotine gum works via buccal mucosal absorption. The combined use of nicotine patches with the nonnicotine medication bupropion shows higher success rates for smoking cessation than by using either therapy alone. Certain beverages, such as coffee, juice, and soft drinks, interfere with nicotine absorption from the gum, so patients should avoid eating or drinking 15 minutes prior

TABLE 16-1 Effectiveness of Nicotine Replacement Therapies

Type of Nicotine Replacement Therapy (NRT)	Ranking of Effectiveness
Nicotine nasal spray (0.5 mg per spray)	1
Nicotine gum (polacrilex; in doses ranging from 2 to 14 mg per dose)	2 (tie)
Nicotine inhaler (4 mg per puff)	2 (tie)
Nicotine patch (doses ranging from 5 mg to 21 mg per patch)	3

TABLE 16-2 Nicotine Replacement Agents

Generic Name	Trade Name	Average Adult Dosage
nicotine polacrilex	Nicorette Gum	PO: 2–4 mg q1–2h p.r.n. (max: 24 pieces/day)
nicotine polacrilex	Nicotrol Inhaler	Nasal inhalation: 4 mg p.r.n. (max: 64 mg/day)
nicotine polacrilex	Commit Lozenge	PO: 4 mg q1–2h p.r.n.
nicotine polacrilex	Nicotrol NS	Nasal instillation: 1–2 sprays per nostril/hour (max: 40 sprays per nostril/day)
nicotine polacrilex	Nicotrol, NicoDerm CQ	Topical(transdermal patch): 7–21 mg/day

to or while chewing it. Patients who previously smoked fewer than 25 cigarettes per day should chew one piece of nicotine gum (with a 2 mg dose of nicotine per piece) every 1 to 2 hours when beginning use of this product. The required number of pieces of gum taper off during the 7th week and beyond. Those who smoked more than 25 cigarettes per day should use the gum that contains 4 mg of nicotine per piece.

Nicotine gum requires a technique known as chew and park. The gum should be chewed slowly, about 15 chews, and then placed between the cheek and gum until its tingling sensation disappears. The gum should then be chewed another 15 times, and the entire process should be repeated until the tingling sensation does not return. Each piece of gum should last 20 to 30 minutes. Within 12 weeks (approximately 3 months), as the gum is used less and less, the need to smoke should subside. Using nicotine gum for more than 3 months is not recommended. It should not be used for more than 6 months without consulting a physician.

Adverse reactions to nicotine gum include headache, indigestion, mouth irritation or ulcers, and nausea. If gastrointestinal effects occur, patients should chew more slowly and for shorter periods of time. The gum does not adversely affect cardiovascular conditions, but it may

stick to dental work. The use of nicotine gum and other NRTs should be accompanied by counseling.

Transdermal Nicotine Patches

Transdermal nicotine patches introduce the drug very slowly through the skin. This type of treatment may fail due to the fact that there is little or no behavioral reinforcement. The hand-to-mouth need that the act of smoking fulfills is completely absent, with only the slow administration of nicotine helping to reduce cravings. Transdermal patches are the only long lasting type of NRT. Treatment beyond 3 months is not recommended. Patients should begin using transdermal nicotine after they have stopped smoking cigarettes. They should not be used concurrently. Doses range from 7 mg to 21 mg.

Transdermal patches should be applied to a portion of skin on the trunk or arm that does not have hair. They should be firmly pressed onto the skin for 10 seconds, and patients should wash their hands after each application. The patch should remain in place for 24 hours to transfer the nicotine and not cause skin irritation. The next patch should be placed in a different area to avoid irritation to the same spot. Normal showering or bathing does not affect the patch. However, heating pads should not be used over the patch. When each patch is ready to be discarded, the patient should fold the adhesive parts together and make sure the patch is discarded away from children and pets. Patches should not be cut in half or altered in any way.

Adverse reactions to transdermal nicotine patches include local skin reactions, such as itching, redness, burning, or rash. Gastrointestinal effects may include diarrhea, heartburn, and dry mouth. Uncommon effects include joint or muscle pain, drowsiness, sweating, and abnormal dreams. To minimize insomnia and other sleep disturbances, the patch can be removed before bedtime and replaced in the morning.

> **POINT TO REMEMBER**
>
> Nicotine transdermal patches should be used with caution in patients who have had a myocardial infarction within the past 2 weeks.

Nicotine Nasal Sprays

Nicotine nasal sprays must be correctly instilled to work effectively. The head should be tilted back slightly as the spray is instilled into each nostril without inhaling or swallowing. The medication is absorbed via the nasal mucosa and throat. Nicotine nasal sprays provide the most rapid nicotine administration of all forms of nicotine replacement therapy; peak effects occur within 4 to 15 minutes. Each dose should consist of one spray into each nostril for a total of 1 mg of nicotine to be absorbed. Patients are usually started at one to two doses per hour, up to a maximum daily dose of 40 mg (80 sprays). Patients should not smoke while using nicotine nasal sprays. Adverse effects of nicotine nasal sprays include local nasal or throat irritation, sneezing, runny nose, watery eyes, and coughing. Less common effects include chest tightness, numbness in the limbs, constipation, and mouth sores.

Nicotine Inhalers

Nicotine inhalers provide the hand-to-mouth satisfaction of cigarettes. These devices utilize a plastic mouthpiece into which a cartridge containing a porous plug of 10 mg of nicotine is inserted. Added menthol reduces the irritant effects of the drug. Intensive inhalation (80 breaths over 20 minutes) releases approximately 4 mg of nicotine per cartridge, with peak concentrations reached within 15 minutes after inhalation ends. Patients should not smoke when using nicotine inhalers.

Nicotine inhalers should be held between the fingers so that three to four puffs per minute can be instilled. The medication is absorbed in the mouth and throat. Adverse effects of nicotine inhalers include local throat irritation, coughing, and inflammation of the nasal passages. Other effects include heartburn and headache.

> **POINT TO REMEMBER**
>
> Nicotine inhalers should be used with caution in patients who have reactive airway disease and have had a myocardial infarction within the last 2 weeks.

Nicotine Lozenges

Nicotine lozenges were first approved by the FDA in 2002 and are available in 2 mg and 4 mg strengths. They are available in a variety of flavors and are sugar free. The lozenges dissolve completely and deliver approximately 25% more nicotine than gums because there is no residual nicotine left over. Peak concentrations are achieved in 30 to 60 minutes. Higher dosages are recommended for smokers who previously smoked their first cigarette of each day within 30 minutes of awakening. The lozenges take between 20 and 30 minutes to dissolve. Patients should use one lozenge every 1 to 2 hours for the first 6 weeks and taper off through weeks 7 to 12. The lozenges should not be chewed or swallowed whole, and they should be periodically rotated to different areas of the mouth. Acidic beverages should be avoided during and 15 minutes prior to use.

Adverse reactions to nicotine lozenges include gastrointestinal events, such as heartburn, hiccups, and nausea. The 4 mg dose may also cause coughing. Other adverse effects include flatulence, headache, and sore throat.

Nonnicotine Replacement Therapy

Bupropion is a nonnicotine replacement strategy for smoking cessation. This drug is an antidepressant that has been available in the United States since 1989. Sustained-release bupropion first appeared for use in smoking cessation in 1997. It works by inhibiting the uptake of norepinephrine, serotonin, and dopamine in the brain, and it is rapidly absorbed from the gastrointestinal tract. For the first 3 days, 150 mg of sustained-release bupropion should be taken once a day, then twice a day for approximately 7 to 12 weeks (with or without NRT). Doses should be taken at least 8 hours apart. Patients should stop smoking during the second week of treatment because the drug takes 1 week to reach adequate blood concentrations. If significant progress has not been made toward quitting smoking by the 7th week, this type of therapy will probably not be successful for the patient.

Adverse effects of bupropion include dose-dependent seizures, depression, suicidal thoughts, tremor, skin rash, agitation, and insomnia. Other adverse effects include dry mouth and coughing. Bupropion is contraindicated in patients with seizure disorders.

> **POINT TO REMEMBER**
>
> The cost of each type of smoking cessation product is ranked, from most expensive to least expensive, as follows: bupropion, transdermal patch, varenicline, nasal spray, inhaler, gum, and lozenge.

The newest medication on the market is varenicline (Chantix), which contains no nicotine. It works by targeting nicotine receptors in the brain and blocking nicotine from reaching them. It has a higher percentage of success in helping people to quit smoking permanently. Varenicline was approved in 2006. Doses of this drug should be gradually increased over 1 week from 0.5 mg per day to 0.5 mg twice per day. The recommended length of treatment is 12 weeks. Patients should begin taking this agent 1 week before their actual quit date, and it should be taken after a meal with a full glass of water.

The most common adverse effects (associated with 1 mg doses) include nausea, insomnia, abnormal dreams, flatulence, constipation, and vomiting. Additional but less common effects include agitation, depression, and suicidal thoughts.

Combination Therapies

Combination therapies have been shown to increase the success rates of patients who are trying to quit smoking. These involve combining first-line therapies with other types of therapy to increase the chances for a patient to quit smoking, and they are usually better than using first-line therapies alone. For example, the use of the nicotine patch along with another type of NRT, such as a nicotine inhaler, may double the patient's chance of quitting. Additionally, a third agent (such as bupropion SR, which is the form of bupropion that is more slowly released) may be added. The FDA approved the use of the nicotine patch with bupropion SR for smoking cessation.

Other Smoking Cessation Therapies

The FDA approved bupropion and varenicline in 2008 as first-line agents for smoking cessation. FDA-approved second-line therapies include the tricyclic antidepressant nortriptyline and the antihypertensive agent clonidine. These two second-line agents are available by prescription only and should be monitored by a physician.

Behavioral Intervention

Behavioral intervention methods for smoking cessation include advice from a physician, individual counseling by a nurse (or other nonphysician), group counseling, telephone counseling, and self-help. The five A's of smoking cessation intervention include the following:

- asking about tobacco use and documenting how often the patient used to smoke, and whether smoking has ceased completely or if not, how often it now occurs
- advising the patient to quit in a clear, strong, and personalized manner
- assessing the patient's willingness to quit and the patient's level of support systems
- assisting the patient to quit by developing a plan, providing problem-solving techniques and skills training, providing treatment and social support, helping to obtain extra treatment and social support, recommending pharmacotherapy, and providing supplementary educational materials
- arranging follow-ups that are scheduled on a weekly, then monthly, basis; follow-up meetings should consist of reviewing, congratulating successes, stressing the importance of cessation, addressing lapses that may have occurred, identifying potential problem areas, assessing the pharmacotherapy being used, and considering increased intervention levels if needed

The five R's used to enhance the motivation to quit tobacco use include the following:

- relevance to the patient and his or her family
- risks of continued smoking
- rewards of being tobacco free
- roadblocks to successfully quitting
- repetition of the previous steps

Tobacco users who have failed to quit using tobacco in the past must be instructed that most users require many attempts before they finally succeed in quitting. The most successful types of behavior interventions are summarized in **Table 16-3**.

Patient Education

Respiratory therapists often have good opportunities to encourage smoking cessation. Most therapists agree that encouraging the cessation of smoking is part of their job requirements. Only a few studies have been

TABLE 16-3 Behavioral Interventions

Type of Intervention	Ranking of Effectiveness
Group intervention	1
Counseling by a nonphysician healthcare professional (such as a respiratory therapist)	2
Individual counseling with a specialist trained in smoking cessation	3
Telephone counseling	4
Brief physician contact	5
Nursing intervention	6 (tie)
Self-help	6 (tie)

undertaken, however, to determine the effectiveness of respiratory therapists in this regard. The access that respiratory therapists have to patients who smoke makes them good candidates to offer smoking cessation interventions.

SUMMARY

Stopping smoking has many long-term health benefits. Because every body system is affected in varying degrees by the use of tobacco products, morbidity and mortality are greatly affected by the cessation of smoking (or the use of other tobacco products). Studies show that the most effective ways of quitting include combining various behavioral and pharmacologic interventions. Counseling, when combined with nicotine replacement therapy (NRT) and bupropion or other agents, is the best way to quit the smoking habit forever. The biggest obstacle to smoking cessation is the intensity of nicotine addiction. Many patients attempt to quit several times before they finally succeed. Respiratory therapists may play a key role in helping smokers because of the opportunities that their jobs provide to discuss respiration and the positive effects of smoking cessation.

LEARNING GOALS

These learning goals correspond to the objectives at the beginning of the chapter, providing a clear summary of the chapter's most important points.

1. Cigarette smoking increases the risk of lung cancer by more than 10 times compared to lung cancer risks in nonsmokers during late middle age. Individuals with chronic bronchitis or COPD usually have a history of smoking, and COPD is primarily caused by smoking. Also, when nonsmokers inhale secondhand smoke, their risk of cancer is increased.

2. Smoking appears to increase vasoconstriction and heart rate, increasing the workload on the heart. It also increases platelet adhesion and the risk of thrombus formation, as well as serum lipid levels. Carbon monoxide from smoking displaces oxygen from hemoglobin.

3. Nicotine is highly addictive. It increases heart rate, blood pressure, and mental alertness and reduces appetite. When cigarettes are smoked, the affect of nicotine on the brain take as little as 10 to 15 seconds.

4. Withdrawal symptoms from stopping smoking can occur in as little as 24 hours. Symptoms of nicotine withdrawal include depression, difficulty concentrating, drowsiness, headache, hostility, frustration, insomnia, anxiety, craving for tobacco, decreased blood pressure and heart rate, gastrointestinal problems, and weight gain.

5. Behavioral intervention methods for smoking cessation include advice from a physician, individual counseling by a nurse (or other nonphysician), group counseling, telephone counseling, and self-help.

6. Pharmacologic interventions for smoking cessation include first-line methods, such as nicotine replacement therapy (transdermal patches, gums, inhalers, and nasal sprays), as well as the antidepressant bupropion. Second-line methods include the use of clonidine or nortriptyline.

7. Nicotine replacement therapy (NRT) commonly involves the use of nicotine gums, patches, nasal sprays, inhalers, and sustained-release bupropion. NRT offsets the craving for nicotine. Bupropion is an antidepressant that reduces the impact of nicotine withdrawal.

8. The adverse effects of nicotine nasal spray primarily involve nasal irritation. Nasal spray should be used with caution in patients who have had a myocardial infarction within the past 2 weeks.

9. Bupropion is an antidepressant that appears to reduce the impact of nicotine withdrawal by diminishing the uptake of dopamine and norepinephrine.

10. When a patient is being assessed about his or her smoking, the five A's and five R's are essential tools that can help the respiratory therapist determine a specific patient's needs. The five A's facilitate smoking cessation interventions, and the five R's are used to enhance the motivation to quit smoking:

   ▪ The five A's: The therapist should *ask* the patient about tobacco use and *advise* quitting while *assessing* how willing the patient is to quit. The patient can then be *assisted* by developing a plan that will help him or her quit smoking, and follow-ups should be *arranged* to monitor the patient's ongoing progress.

   ▪ The five R's: The *relevance* of quitting to both the patient and his or her family should be addressed, along with the *risks* of continued smoking. The therapist should describe the *rewards* of being tobacco free and also identify the potential *roadblocks* that may be encountered during the process of quitting. Finally, the previous steps need to be *repeated* for the smoking cessation process to be effective.

CRITICAL THINKING QUESTIONS

1. Exlain why nicotine causes addiction.
2. Why do many people who quit smoking experience weight gain?

WEB SITES

http://www.aafp.org/afp/20060715/262.html
http://www.acsh.org/publications/pubID.377/pub_detail.asp
http://www.americanheart.org/presenter.jhtml?identifier=4615
http://www.ehow.com/video_4766940_facts-second-hand-smoking.html
http://www.medicinenet.com/bupropion/article.htm
http://www.nida.nih.gov/ResearchReports/Nicotine/Nicotine.html
http://www.nlm.nih.gov/medlineplus/quittingsmoking.html
http://www.virtualcancercentre.com/healthandlifestyle.asp?sid=3

REVIEW QUESTIONS

Multiple Choice

Select the best response to each question.

1. Which of the following is the primary disorder of the respiratory system that is caused by cigarette smoking?
   A. respiratory distress syndrome
   B. chronic obstructive pulmonary disease
   C. bronchial asthma
   D. cancer of the larynx

2. Which of the following cancers occur predominantly in people with a history of alcohol and cigarette smoking?
   A. esophageal
   B. rectal
   C. renal
   D. bronchial

3. Which of the following is the most frequent form of urinary tract cancer related to nicotine?
   A. kidney
   B. urethra
   C. bladder
   D. ureter

4. Approximately how many people smoke cigarettes worldwide?
   A. 50 million
   B. 100 million
   C. 600 million
   D. 1 billion
5. Cigarette smoking during pregnancy can cause all of the following complications except
   A. placenta previa
   B. vaginal bleeding
   C. stillbirth
   D. sudden infant death syndrome
6. Which of the following statements is true about the effects of cigarette smoking on the cardiovascular system?
   A. It increases platelet adhesion and the risk of thrombus formation.
   B. It decreases serum lipid levels in the blood circulation.
   C. It decreases the risk of stroke.
   D. It increases oxygen in the hemoglobin and decreases carbon monoxide in the blood circulation.
7. Which of the following is *not* considered to be a first-line agent for smoking cessation?
   A. nicotine nasal spray
   B. clonidine
   C. varenicline
   D. bupropion SR
8. Smoking cessation should begin with
   A. physical examination of the heart and lungs
   B. assessment of the smoker's desire to quit
   C. assessment of the smoker's income
   D. the prescribing of nicotine gums or nasal sprays
9. Absorption of nicotine when chewing nicotine gum occurs via which of the following portions of the digestive tract?
   A. the buccal mucosa
   B. the stomach mucosa
   C. the intestine mucosa
   D. none of the above
10. The adverse effects of nicotine gum include
    A. hiccups and jaw fatigue
    B. runny nose and coughing
    C. low-grade fever and nosebleed
    D. insomnia and seizures

11. Which of the following are the adverse effects of bupropion?
    A. mouth and throat irritation
    B. angina pectoris
    C. insomnia and dry cough
    D. nausea and hiccups
12. Which of the following smoking cessation agents does *not* contain nicotine?
    A. NicoDerm
    B. Wellbutrin SR
    C. ProStep
    D. Habitrol
13. Which of the following is a major nicotine metabolite?
    A. calcium
    B. cotinine
    C. carcinogen
    D. zinc
14. Which of the following disorders or conditions may increase in severity when children are exposed to parental cigarette smoking indoors?
    A. vomiting
    B. apnea
    C. asthma
    D. pneumonia
15. The five A's is an effective strategy to provide counseling for smoking cessation. Which of the following is the first step for every patient when using this model?
    A. assess
    B. arrange
    C. advise
    D. ask

CASE STUDY

A 77-year-old man with a 37-year history of smoking presents with puffiness of the face, arms, and shoulders associated with a bluish to purplish discoloration of the skin. In addition, he complains of dizziness, dyspnea, and coughing. Neck vein distention is noted on physical examination. Chest X-rays show a mass in the middle lobe of the right lung, and blood tests show bacterial pneumonia in both lungs.

1. What is the primary diagnosis likely to be?
2. What type of treatment should be started first?

CHAPTER 1

Antitussives, Expectorants, Mucolytics, and Decongestants

OUTLINE

Introduction
Antitussives
    Method of Action
    Clinical Implications
    Adverse Effects
    Contraindications
    Precautions
Expectorants and Mucolytics
    Method of Action
    Clinical Implications
    Adverse Effects
    Contraindications
    Precautions
Decongestants
    Method of Action
    Clinical Implications
    Adverse Effects
    Contraindications
    Precautions
Patient Education
Summary

OBJECTIVES

Upon completion of this chapter, the reader should be able to do the following:
1. Explain drug therapy for coughing.
2. Describe various types of antitussives.
3. Explain the indications of mucolytic drugs.
4. Discuss adverse effects of decongestants.
5. Define expectorants and mucolytic agents.
6. Explain the contraindications of antitussives.
7. List the most common mucolytic drugs.
8. Explain the contraindications of expectorants.
9. Discuss the mechanism of action of decongestants.
10. List common respiratory system disorders that may cause mucus.

KEY TERMS

Antitussives	Mucolytics
Atelectasis	Rebound congestion
Decongestants	Tracheostomy
Expectorants	

INTRODUCTION

Coughing is a natural reflex mechanism that forcibly removes excess secretions and foreign material from the respiratory system. Coughing is often described as productive or nonproductive. Productive coughing brings up fluid or mucus from the lungs. Nonproductive coughing is a sudden ejection of air from the lungs, through the mouth, that does not expel (produce) mucus or fluid from the throat or lungs. Mucus is a sticky fluid that normally cleans and protects air passages by trapping debris and bacteria. It also helps the air passages to remain clean and lubricated. Certain conditions, such as asthma or cystic fibrosis, cause mucus to build up and thicken. This can cause difficulty breathing because the debris and bacteria can no longer be removed.

Many respiratory disorders may be treated with various agents that include antitussives, expectorants, mucolytics, and decongestants. These are commonly prescribed agents, and some of them are available over the counter (OTC). These agents may be used to treat conditions including the common cold, flu, acute and chronic bronchitis, emphysema, cystic fibrosis, and others.

Antitussives

Antitussives are also known as cough suppressants because they are used to reduce coughing. Many disorders of the upper and lower respiratory tracts are accompanied by an uncomfortable, nonproductive cough. These disorders include the common cold, pharyngitis, pneumonia, and sinusitis. Persistent coughing can be exhausting, causing muscle strain and further irritation of the respiratory tract. Antitussives may be in one of two main groups: opioid and nonopioid. **Table 17-1** summarizes major types of antitussives.

Method of Action

Opioid antitussives may cause respiratory depression, similar to the effects of morphine. The antitussive effects are mediated through direct action on receptors in the cough center of the medulla oblongata in the brain (see Chapter 21). Codeine also has a drying effect on the respiratory tract. This increases the viscosity of bronchial secretions. However, antitussive action requires lower doses than those needed for analgesia. Nonopioid antitussives do not suppress respiration, but they do reduce peripheral cough receptor activity. They also appear to increase the threshold of the central cough center.

Clinical Implications

Opioid antitussives suppress nonproductive cough but have unwanted side effects. Codeine and hydrocodone elevate the cough threshold but are not as effective as other opioids. Nonopioid antitussives are used for temporary relief of coughing spasms in nonproductive coughs from colds, influenza, and pertussis. Many nonopioid antitussives are OTC medications. The most commonly used nonopioid antitussive is dextromethorphan. This agent is chemically similar to the opioids and also acts on the CNS to raise the cough threshold.

> **POINT TO REMEMBER**
>
> Opioid analgesics at low doses are among the most effective drugs used as cough suppressants.

Adverse Effects

Common adverse effects of antitussives include breathing difficulties, drowsiness, itching, skin rash, constipation, dizziness, nausea, nervousness, and restlessness.

> **POINT TO REMEMBER**
>
> Dextromethorphan is not as effective as codeine. However, dextromethorphan carries no risk of dependence.

Contraindications

Antitussives are contraindicated with known hypersensitivity, asthma, diabetes, emphysema, heart disease, seizures, thyroid conditions, chronic bronchitis, and liver disease. They should not be taken with alcohol, monoamine oxidase (MAO) inhibitors, hypnotics and sedatives, allergy and cold medications, analgesics, or muscle relaxants.

Precautions

Antitussives should be used with caution in pregnant or lactating women. If coughing persists, lasts more than 7 days, or produces mucus, the patient should contact his or her physician. The patient should also contact his or her physician if symptoms of fever, persistent headache, rash, sore throat, or vomiting occur.

Expectorants and Mucolytics

Expectorants are drugs that liquefy lower respiratory tract secretions. Therefore, they reduce the thickness and viscosity of bronchial mucus. This action increases mucus flow so that coughing can help remove it from the bronchi. Expectorants are available in many OTC preparations, making them widely available to patients without consulting a healthcare provider. Mucolytics differ from expectorants because they directly loosen thick, high-viscosity mucus by breaking down its molecules and thinning it. Mucolytics help high-risk respiratory patients cough up thick, sticky secretions. This improves breathing and airflow. Mucolytics can be administered by a nebulizer or by direct instillation into the trachea through

TABLE 17-1 Major Types of Antitussives

Generic Name	Trade Name	Average Adult Dosage
Opioids		
• chlorpheniramine–hydrocodone	Tussionex	PO: 5 mL b.i.d.
• codeine	Generic only	PO: 10–20 mg q4–6h PRN (max: 120 mg/day)
• hydrocodone	Hycodan, Robidone A	PO: 5–10 mg q4–6h PRN (max: 15 mg/dose)
Nonopioids		
• benzonatate	Tessalon Perles	PO: 100–200 mg t.i.d. (max: 600 mg/day)
• dextromethorphan	Robitussin DM, Romilar CF	PO: 10–20 mg q4h or 30 mg q6–8h (max: 120 mg/day) or 60 mg of sustained-action liquid b.i.d.
• diphenhydramine	Benadryl, Benahist	PO: 25 mg q4–6h (max: 100 mg/day)

TABLE 17–2 Expectorants and Mucolytics

Generic Name	Trade Name	Average Adult Dosage
acetylcysteine	Mucomyst	Inhalation: 10 mL of 20% solution or 2–20 mL of 10% solution q2–6h
dornase alfa	Pulmozyme	Inhalation: 2.5 mg/day inhaled through nebulizer
guaifenesin	Fenesin, Humibid	PO: 100–400 mg q4h
potassium iodide	Pima, SSKI	PO: 300–1000 mg after meals b.i.d.–t.i.d. up to 1.5 g t.i.d.

an endotracheal tube (tracheostomy). Mucolytics are usually reserved for patients who have major difficulty in coughing up secretions. These drugs loosen mucus that has built up in the lungs because of various chronic respiratory ailments. Certain mucolytic agents contain a chemical that enhances the production of an enzyme called glutathione, which breaks down and thins mucus. Expectorants and mucolytics are listed in **Table 17–2**. Another substance that is sometimes used as a mucolytic agent is sodium bicarbonate.

Method of Action

> **POINT TO REMEMBER**
>
> Wild cherry bark acts as an expectorant and a mild sedative. It is available in syrup and tincture forms.

In general, expectorants increase the outflow of respiratory tract fluids by irritating the gastric mucosa. Mucolytics act by lowering viscosity to make the removal of secretions easier.

Clinical Implications

> **POINT TO REMEMBER**
>
> Wild cherry bark should not be used during pregnancy.

Expectorants and mucolytics are used for abnormal, sticky, or thickened mucus secretions as seen in bronchopulmonary disease. They are also used for the pulmonary complications of atelectasis, cystic fibrosis, chronic bronchitis, and after a tracheostomy procedure. Acetylcysteine is one of the few drugs available to directly loosen thick, viscous bronchial secretions. This agent is delivered by the inhalation route and is not available OTC.

Adverse Effects

Expectorants and mucolytics have few significant adverse effects, but occasional drowsiness and nausea may occur depending on the dosage. A less common adverse effect of mucolytics is uterine mucosal thinning.

Contraindications

Expectorants and mucolytics are contraindicated in known hypersensitivity, pulmonary tuberculosis, and during pregnancy or lactation. The expectorant known as guaifenesin may interact with heparin therapy to increase the risk of hemorrhage.

Precautions

While taking expectorants and mucolytics, patients should drink at least eight glasses of water or other fluids per day. Coughing that persists beyond 7 days should prompt the patient to contact his or her physician. Women should not breastfeed while taking these medications without the approval of their physician.

> **POINT TO REMEMBER**
>
> Acetylcysteine is given by the oral or intravenous routes to patients who have received an overdose of acetaminophen.

Decongestants

Decongestants are drugs taken to decrease nasal congestion related to the common cold, allergic rhinitis, and sinusitis. Allergic rhinitis is caused by an inflammatory response in the upper respiratory tract. Nasal decongestants constrict nasal arterioles, thereby decreasing the swelling nasal membranes. These drugs can be administered orally or topically into the nostrils. When taken orally, decongestants are absorbed into the body, thus increasing the chance of adverse effects. When used as nasal drops or sprays, they have the same therapeutic effects but with lowered potential for adverse effects. Decongestants reverse congestion (excessive blood flow) in an area. They are available in nasal and oral preparations. **Table 17–3** shows commonly used decongestants.

Method of Action

Decongestants are vasoconstrictors that shrink nasal airway mucous membranes. Most oral decongestants are adrenergic in action, meaning that they mimic the effects of the sympathetic nervous system.

Clinical Implications

Decongestants are indicated for the relief of nasal congestion as caused by the common cold, sinusitis, and upper respiratory allergies.

Adverse Effects

The adverse effects of decongestants include insomnia, nervousness, dizziness, headache, irritability, and restlessness. They may also cause blurred vision, nausea, tachycardia, and vomiting. The most serious, limiting adverse effect of intranasal preparations is rebound congestion. Prolonged use causes hypersecretion of mucus,

TABLE 17-3 Decongestants

Generic Name	Trade Name	Average Adult Dosage
Nasal decongestants		
• oxymetazoline 0.05%	Afrin	Nasal: 2–3 drops or sprays in each nostril b.i.d. up to 3–5 days
• phenazoline 0.05%	Allerest	Nasal: 2 drops or sprays in each nostril q3–6h up to 3–5 days
• phenylephrine 1%	Neo-Synephrine, Sinex	Nasal: 1–2 drops in each nostril q3–4h
• tetrahydrozoline 0.1%	Tyzine	Nasal: 2–4 drops in each nostril q3h p.r.n.
Oral Decongestants		
• pseudoephedrine	Sudafed	PO: 60 mg q4–6h or 120 mg sustained release q12h
Combination decongestants–antihistamines		
• cetirizine–pseudoephedrine	Zyrtec-D	PO: 5–10 mg once/day
• clemastine fumarate	Tavist	PO: 1.34 mg b.i.d., may increase to 8.04 mg/day
• fexofenadine–pseudoephedrine	Allegra D	PO: 60 mg t.i.d.
• loratadine–pseudoephedrine	Claritin-D, etc.	PO: 10 mg/day on empty stomach
• naproxen–pseudoephedrine	Aleve Cold & Sinus	PO: 275–1100 mg/day

worsening nasal congestion when the drug effects wear off. This may lead to increased use of the medication as the condition worsens.

Contraindications

Decongestants are contraindicated in patients taking other sympathomimetic drugs and in patients with diabetes, heart disease, uncontrolled hypertension, hyperthyroidism, pneumonia, and prostatic hypertrophy. Nasal decongestants are contraindicated for use with certain MAO inhibitors, methyldopa, reserpine, and urine acidifiers.

Precautions

Decongestants should not be taken within 2 hours of bedtime. Patients should contact their physician if they experience extreme restlessness or signs of sensitivity to decongestants, and women should not breastfeed while taking decongestants.

Patient Education

Patients should avoid operating machinery or performing other tasks that require alertness when taking antihistamines for the first time because drowsiness may occur. Alcohol should be avoided while taking antihistamines. The patient should use ice chips, hard candies, or chewing gum to reduce mouth dryness caused by some decongestants and antihistamines.

SUMMARY

Various disorders may cause coughing and congestion or produce mucus. The drugs used for this purpose are available by prescription or over the counter. Antitussives are drugs used to suppress the cough reflex when dry, nonproductive coughing is tiring or irritating to the respiratory system. Expectorants and mucolytics are drugs used to increase the viscosity and volume of respiratory tract secretions, which helps the patient to clear the lower respiratory tract of tenacious secretions. Decongestants are drugs used to decrease the swelling and blood flow to the mucosa of the respiratory tract. Oral decongestants have a greater potential for systemic adverse effects than topical decongestants, which are applied directly to the mucosa. However, topical decongestants are more likely to cause rebound congestion if they are used longer than 5 consecutive days.

LEARNING GOALS

These learning goals correspond to the objectives at the beginning of the chapter, providing a clear summary of the chapter's most important points.

1. Drugs used to relieve coughing are known as antitussives. They are also called cough suppressants. Antitussives may be either opioid or nonopioid in nature.

2. Opioid antitussives include chlorpheniramine–hydrocodone, codeine, and hydrocodone. Nonopioid antitussives include benzonatate, dextromethorphan, and diphenhydramine.

3. Mucolytic drugs are indicated to reduce abnormal, sticky, or thickened mucus secretions from bronchopulmonary disease. They are also used for atelectasis, cystic fibrosis, and following tracheostomy procedures.

4. The adverse effects of decongestants include insomnia, nervousness, dizziness, headaches, irritability, restlessness, blurred vision, nausea, tachycardia, and vomiting. More adverse effects

occur from oral decongestants than from nasal decongestants.

5. Expectorants are drugs that liquefy lower respiratory tract secretions, helping to bring up secretions by coughing. Mucolytics directly loosen thick, high-viscosity mucus by thinning it.

6. Antitussives are contraindicated in known hypersensitivity, asthma, diabetes, emphysema, heart disease, seizures, thyroid conditions, chronic bronchitis, and liver disease.

7. The most common mucolytic drugs include acetylcysteine and dornase alfa.

8. Expectorants are contraindicated in known hypersensitivity and during pregnancy or lactation. Guaifenesin should not be used with heparin.

9. Decongestants work by mimicking the effects of the sympathetic nervous system. They are vasoconstrictors that shrink nasal airway mucous membranes.

10. Common respiratory disorders that may cause mucus include the common cold, influenza, bronchitis, emphysema, cystic fibrosis, atelectasis, and other bronchopulmonary conditions.

CRITICAL THINKING QUESTIONS

1. What is the reason that expectorants should not be used in patients with tuberculosis?
2. What genetic disease requires mucolytic drugs for treatment?

WEB SITES

http://familydoctor.org/online/famdocen/home/
   otc-center/otc-medicines/859.html
http://video.about.com/asthma/Mucolytics.htm
http://www.drugs.com/drug-class/antitussives.html
http://www.merck.com/mmhe/sec04.html
http://www.uihealthcare.com/topics/medications/
   medi4757.html
http://www.webmd.com/cold-and-flu/tc/coughs-
   topic-overview

REVIEW QUESTIONS

Multiple Choice

Select the best response to each question.

1. Which of the following is the generic name of Benadryl?
   A. benzonatate
   B. dextromethorphan
   C. diphenhydramine
   D. chlorpheniramine

2. Which of the following antitussives may elevate the cough threshold?
   A. codeine
   B. diphenhydramine
   C. dextromethorphan
   D. benzonatate

3. Decongestants are contraindicated in patients with all of the following disorders except
   A. diabetes
   B. prostatic hypertrophy
   C. uncontrolled hypertension
   D. sinusitis

4. Allerest is the trade name of
   A. oxymetazoline
   B. phenazoline
   C. phenylephrine
   D. tetrahydrozoline

5. Drugs that help to bring up mucus from the respiratory tract are referred to as
   A. decongestants
   B. antitussives
   C. mucolytics
   D. expectorants

6. Which of the following is *not* in the class of antitussives?
   A. codeine
   B. potassium iodide
   C. hydrocodone
   D. chlorpheniramine

7. Mucolytic agents are indicated for which of the following disorders?
   A. cystic fibrosis
   B. asthma
   C. pharyngitis
   D. sinusitis

8. In which of the following parts of the brain is the cough center?
   A. medulla oblongata
   B. cerebellum
   C. spinal cord
   D. cerebrum

9. Allegra is the trade name of
   A. clemastine
   B. cetirizine and pseudoephedrine
   C. fexofenadine and pseudoephedrine
   D. naproxen and clemastine

10. Decongestants are prescribed for all of the following except
   A. upper respiratory allergies
   B. the common cold
   C. pneumonia
   D. sinusitis

11. What are the common adverse effects of expectorants and mucolytics?
   A. hypotension and respiratory depression
   B. drowsiness and nausea
   C. urinary retention
   D. tremor and diarrhea
12. Decongestants are
   A. vasodilators
   B. vasoconstrictors
   C. both
   D. neither
13. Which of the following is the most serious, limiting adverse effect of intranasal decongestant preparations?
   A. rebound congestion
   B. insomnia
   C. headache
   D. fever
14. Acetylcysteine is an example of
   A. a decongestant
   B. an antitussive
   C. an expectorant
   D. a mucolytic

15. Which of the following is *not* a decongestant?
   A. oxymetazoline (Afrin)
   B. phenazoline (Allerest)
   C. hydrocodone (Hycodan)
   D. phenylephrine (Neo-Synephrine)

CASE STUDY

A teenage girl was involved in a car accident and brought to the emergency department with a fractured leg and facial lacerations. After her history was taken, it was discovered that she had a history of seasonal allergies and sinusitis.
1. What medication related to her allergies may have been involved in this car accident?
2. What are the adverse effects of the most common anti-allergy drugs?

Antimicrobial Medications

OBJECTIVES

Upon completion of this chapter, the reader should be able to do the following:
1. Describe the way that antimicrobial drugs are classified.
2. Explain how bacteria are described and classified.

3. Describe the primary therapeutic uses for sulfonamides.
4. Contrast bacteriostatic and bactericidal actions.
5. Describe the mechanism of action for antiviral agents.
6. Contrast macrolides and sulfa drugs.
7. List the first-line antitubercular agents.
8. Define HAART and explain its indications.
9. Describe the general drug actions and indications of antifungal agents.
10. Discuss drugs used to treat protozoal infections.

KEY TERMS

Acne rosacea	Candidemia
Antibiotic	Conjunctivitis
Anti-infective	Fungi
Antivirals	Gram-negative bacteria
Bacteremia	Gram-positive bacteria
Bactericidal	Protozoa
Bacteriostatic	Spores
Beta-lactam antibiotics	Trichomoniasis
Blepharitis	Viruses
Broad spectrum	

INTRODUCTION

There have been many discoveries of antimicrobial agents in recent years, with continued improvement of technology to diagnose microbial pathogens. In developing countries, infectious disease is still one of the leading causes of morbidity and mortality. The risk for infectious disease is increased by conditions of poverty, lack of clean water, inadequate housing, malnutrition, and poor sanitation. In developed or industrialized countries, chronic and noninfectious diseases are now a leading cause of disability and death. However, infectious diseases remain the third most common cause of death in the United States and the *most* common cause of death in the rest of the world. In this chapter, antibacterials, antifungals, antiprotozoals, and antivirals will be discussed.

Classifications of Bacteria

Bacteria are commonly classified by using a crystal violet Gram stain. Bacteria that have thicker cell walls retain this purple stain and are known as Gram-positive bacteria. This type includes staphylococci, streptococci, and enterococci. Gram-negative bacteria have thinner cell walls and do not retain the Gram stain. This type includes *Bacteroides, Escherichia coli, Klebsiella, Pseudomonas,* and *Salmonella*. Gram-positive and Gram-negative bacteria are biochemically and physiologically different. Certain antibacterial agents are effective against only one of these two types.

Bacteria are also classified because of their shapes. Bacilli are rod shaped, cocci are sphere shaped, and spirilla are spiral shaped (see **Figure 18–1**). A third method of bacteria classification is their ability to use oxygen. Aerobic bacteria live and grow in an oxygen-rich environment, and anaerobic bacteria live and grow when oxygen is not present. Antibacterial drugs are designed to specifically treat aerobic or anaerobic bacteria.

An anti-infective is an agent that may be used to treat an infection caused by a microorganism. This term encompasses antibacterial, antiviral, and antifungal agents. Technically, an antibiotic is an antibacterial drug that is derived from a natural rather than a synthetic source. The most common sources of antibiotics are molds and other bacteria. Although they are effective for treating many bacterial infections, sulfa drugs are not truly antibiotics because they are derived from synthetic sources. This distinction is rarely made in common usage of the term. Anti-infective agents are also classified by their mechanism of action, based on whether they inhibit cell walls, protein synthesis, folic acid, or reverse transcriptase.

> **POINT TO REMEMBER**
>
> The widespread and sometimes unwarranted use of antibiotics has led to a large number of resistant bacterial strains.

Bactericidal Versus Bacteriostatic

The term bactericidal (also written *bacteriocidal*) describes a substance that actually kills bacteria, and it usually refers to antiseptics, disinfectants, or antibiotics. Bacteriostatic agents are capable of stopping the growth and reproduction of bacteria. This term is typically used to describe antibiotics that inhibit bacterial growth without killing the bacteria. Bacteriostatic antibiotics suppress reproduction and growth of bacteria until the body's immune system can kill the bacteria.

Antibacterials

Antibacterials are drugs or chemicals used to kill or inhibit the growth and reproduction of bacteria. Antibacterial agents exist in many different types. They include penicillins, cephalosporins, aminoglycosides, fluoroquinolones, tetracyclines, macrolides, sulfonamides, and miscellaneous agents.

> **POINT TO REMEMBER**
>
> It is common for patients to discontinue taking their antibiotics when they begin to feel better.

Penicillins

Although it was not the first anti-infective to be discovered, penicillin was the first mass-produced antibiotic. Penicillins are a class of antibiotics derived in whole or in part from the mold *Penicillium notatum*. Therefore, penicillins are true antibiotics. Penicillin G was the first purified antibiotic to be used clinically. Chemical

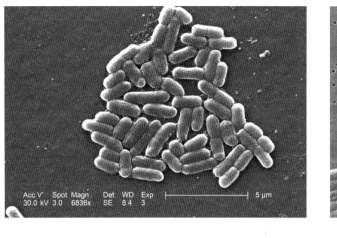
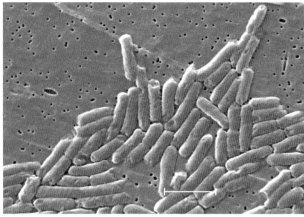
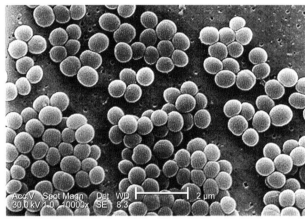
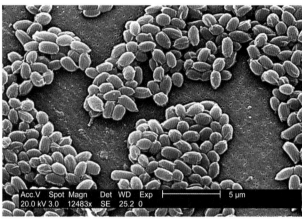
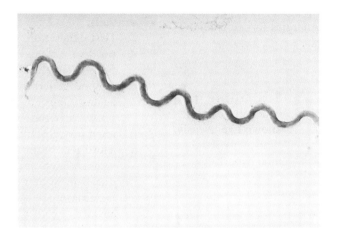

FIGURE 18–1 Various shapes of bacteria.

derivatives of penicillin G are widely used in medicine. **Table 18–1** lists commonly used forms of penicillin.

Method of Action

Penicillins are beta-lactam antibiotics. They inhibit the synthesis of bacterial cell walls. This disruption allows water to enter and kill the microorganism. The actions of penicillins are specific to bacterial cells because human cells do not contain cell walls.

Clinical Implications

Oral penicillins are used to treat many infections, including otitis media, strep throat, and skin infections. They are also prescribed to prevent recurrent rheumatic fever. Penicillins are also indicated for the treatment of meningitis, pneumonia, and infections of the bones, joints, and stomach, as well as for bacteremia. They are indicated for gas gangrene, tetanus, anthrax, and sickle cell anemia in infants.

TABLE 18-1 Commonly Used Penicillins

Generic Name	Trade Name	Average Adult Dosage
Broad spectrum (aminopenicillins)		
• amoxicillin	Amoxil, Trimox, Wymox	PO: 250–500 mg t.i.d.
• amoxicillin–clavulanate	Augmentin	PO: 250–500 mg amoxicillin with 125 mg clavulanate q8–12h
• ampicillin	Polycillin, Omnipen	PO: 250–500 mg b.i.d.
• bacampicillin	Spectrobid	PO: 400–800 mg b.i.
Extended spectrum (antipseudomonal)		
• carbenicillin	Geocillin, Geopen	PO: 382–764 mg q.i.d.
• piperacillin sodium	Pipracil	IM: 2–4 g t.i.d.–q.i.d. (max: 24 g/day)
• piperacillin tazobactam	Zosyn	IM: 3.375 g q.i.d. over 30 minutes
• ticarcillin	Ticar	IM: 1–2 g q.i.d. (max: 40 g/day)
Narrow spectrum–penicillinase sensitive		
• penicillin G benzathine	Bicillin	IM: 1.2 million units as a single dose
• penicillin G procaine	Crysticillin, Wycillin	IM: 600,000–1.2 million units/day
• penicillin G sodium–potassium	Pentids	PO: 400,000–800,000 units/day
• penicillin V	Pen-Vee K, Veetids, Betapen	PO: 125–250 mg q.i.
Penicillinase resistant		
• cloxacillin	Tegopen	PO: 250–500 mg b.i.d.
• dicloxacillin	Dynapen	PO: 125–500 mg q.i.d.
• nafcillin	Nafcil, Unipen	PO: 250 mg–1 g q.i.d. (max: 12 g/day)
• oxacillin	Prostaphlin, Bactocill	PO: 250 mg–1 g q.i.d. (max: 12 g/day)

Adverse Effects

Penicillins may cause serious adverse effects, including anaphylaxis symptoms such as angioedema, cardiac arrest, and circulatory collapse. Another serious adverse effect is nephrotoxicity. Additional adverse effects include pruritus (itching), rash, diarrhea, fever, nausea, and superinfections. Allergies to penicillin are the most serious adverse effects.

Contraindications

> **POINT TO REMEMBER**
>
> After parenteral administration of penicillin, observe the patient for possible allergic reactions for 30 minutes, especially following the first dose.

Penicillins are contraindicated in known hypersensitivity, hypernatremia, hyperkalemia, and heart failure.

Precautions

Penicillins should be used with caution in patients who have impaired renal function, are taking high doses of anticoagulants, or are lactating. Patients should be monitored for any signs of antibiotic-associated pseudomembranous colitis, which may become life threatening. Patients who are allergic to penicillins should wear a medical alert bracelet. Many penicillins should be taken with a full glass of water 1 hour before or 2 hours after meals to increase absorption.

Cephalosporins

Cephalosporins are a class of antibiotics that are effective against both Gram-positive and Gram-negative organisms but also have a beta-lactam component. The cephalosporins share many properties with the penicillins, including the potential for allergic reactions. Cephalosporins affect a wider range of bacteria than penicillins.

Cephalosporins work in a manner similar to penicillins. They are available in the following four generations:

1. First generation: most effective against Gram-positive organisms, but bacteria that produce beta-lactamase are usually resistant to them
2. Second generation: have a broader spectrum against Gram-negative organisms and are more potent than the first-generation agents, and they are more resistant to beta-lactamase
3. Third generation: have an even broader spectrum against Gram-negative organisms with a longer duration of action and are resistant to beta-lactamase; are sometimes the drugs of choice against klebsiella, neisseria, pseudomonas, salmonella, proteus, and *Haemophilus influenza* infections; can enter the cerebrospinal fluid to treat CNS infections
4. Fourth generation: effective against organisms that have become resistant to other cephalosporins; can also enter the cerebrospinal fluid to treat CNS infections

Table 18-2 lists commonly used forms of cephalosporins.

Method of Action

Cephalosporins work similarly to penicillins by affecting the bacterial cell wall. They are bactericidal and destroy bacteria.

TABLE 18-2 Commonly Used Cephalosporins

Generic Name	Trade Name	Average Adult Dosage
First generation		
• cefazolin	Generic only	Injection: 10–20 mg/mL or 0.5–10 g powder for injection
• cefadroxil	Duricef	PO: 500 mg–1 g or 250–500 mg/5 mL
• cephalexin	Keflex	PO: 250–500 mg or 125–250 mg/5 mL
Second generation		
• cefaclor	Generic only	PO: 250–500 mg or 125–375 mg/5 mL
• cefotetan	Cefotan	Injection: 1–10 g or 1 g/50 mL
• cefoxitin	Mefoxin	Injection: 1–10 g or 1–2 g/50 mL
• cefuroxime	Ceftin, Zinacef	Injection: 750 mg–1.5 g; PO: 250–500 mg or 125–250 mg/5 mL
Third generation		
• cefotaxime	Claforan	Injection: 500 mg–10 g or 20–40 mg/mL
• ceftazidime	Fortaz, Tazicef	Injection: 500 mg–6 g
• ceftizoxime	Cefizox	Injection: 1–2 g
• ceftriaxone	Rocephin	Injection: 250 mg–10 g
• cefixime	Suprax	PO: 400 mg or 100–200 mg/5 mL
• cefpodoxime	Vantin	PO: 100–200 mg or 50–100 mg/5 mL
• ceftibuten	Cedax	PO: 400 mg or 90 mg/5 mL
Fourth generation		
• cefepime	Maxipime	Injection: 500 mg–2 g/day

Clinical Implications

Cephalosporins are used to treat many different conditions based upon their generation. First- and second-generation cephalosporins are used for prophylaxis during surgeries, with cefazolin being the drug of choice. Many second- and third-generation cephalosporins are also used during surgical procedures to prevent infection. In general, these agents are not used initially for bacterial infections due to cost and effectiveness.

Adverse Effects

Cephalosporins may cause hypersensitivity reactions, including fever, rash, serum sickness, hives, anaphylaxis, neutropenia, and nephritis. Other adverse effects include pain, sterile abscess, nausea, vomiting, diarrhea, glossitis, and abdominal pain.

Contraindications

Cephalosporins should not be used with other antibiotics that can cause nephrotoxicity or ototoxicity. Other agents that should be avoided include ethacrynic acid, furosemide, and estrogen-containing oral contraceptives.

Precautions

Patients must be instructed to take cephalosporins on an empty stomach, but they may be taken with food if gastric irritation occurs.

Aminoglycosides

Aminoglycosides are a class of antibiotics that are most commonly used against Gram-negative bacteria. Streptomycin was the first aminoglycoside ever discovered,

TABLE 18-3 Commonly Used Aminoglycosides

Generic Name	Trade Name	Average Adult Dosage
amikacin	Amikin	Injection: 50–250 mg/mL
gentamicin	Genoptic S.O.P., Gentak	Injection: 60–100 mg/vial or 0.6–40 mg/mL; ophthalmic ointment: 0.3%
kanamycin	Generic only	Injection: 333 mg/mL
neomycin	Generic only	PO: 500 mg
streptomycin	Generic only	Injection: 1 g
tobramycin	TOBI, Tobrex OS	Injection: 1.2 g or 0.8–40 mg/mL or 60 mg/50 mL; inhalation: 500 mg/5 mL; ophthalmic solution: 0.3%

found in *Streptomyces griseus*, an organism found in soil. Its use is now limited against tuberculosis because of many resistant bacteria strains. Aminoglycosides have higher levels of toxicity than other antibiotics but are important in treating aerobic Gram-negative bacteria, mycobacteria, and certain protozoans. Aminoglycosides are listed in **Table 18–3**.

Method of Action

Aminoglycosides work by combining with bacterial ribosomes, which stop protein synthesis to prevent the bacteria from reproducing. When this occurs, the bacteria die.

TABLE 18–4	Commonly Used Fluoroquinolones	
Generic Name	Trade Name	Average Adult Dosage
Classical fluoroquinolones		
• ciprofloxacin	Cipro	PO: 500–750 mg q12h; injection: 400 mg q12h
• enoxacin	Penetrex	PO: 200–400 mg q12h for 1–2 weeks
• levofloxacin	Levaquin	PO: 250–500 mg/day; injection: 25 mg/mL
• lomefloxacin	Maxaquin	PO: 400 mg/day for 2 weeks
• nalidixic acid	NegGram	PO: 500 mg (tablet form) or 300 mg/5 mL (suspension form)
• norfloxacin	Noroxin	PO: 400 mg q12h for 3 days
• ofloxacin	Floxin	PO: 200–400 mg q12h
Newer fluoroquinolones		
• gatifloxacin	Tequin	PO: 400 mg/day for 7–14 days; injection: 400 mg/40 mL
• moxifloxacin	Avelox	PO: 400 mg/day for 5–10 days
• sparfloxacin	Zagam	PO: loading dose 400 mg on day 1, then 200 mg/day for 10 days
• trovafloxacin	Trovan	PO: 100 mg

Clinical Implications

Aminoglycosides are commonly given orally in large doses before abdominal surgery to reduce the amounts of intestinal bacteria. They are usually administered by injection (IM or IV), although they may be administered via drops into the eyes or ears for localized infections. Aminoglycosides are prescribed in the treatment of serious infections of the urinary tract, reproductive system, kidneys, bones, brain, abdomen, and heart. The topical forms are also used for the treatment of conjunctivitis and blepharitis.

Adverse Effects

> **POINT TO REMEMBER**
>
> Elderly patients are at high risk of nephrotoxicity and ototoxicity from aminoglycosides because of reduced renal function, and they may require lower doses.

Aminoglycosides may cause serious adverse effects, such as nephrotoxicity or ototoxicity. These adverse effects limit their use to serious infections. Prolonged use may cause superinfections.

Contraindications

Aminoglycosides are contraindicated during pregnancy due to great potential for harm to the fetus. When used with penicillins, their effectiveness decreases greatly; therefore, if their use is required, they should be administered several hours before or after the penicillin.

Precautions

Aminoglycoside dosages must be very closely monitored in pediatric and geriatric patients. They should be used with caution along with warfarin or ethacrynic acid.

Fluoroquinolones

Fluoroquinolones are a group of broad-spectrum antibacterial drugs (see **Table 18–4**). Fluoroquinolones have high levels of toxicity in general, but newer forms have been developed with lower toxicities. Previously they were indicated for only urinary tract infections, but now they are used for a variety of infections, such as sexually transmitted infections and infectious diarrhea.

Method of Action

Fluoroquinolones interfere with an enzyme, called DNA gyrase, that bacteria need to synthesize DNA. This affects cell reproduction, killing the bacteria (bactericidal).

Clinical Implications

Fluoroquinolones have a broad spectrum of activity and are used for prostatitis, urinary tract infections (UTIs), anthrax, gonorrhea, respiratory infections (such as pneumonia), and bone or joint infections. The newer ones are significantly more effective against Gram-positive microbes, such as staphylococci, streptococci, and enterococci.

> **POINT TO REMEMBER**
>
> A major advantage of the fluoroquinolones is that most are well absorbed orally and may be administered either once or twice a day.

Adverse Effects

Fluoroquinolones usually have only mild, transient effects. These include nausea, vomiting, diarrhea, flatulence, abdominal discomfort, rash, photosensitivity, and nephrotoxicity. Rare adverse effects include cardiac abnormalities, neuropsychiatric effects, and liver dysfunction. With caffeine, they may cause insomnia or hyperactivity.

Contraindications

Fluoroquinolones are contraindicated in children younger than age 18 years and in pregnant or lactating women.

Precautions

Patients taking fluoroquinolones should avoid dairy products, antacids, magnesium laxatives, and iron

TABLE 18-5 Commonly Used Tetracyclines

Generic Name	Trade Name	Average Adult Dosage
demeclocycline	Declomycin	PO: 150–300 mg
doxycycline hyclate	Doryx, Periostat, Vibra-Tabs, Vibramycin	PO: 100 mg capsule, 20–100 mg tablet, 75–100 mg delayed-release tablet, 50 mg/5 mL syrup, or 25 mg/5 mL powder for suspension
doxycycline monohydrate	Adoxa, Adoxa Pak, Monodox	PO: 50–150 mg tablet
minocycline	Cleeravue-M Kit, Dynacin, Minocin	PO: 50–100 mg capsule, 50–100 mg tablet, or 45–135 mg extended-release tablet
tetracycline	Emtet, Sumycin	PO: 500 mg capsule, 125 mg/mL syrup, or 250–500 mg tablet; ophthalmic ointment: 1%

TABLE 18-6 Commonly Used Macrolides

Generic Name	Trade Name	Average Adult Dosage
azithromycin	Zithromax	PO: 500–2000 mg
clarithromycin	Biaxin	PO: 250–500 mg
dirithromycin	Dynabac	PO: 250 mg
erythromycin base	Eryc, E-Mycin	PO: 250 mg
erythromycin estolate	Ilosone	PO/IM/IV: 30 mg–1 g
erythromycin stearate	Erythrocin	PO/IV: 30 mg–1 g
troleandomycin	Tao	PO: 125–500 mg

supplements. Patients should drink adequate amounts of fluids to prevent crystalluria. They should report any visual disturbances, dizziness, light-headedness, or depression to their physician to avoid potential CNS toxicity. Patients should avoid driving or operating heavy machinery and avoid alcoholic beverages.

Tetracyclines

Tetracyclines, like the aminoglycosides, were first discovered in a *Streptomyces* soil organism. These broad-spectrum agents are useful in treating a wide variety of conditions (see **Table 18–5**). Tetracyclines may be bactericidal or bacteriostatic.

Method of Action

Tetracyclines are primarily bacteriostatic and work by binding to bacterial ribosomes to prevent protein synthesis. They affect both Gram-positive and Gram-negative bacteria, as well as mycobacteria, chlamydiae, and rickettsia.

Clinical Implications

Tetracyclines are indicated for Rocky Mountain spotted fever, typhus fever, chlamydial infections, brucellosis, cholera, amebiasis, traveler's diarrhea, and tularemia. They are also prescribed as alternative treatments to penicillin for gonorrhea, syphilis, anthrax, Lyme disease, and *Haemophilus influenzae* respiratory infections.

Adverse Effects

Tetracyclines have many adverse effects, including GI toxicity (such as heartburn, nausea, vomiting, and diarrhea), photosensitivity, superinfections (such as candidiasis), hypersensitivity reactions, and hepatotoxicity.

Contraindications

Tetracyclines should be avoided in hypersensitive patients, patients with liver disease, pregnant or lactating women, and in children younger than age 8 years (due to potential graying of their developing teeth, as well as impaired bone growth). Because they can interact with various foods (such as dairy products) and drugs (that contain aluminum, calcium, and ferrous supplements), tetracyclines should be taken on an empty stomach.

Precautions

Patients should be instructed to avoid exposure to the sun as much as possible to avoid photosensitivity reactions. These medications must be stored away from light and extreme heat and must be disposed of immediately when they expire.

Macrolides

Macrolides were first discovered similarly to the aminoglycosides and tetracyclines. They are very safe alternatives to using penicillin, although they are not usually the first drugs of choice. Macrolides are listed in **Table 18–6**.

Method of Action

Macrolides work by inhibiting bacterial protein synthesis via binding to the bacterial ribosome to stop bacterial growth. Macrolides equally affect Gram-positive and Gram-negative bacteria.

Clinical Implications

Macrolides are indicated for chronic obstructive pulmonary disease (COPD), skin infections, pharyngitis, tonsillitis, bronchitis, sinusitis, other respiratory tract infections, acute otitis media, pneumonia, duodenal ulcers, pelvic inflammatory disease, intestinal amebiasis, rheumatic fever, soft-tissue infections, urethritis, legionnaires disease, syphilis, UTIs, and rectal infections.

TABLE 18-7 Commonly Used Sulfonamides

Generic Name	Trade Name	Average Adult Dosage
mafenide	Sulfamylon	Topical: 1–2 times/day
silver sulfadiazine	Silvadene, Flamazine	Topical: 1–2 times/day; PO: 500 mg
sulfamethizole	Thiosulfil Forte	PO: 0.5–1 g t.i.d.–q.i.
sulfamethoxazole	Gantanol	PO: initial dose 2 g; maintenance dose 1 g b.i.d.–t.i.
sulfasalazine	Azulfidine	PO: initial dose 1–4 g/day in divided doses; maintenance dose 2 g/day in evenly spaced doses of 500 mg q.i.
sulfisoxazole	Gantrisin	PO: loading dose 2–4 g; maintenance dose 4–8 g/day in 4–6 divided doses
trimethoprim (TMP) and sulfamethoxazole (SMZ)	Bactrim, Septra	PO: 160 mg TMP with 800 mg SMZ q12h; injection: 8–10 mg/kg/day (based on TMP) in 2–4 divided doses

Adverse Effects

Macrolides are generally safe to use, although common adverse effects include GI discomfort, abdominal pain, nausea, and vomiting. The older macrolides cause more adverse effects than the newer agents. In rare cases, severe hepatotoxicity can occur.

Contraindications

Macrolides are contraindicated in hypersensitive patients, erythromycin-associated hepatitis, and liver dysfunction. They should not be taken with cyclosporine.

Precautions

Patients should be instructed to take oral macrolides with a full glass of water on an empty stomach. Enteric-coated or sustained-release macrolides can be administered with food. Patients should not take macrolides with fruit juices.

Sulfonamides

Sulfonamides are a class of drugs that interfere with bacterial growth and development (see **Table 18–7**). They are the oldest anti-infective drugs. Sulfonamides are frequently called sulfa drugs. They are commonly used to treat a wide variety of infections.

Method of Action

Sulfonamides work by blocking a specific step in the folic acid biosynthetic pathway, slowing the multiplication of bacteria. They interfere with para-aminobenzoic acid (PABA) and folic acid formation to destroy bacteria. Therefore, these agents are primarily bacteriostatic with some bactericidal actions.

Clinical Implications

Sulfonamides are now used primarily to treat relatively minor infections, including most urinary tract infections, otitis media (usually in children), sinusitis, certain lower respiratory infections, and ulcerative colitis. They are also prescribed for treatment of AIDS-related pneumonia (*Pneumocystis carinii*).

Adverse Effects

The older sulfonamides are primarily responsible for causing blood dyscrasias, crystalluria, life-threatening hepatitis, and hematuria. Newer sulfa drugs do not cause nearly the number of adverse effects as the older drugs. Other adverse effects may include aplastic anemia, leukopenia, agranulocytosis, and thrombocytopenia. Minor adverse effects include loss of appetite, nausea, vomiting, diarrhea, fever, photosensitivity, and stomatitis.

Contraindications

Sulfonamides are contraindicated in hypersensitive patients, in the final stages of pregnancy, during lactation, and in children younger than age 2 years. They may interact with oral anticoagulants, methotrexate, and hydantoin.

Precautions

Patients taking sulfonamides should be instructed to take them on an empty stomach with a full glass of water. They should also avoid exposure to sunlight and complete the full course of therapy.

> **POINT TO REMEMBER**
>
> Encourage patients to drink 3 liters of fluids per day to achieve a urinary output of 1500 milliliters every 24 hours to decrease the possibility of crystalluria.

Miscellaneous Antibacterials

Miscellaneous antibacterials exist outside of the previously discussed classes, but they are still important in the treatment of various types of infections. **Table 18-8** lists commonly used miscellaneous antibacterials.

Chloramphenicol is a broad-spectrum antibacterial that inhibits protein synthesis. It is very toxic in comparison to other antibacterials and is not the drug of first choice. It should be avoided in children. Chloramphenicol is commonly used to treat bacterial meningitis, brain abscess, and Rocky Mountain spotted fever. Clindamycin is primarily used for acne and vaginosis; however, patients should drink large amounts of fluids because clindamycin has the potential to cause the development of the *Clostridium difficile* bacteria, which causes diarrhea and colitis. Isoniazid is used for tuberculosis, but it has the potential to cause liver disease and nerve damage. It should be administered concurrently with vitamin B$_6$ to prevent neurotoxicity. Metronidazole is an amoebicide that is used for giardiasis and trichomoniasis, and it is the drug of choice for *Clostridium difficile* enteritis. It may also be used topically to treat acne rosacea and other conditions. Metronidazole should not be used with alcohol. Mupirocin is used topically as an anti-infective against staphylococcal skin infections (such as impetigo).

TABLE 18–8 Miscellaneous Antibacterials

Generic Name	Trade Name	Average Adult Dosage
chloramphenicol	Chloromycetin	Injection: 1 g powder
clindamycin	Cleocin, Cleocin Pediatric	PO: 75–300 mg capsule
isoniazid	Nydrazid	PO: 100–300 mg tablet
metronidazole	Flagyl, Flagyl ER, MetroCream, MetroGel, MetroLotion, Noritate, Vandazole	PO: Extended-release tablet 750 mg, 375 mg capsule, 250–500 mg tablet
mupirocin	Bactroban Cream, Centany	Cream or ointments: 2%

Classifications of Fungi

Fungi play a valuable role in the world's ecosystems. They assist in the decay process of dead plants and animals, but some fungi are also able to infect living tissue. Fungi may produce diseases that range from athlete's foot and diaper rash to serious diseases, such as pneumonia and meningitis. Fungi may have either one or many cells and include mushrooms, molds, and yeasts. They may be classified according to their systemic or superficial nature. The most common diseases related to fungal infections are listed in **Table 18–9**.

Fungal Infections

A few species of fungi grow on the skin and mucosal surfaces as part of the normal host flora. Many fungal infections involve the skin, hair, nails, and respiratory tract. The lungs serve as a route for invasive fungi to enter the body and infect the internal organs. An additional common source of fungal infections, especially of the mouth or vagina, is overgrowth of normal flora. Fungal diseases are called mycoses and are classified as either superficial or systemic. Superficial mycoses affect the skin, nail, scalp, and mucous membranes in areas such as the oral cavity and vagina. In most infections, the fungus invades only the surface layers of these regions.

Systemic fungal infections can affect nearly the entire body, including the internal organs such as the brain, digestive organs, and lungs. Although they are not as common as superficial fungal infections, systemic fungal infections can be fatal in patients with suppressed immune systems. Most systemic fungal infections are treated with oral and parenteral medications that cause more adverse effects than topical antifungals.

TABLE 18–9 Classifications of Fungi

Type of Fungi	Infections and Affected Areas
Superficial	
• *Candida albicans*, etc.	Candidiasis: skin, nails, oral cavity (thrush), vagina
• *Epidermophyton floccosum*	Tinea pedis (athlete's foot), Tinea cruris (jock itch), other dermatophytoses: feet, groin, or other sites
• *Microsporum audouini*, etc.	Tinea capities (ringworm): scalp
• *Sporothrix schenckii*	Sporotrichosis: usually the skin and superficial lymph nodes
• *Trichophyton* (various types)	Trichophyton infection: scalp, skin, and nails
Systemic	
• *Aspergillus fumigatus*, etc.	Aspergillosis (opportunistic): usually lungs, can spread to other organs
• *Blastomyces dermatitidis*	Blastomycosis: begins in lungs and spreads to other organs
• *Candida albicans*, etc.	Candidiasis (the most opportunistic fungal infection): most organs
• *Coccidioides immitis*	Coccidioidomycosis: begins in lungs and spreads to other organs
• *Cryptococcus neoformans*	Cryptococcosis (opportunistic): begins in lungs; the most common cause of meningitis in AIDS patients
• *Histoplasma capsulatum*	Histoplasmosis: begins in lungs and spreads to other organs
• *Mucorales* (various types)	Mucormycosis (opportunistic): blood vessels, sinuses, stomach (ulcers), etc.
• *Pneumocystis carinii* (*Pneumocystis jiroveci*)	*Pneumocystis* pneumonia (opportunistic): lungs (pneumonia) but can spread to other organs; was once believed to be a protozoan

Antifungals

There are many over-the-counter (OTC) antifungal medications that treat a variety of fungal infections, including athlete's foot, jock itch, and vulvovaginal candidiasis. In this chapter, only drugs for systemic fungal infections will be discussed. Various antifungals are shown in **Table 18–10**.

Method of Action

The method of action of systemic antifungals, such as amphotericin B, is the destruction of the cell membrane of the fungus. This is accomplished by binding to the ergosterol in the fungal cell membrane.

Clinical Implications

Amphotericin B has a broad spectrum of activity. It is the drug of choice for most severe systemic fungal infections, and it may be used as a prophylactic antifungal for patients with severe immunosuppression. Anidulafungin is used to treat candidemia and other *Candida* infections. It is also indicated for the treatment of esophageal candidiasis. Caspofungin is used to treat aspergillosis and candidemia due to *Candida*. Flucytosine is used alone or in combination with amphotericin B for serious systemic infections caused by *Cryptococcus* and *Candida* species.

Adverse Effects

> **POINT TO REMEMBER**
>
> Infuse amphotericin B slowly because cardiovascular collapse may result when the mediation is infused too rapidly.

The adverse effects of systemic antifungals can be very serious, including imbalances of electrolytes (hypokalemia and hypomagnesemia), dysrhythmias, cardiac arrest, hypotension, and nephrotoxicity. Many patients develop headache, vomiting, chills, and fever. Phlebitis is common during IV therapy.

Contraindications

Hypersensitivity is the only contraindication of drugs used for systemic mycoses.

Precautions

Systemic antifungal drugs must be used with caution in patients with hepatic or renal dysfunction and in older adults.

Protozoal Infections

The single-celled animals known as protozoa are capable of causing disease in humans, although most of these animals are harmless. They are found in the soil and live on dead or decaying material. Infection occurs by ingestion of spores or by bites from infected insects. Protozoa are parasitic creatures commonly found in areas with poor sanitation and personal hygiene. Immunocompromised patients are often the victims of protozoal infections. Protozoal infections include malarial and nonmalarial types. Malaria is spread by mosquitos and is the most common protozoal infection worldwide. However, it is uncommon in the United States. The protozoa that cause malaria live in and destroy the red blood cells of the host. Nonmalarial protozoal infections include amebiasis, cryptosporidiosis, giardiasis, leishmaniasis, trichomoniasis, and trypanosomiasis (see **Table 18–11**).

TABLE 18–10 Commonly Used Systemic Antifungals

Generic Name	Trade Name	Average Adult Dosage
amphotericin B	Fungizone, Abelcet, Amphotec, AmBisome	IV: 0.25 mg/kg/day, may increase to 1 mg/kg/day or 1.5 mg/kg every other day (max: 1.5 mg/kg/day)
anidulafungin	Eraxis	IV: loading dose 100 mg (day 1), followed by 50 mg/day
caspofungin acetate	Cancidas	IV: loading dose 70 mg (infused over 1 hour)
flucytosine	Ancobon	PO: 50–150 mg/kg in divided doses
micafungin	Mycamine	IV: 150 mg/kg/day over 1 hour for active *Candida* infection; for *Candida* prophylaxis, administer 50 mg/kg/day over 1 hour

TABLE 18–11 Nonmalarial Protozoal Infections

Protozoan	Infections and Affected Areas
Cryptosporidium (various types)	Cryptosporidiosis: intestines (often in immunocompromised patients)
Entamoeba histolytica	Amebiasis: large intestine (causes liver abscesses); sometimes travels to the brain, lungs, or kidneys
Giardia lamblia	Giardiasis: intestines (causes abdominal distention, gas, and malabsorption)
Leishmania (various types)	Leishmaniasis: various body systems (skin, liver, spleen, or blood)
Toxoplasma gondii	Toxoplasmosis: brain (causes fatal encephalitis in immunocompromised patients)
Trichomonas vaginalis	Trichomoniasis: vagina and urethra (spreads through sexual contact)
Trypanosoma brucei	Trypanosomiasis: CNS (may cause African sleeping sickness) or heart (causes Chagas disease in the United States)

TABLE 18-12 Antiprotozoal Agents

Generic Name	Trade Name	Average Adult Dosage
Antimalarial antiprotozoal agents		
• atovaquone–proguanil	Malarone	PO: 1 tablet/day (1–2 days before travel, continuing until 7 days after returning)
• chloroquine	Aralen	PO: Initial dose 600 mg, then 300 mg/week
• hydroxychloroquine sulfate	Plaquenil	PO: Initial dose 620 mg, then 310 mg/week
• mefloquine	Lariam	PO: For prevention, 250 mg once/week for 4 weeks, then 250 mg every other week; for treatment: 1250 mg single dose
• primaquine	Generic only	PO: 15 mg/day for 2 weeks
• pyrimethamine	Daraprim	PO: 25 mg once/week for 10 weeks
• quinine	Quinamm	PO: 260–650 mg t.i.d. for 3 days
Nonmalarial antiprotozoal agents		
• iodoquinol	Yodoxin	PO: 630–650 mg t.i.d. for 20 days (max: 2 g/day)
• metronidazole	Flagyl	PO: 250–750 mg t.i.d.
• paromomycin	Humatin	PO: 25–35 mg/kg in 3 divided doses for 5–10 days
• pentamidine	Pentam 300, NebuPent	IV: 4 mg/kg/day for 14–21 days (infuse over 60 minutes)
• sodium stibogluconate	Pentostam	IM: 20 mg/kg/day
• tinidazole	Tindamax	PO: 50 mg/kg single dose (max: 2 g) for giardiasis; 2 g/day for 3–5 days for amebiasis
• trimetrexate	Neutrexin	IV: 45 mg/m^2 daily

Antiprotozoals

There are two classes of antiprotozoals: antimalarial drugs and nonmalarial drugs. Both of these types are antiprotozoal agents (see **Table 18–12**).

Antimalarial Agents

The main drugs used for antimalarial drug therapy include proguanil and chloroquine, as shown in Table 8–12. The three goals of antimalarial therapy include prevention, treatment of acute attacks, and prevention of relapse. According to the Centers for Disease Control and Prevention (CDC), the prevention of malaria should involve travelers receiving proguanil as a prophylactic antimalarial for 1 week. Chloroquine is the classic antimalarial for treating acute malaria. Primaquine phosphate can cure malaria completely.

Classification of Viruses

Viruses differ from other types of microorganisms in that they are not alive. Viruses may infect bacteria, animals, and plants. A virus is protected by a coat of protein and contains a few dozen genes (either RNA or DNA) that are used to help the virus replicate. When an infective viral particle matures, it is called a virion. Viruses enter a host's target cell and use the cell's components to replicate. This means that viruses are actually intercellular parasites. They cannot cause an infection unless they are inside a host cell. Enzymes that are present in viruses are being used to design antiviral drugs that can actively destroy the viruses. Viruses are the smallest type of microorganism in comparison with bacteria, fungi, and protozoans. Viral infections include the common cold, herpes, and HIV–AIDS.

HIV–AIDS

Human immunodeficiency virus (HIV) infects patients via exposure to contaminated body fluids (primarily blood and semen). Transmission of HIV can occur through sexual activity, infected fluids that contact skin or mucous membranes, or because of needlesticks. Also, the virus can be passed to infants during birth or breastfeeding. After the HIV virus invades a host's RNA, it converts the RNA strands into DNA to produce more viral particles.

Classification of Drugs for HIV–AIDS

Antiretroviral drugs used to treat HIV–AIDS involve the use of multiple agents in a drug regimen called highly active antiretroviral therapy (HAART). The goal of HAART is to eliminate or greatly reduce HIV RNA from the blood, although it is also present in the lymph nodes and other areas of the body. Therefore, HAART is not a cure, but it can greatly decrease progression of the virus. Multiple-drug therapy decreases the likelihood of viral resistance, but it must continue for the remainder of the patient's life. These agents are classified in **Table 18–13**.

Antivirals

Antivirals are designed to inhibit the replication of viruses. They achieve their optimal effects when the patient has a normal, healthy immune system. These agents do not actually destroy viruses; they allow immune system cells to attack them. Effective treatment of viral infections relies on factors concerning the host, the drugs being used, and the virus itself. **Table 18–14** lists common antiviral agents that are primarily used for herpesviruses.

TABLE 18–13 Antiretroviral Drugs Used for HIV–AIDS

Generic Name	Trade Name	Average Adult Dosage
Nucleoside and nucleotide reverse transcriptase inhibitors (NRTIs and NtRTIs)		
• abacavir	Ziagen	PO: 300 mg b.i.d.
• didanosine	Videx, DDI	PO: 125–300 mg b.i.d.
• emtricitabine	Emtriva	PO: 200 mg/day
• lamivudine	Epivir, 3TC	PO: 150 mg b.i.d.
• stavudine	Zerit, D4T	PO: 40 mg b.i.d.
• tenofovir disoproxil fumarate	Viread	PO: 300 mg/day
• zalcitabine	Hivid, DDC	PO: 0.75 mg t.i.d.
• zidovudine	Retrovir, AZT	PO: 200 mg q4h (1200 mg/day), after 1 month may reduce to 100 mg q4h (600 mg/day); IV: 1–2 mg/kg q4h (1200 mg/day)
Nonnucleoside reverse transcriptase inhibitors (NNRTIs)		
• delavirdine	Rescriptor	PO: 400 mg t.i.d.
• efavirenz	Sustiva	PO: 600 mg/day
• nevirapine	Viramune	PO: 200 mg/day for 14 days, then increase to b.i.d.
Protease inhibitors (PIs)		
• amprenavir	Agenerase	PO: 1200 mg b.i.d.
• atazanavir	Reyataz	PO: 400 mg/day
• darunavir	Prezista	PO: 600 mg taken with ritonavir 100 mg b.i.d.
• fosamprenavir	Lexiva	PO: 700–1400 mg b.i.d. in combination with ritonavir 100–200 mg b.i.d.
• indinavir	Crixivan	PO: 800 mg t.i.d.
• lopinavir with ritonavir	Kaletra	PO: 400 mg lopinavir with 100 mg ritonavir (3 capsules or 5 mL suspension) b.i.d.; increase to 533 mg with 133 mg (4 capsules or 6.5 mL) b.i.d.; use concurrently with efavirenz or nevirapine
• nelfinavir	Viracept	PO: 750 mg t.i.d.
• ritonavir	Norvir	PO: 600 mg b.i.d.
• saquinavir	Invirase, Fortovase	PO: 600 mg t.i.d.
• tipranavir	Aptivus	PO: 500 mg with ritonavir 200 mg b.i.d.
Fusion (entry) inhibitor		
• enfuvirtide	Fuzeon	SC: 90 mg b.i.d.

TABLE 18–14 Drugs Used for the Treatment of Systemic Viral Conditions

Generic Name	Trade Name	Average Adult Dosage
For cytomegalovirus		
• cidofovir	Vistide	IV: 5 mg/kg once per week for 2 weeks with probenecid; for prophylaxis: 5 mg/kg IV once every other week
For influenza		
• oseltamivir	Tamiflu	IV: 75 mg twice daily for 5 days (for acute infection); once daily for 10 days (for prophylaxis)
• zanamivir	Relenza	Oral inhalation: 2 doses initially, then 2 inhalations twice daily for 5 days; begin within 48 hours of symptoms; for prophylaxis, 2 inhalations daily for 28 days
For herpes virus		
• acyclovir	Zovirax	PO: 400 mg t.i.d.
• famciclovir	Famvir	PO: 500 mg t.i.d. for 7 days
• foscarnet	Foscavir	IV: 40–50 mg/kg infused over 1–2 hours t.i.d.
• ganciclovir	Cytovene	IV: 5 mg/kg infused over 1 hour b.i.d.
• penciclovir	Denavir	Topical: apply every 2 hours for 4 days, starting within 1 hour of onset of symptoms
• trifluridine	Viroptic	Topical: instill 1 drop in affected eye every 2 hours (maximum: 9 drops/day)
• valacyclovir	Valtrex	PO: 1 g t.i.
For hepatitis B or C		
• interferon alfa-2a	Roferon A	Only for hepatitis C—SC: 3 million international units 3 times/week for 12 months, or 6 million international units 3 times/week for 3 months followed by 3 million international units 3 times/week for 9 months
• interferon alfa-2b	Intron A	For hepatitis B—SC/IM: 30 to 35 million international units/week for 16 weeks; for hepatitis C—SC/IM: 3 million international units 3 times/week for up to 18–24 months
• interferon alfacon-1	Infergen	Only for hepatitis C—SC: 9–15 micrograms 3 times/week for 24 weeks, with at least 48 h between doses
• peginterferon alfa-2a	Pegasys	For both hepatitis B and C—SC: 180 micrograms once/week for 48 weeks
• peginterferon alfa-2b	PEG-Intron	Only for hepatitis C—SC: 1 microgram/kg per week for 1 year
• ribavirin	Copegus	Only for hepatitis C—Oral: 600 mg twice/day plus interferon alfa-2b for 24 to 48 weeks

TABLE 18-15   Common Antituberculosis Drugs

Generic Name	Trade Name	Average Adult Dosage
First-line agents		
• ethambutol	Myambutol	PO: 15–25 mg/kg/day
• isoniazid	INH, etc.	PO: 15 mg/kg/day
• pyrazinamide	PZA	PO: 5–15 mg/kg t.i.d.–q.i.d. (max: 2 g/day)
• pyrazinamide with isoniazid and rifampin	Rifater	PO: 6 tablets/day (for clients who weigh more than 121 lb)
• rifampin	Rifadin, Rimactane	PO: 600 mg/day as a single dose
• rifapentine	Priftin	PO: 600 mg twice/week for 2 months, then once/ week for 4 months
• streptomycin sulfate	Streptomycin	IM: 15 mg/kg up to 1 g/day as a single dose
Second-line agents		
• amikacin	Amikin	IM: loading dose 5–7.5 mg/kg, then 7.5 mg/kg b.i.d.
• capreomycin	Capastat Sulfate	IM: 1 g/day (up to 20 mg/kg/day) for 60–120 days, then 1 g 2–3 times/week
• ciprofloxacin	Cipro	PO: 250–750 mg b.i.d.
• cycloserine	Seromycin	PO: 250 mg q12h for 2 weeks, may increase to 500 mg q12h (max: 1 g/day)
• ethionamide	Trecator-SC	PO: 0.5–1 g/day in divided doses q8–12h
• kanamycin	Kantrex	IM: 5–7.5 mg/kg b.i.d.–t.i.d.
• ofloxacin	Floxin	PO: 200–400 mg b.i.d.

Method of Action

In general, these agents interfere with DNA synthesis of the virus to inhibit viral replication.

Clinical Implications

These antivirals are used for herpes genitalis, herpes encephalitis, cold sores, mucocutaneous herpes simplex, influenza, hepatitis, and in immunocompromised patients.

Adverse Effects

Primary adverse effects of these antivirals include headache, nausea, vomiting, and diarrhea. Serious adverse effects include acute renal failure and thrombocytopenic purpura–hemolytic uremic syndrome. Other adverse effects include fatigue, glomerulonephritis, rash, and phlebitis.

Contraindications

In general, these antivirals are contraindicated in hypersensitive patients.

Precautions

These antivirals should be used with caution in patients with renal insufficiency, dehydration, seizure disorders, neurologic diseases, and during pregnancy.

Antitubercular Medications

Tuberculosis is a serious condition that usually affects the lungs, but it may travel to other parts of the body, including the bones (via the blood and lymph fluid). Slowly growing mycobacteria develop inside the tubercles of the lungs. Tuberculosis may develop in as many as 20% of patients with AIDS. Antitubercular medications

must be able to penetrate a protective cell wall characteristic of *Mycobacterium tuberculosis*. Therefore, tubercular medications must be administered continually for 6 to 12 months and sometimes as long as 24 months. Different combinations of drugs are usually used to keep resistance from occurring. **Table 18–15** shows common antituberculosis drugs.

Method of Action

In general, antitubercular medications work by inhibiting bacterial protein synthesis via irreversible binding to the ribosomes of susceptible bacteria.

Clinical Implications

These agents are often used in combination with other antitubercular drugs for all forms of tuberculosis caused by *M. tuberculosis*. Multiple drug therapy is necessary because the mycobacteria grow slowly, and resistance is common. During the 6- to 24-month treatment period, different combinations of drugs may be used.

Adverse Effects

Serious adverse effects of antitubercular medications include anaphylactic shock, CNS depression syndrome in infants, respiratory depression, and exfoliative dermatitis. Other adverse effects include paresthesias, pain and irritation at the injection site, superinfections, hepatotoxicity, blood dyscrasias, optic or otic damage, nephrotoxicity, and encephalopathy.

Contraindications

These agents are contraindicated in history of toxic reaction or hypersensitivity to aminoglycosides, labyrinthine disease, myasthenia gravis, use of other neurotoxic or nephrotoxic agents, and during pregnancy.

Precautions

These agents should be used with caution in patients with impaired kidney function, in older adults, in premature infants or neonates, and in children.

Patient Education

The role of the respiratory therapist in drug therapy with penicillins involves careful monitoring of a patient's condition and providing education as it relates to the prescribed drug treatment. This is because allergies occur more frequently with penicillins than with any other antibiotic class.

Respiratory therapists should instruct patients that many microorganisms still remain even after symptoms disappear. Therefore, patients must take their entire drug regimen. They should increase fluid intake while taking antibiotics. They must immediately report tinnitus, high-frequency hearing loss, persistent headache, or vertigo. Patients must also be advised of the following:

- They must not save antibiotics because toxic effects may occur if they are taken past the expiration date.
- They must not take these medications (especially tetracyclines) with milk products, iron supplements, magnesium-containing laxatives, or antacids.

SUMMARY

Microorganisms are classified as bacteria, fungi, protozoa, and viruses. Antibiotics are used to treat various bacterial infections. Bacteria are categorized by their shape (bacilli, cocci, or spirilla), their ability to utilize oxygen, and by their staining characteristics (Gram positive or Gram negative). Penicillins are most effective against Gram-positive bacteria. Allergies occur most frequently with penicillins. Multiple drugs are used in the treatment of tuberculosis because the complex microbes are slow growing and commonly develop drug resistance. Antifungal medications act by disrupting aspects of growth or metabolism that are unique to these organisms. Systemic mycoses affect internal organs and may required prolonged, aggressive drug therapy. Amphotericin B is the drug of choice for serious fungal infections.

Protozoal infections are caused by single-celled animals in humans. Malaria is the most common protozoal infection. Other protozoal infections include amebiasis, cryptosporidiosis, giardiasis, trichomoniasis, and trypanosomiasis. Viruses are nonliving, intracellular parasites that require host organelles to replicate. Some viral infections are self-limiting, whereas others benefit from drug therapy. Antiretroviral drugs used in the treatment of HIV–AIDS do not cure the disease, but they do help many patients live longer. Antiviral agents can lessen the severity of acute herpes simplex infection. They are available to prevent and treat influenza infections.

LEARNING GOALS

These learning goals correspond to the objectives at the beginning of the chapter, providing a clear summary of the chapter's most important points.

1. Antimicrobial drugs are classified as follows:
   - Antimicrobials: kill or inhibit the growth and reproduction of bacteria
   - Antifungals: kill or inhibit the growth and reproduction of fungi
   - Antiprotozoals: kill or inhibit the growth and reproduction of protozoans; they are divided into antimalarial drugs and nonmalarial drugs
   - Antivirals: eliminate or reduce viruses by impairing their replication
   - Antitubercular medications: inhibit bacterial protein synthesis by binding to ribosomes of bacteria that are susceptible to tuberculosis

2. Bacteria are commonly classified by their shape, ability to use oxygen, and Gram-staining properties:
   - Shape: Bacilli are rod shaped, cocci are sphere shaped, and spirilla are spiral shaped.
   - Oxygen use: Aerobic bacteria live and grow in an oxygen-rich environment, and anaerobic bacteria live and grow when oxygen is not present.
   - Gram-staining properties: Bacteria with thicker cell wells retain the purple Gram stain and are known as Gram-positive bacteria (including staphylococci, streptococci, and enterococci); those with thinner cell walls do not retain the Gram stain (including bacteroides, *Escherichia coli*, klebsiella, pseudomonas, and salmonella).

3. Sulfonamides are primarily used for minor urinary tract infections, otitis media, sinusitis, certain lower respiratory infections, and ulcerative colitis. They are also prescribed for AIDS-related pneumonia.

4. Bacteriostatic agents are capable of stopping the growth and reproduction of bacteria without actually killing the bacteria. Bactericidal agents actually kill bacteria and include antiseptics, disinfectants, and antibiotics.

5. In general, antiviral agents interfere with DNA synthesis to inhibit viral replication.

6. Macrolides inhibit bacterial protein synthesis to stop bacterial growth and are effective against both Gram-positive and Gram-negative bacteria. Sulfa drugs (sulfonamides) interfere with bacterial growth and development and are primarily bacteriostatic with some bactericidal actions. They have been available much longer than macrolides.

7. The first-line antitubercular drugs include the following:
   - ethambutol
   - isoniazid
   - pyrazinamide
   - rifampin
   - rifapentine
   - streptomycin sulfate
8. HAART stands for highly active antiretroviral therapy, and it involves the use of multiple agents to treat HIV–AIDS. It can greatly decrease the progression of the virus but must be continued for the remainder of the patient's life.
9. In general, antifungal agents work by destroying the cell membrane of the fungus via binding to the ergosterol in the fungal cell membrane. They are indicated for severe systemic fungal infections, as prophylactics for patients with severe immunosuppression, for candidemia and other *Candida* infections (such as esophageal candidiasis), for aspergillosis, and for *Cryptococcus* infections.
10. Drugs used to treat protozoal infections include antimalarial drugs and nonmalarial drugs. Antimalarial drugs include atovaquone–proguanil, chloroquine, hydroxychloroquine sulfate, mefloquine, primaquine, pyrimethamine, and quinine. Nonmalarial drugs include iodoquinol, metronidazole, paromomycin, pentamidine, sodium stibogluconate, tinidazole, and trimetrexate.

CRITICAL THINKING QUESTIONS

1. Explain why infectious diseases occur less often than they did 100 years ago.
2. Discuss how many types of HIV exist today.

WEB SITES

http://hubpages.com/hub/Uses-and-Classifications-of-Bacteria

http://student.ccbcmd.edu/courses/bi0141/lecguide/unit3/viruses/classvir.html

http://www.aids.org/

http://www.anaesthetist.com/icu/infect/fungi/Findex.htm#serious.htm

http://www.botany.hawaii.edu/faculty/wong/BOT135/Lect04.HTM

http://www.cdc.gov/flu/professionals/antivirals/

http://www.medicinenet.com/bcg_vaccine-antitubercular/article.htm

http://www.news-medical.net/news/2004/10/21/5741.aspx

http://www.tufts.edu/med/apua/Q&A/Q&A_antibacterials.html

http://www.webmd.com/sexual-conditions/antiprotozoals-for-trichomoniasis

REVIEW QUESTIONS

Multiple Choice

Select the best response to each question.

1. Gemifloxacin is a(n)
   A. local anesthetic
   B. glucocorticoid
   C. anti-infective
   D. sunscreen agent
2. Which of the following is/are true for tetracyclines?
   A. they are bactericidal
   B. they may cause discoloration of the teeth in children
   C. they exhibit a broad spectrum of activity
   D. both b and c
3. Adefovir is a member of which class of anti-infectives?
   A. penicillins
   B. tetracyclines
   C. antivirals
   D. antifungals
4. Nystatin is used to treat
   A. candidiasis
   B. rickettsial infections
   C. *Escherichia coli* infections
   D. all of the above
5. Gentamicin exhibits
   A. significant hepatotoxicity
   B. significant nephrotoxicity
   C. significant cardiotoxicity
   D. all of the above
6. Which of the following drugs is used in treating potentially fatal fungal infections?
   A. miconazole
   B. griseofulvin
   C. nystatin
   D. amphotericin B
7. Atazanavir is usually classified as an
   A. oral antidiabetic
   B. antiviral
   C. antibacterial
   D. antifungal
8. Rifampin is used primarily as an
   A. antiprotozoal
   B. antidepressant
   C. antituberculosis agent
   D. antiviral
9. Which of the following antibiotics may be used for the treatment of AIDS-related pneumonia (*Pneumocystis carinii*)?
   A. penicillins
   B. tetracyclines
   C. sulfonamides
   D. fluoroquinolones

10. Tetracyclines are contraindicated in
    A. children younger than age 8 years
    B. children younger than age 16 years
    C. elderly patients older than age 65 years
    D. patients who have syphilis
11. *Cryptococcus* is classified as a
    A. bacteria
    B. virus
    C. fungus
    D. protozoan
12. Which of the following drugs is classified as a fusion inhibitor (antiretroviral agent for HIV–AIDS)?
    A. enfuvirtide (Fuzeon)
    B. efavirenz (Sustiva)
    C. zidovudine (AZT)
    D. stavudine (D4T)
13. Anti-infective drugs derived from natural substances are referred to as
    A. antifungals
    B. antibiotics
    C. antiprotozoals
    D. antivirals
14. Which of the following antibiotics should *not* be used in children younger than the age of 18 years?
    A. isoniazid and rifampin
    B. chloramphenicol and streptomycin
    C. tetracyclines
    D. ciprofloxacin
15. Which of the following antibiotics may lead to gray baby syndrome?
    A. streptomycin
    B. chloramphenicol
    C. erythromycin
    D. sulfonamide

CASE STUDY

Samantha is 14 years old and has a streptococcal infection. She has a history of mitral valve stenosis. After receiving her 7th in a series of 10 penicillin shots, she left the pediatrician's office with her mother. Shortly after, she had difficulty breathing and a bluish discoloration of her lips and face. Her mother called the office from her cell phone and brought Samantha right back. Upon entering the office, she collapsed. The pediatrician immediately started treatment to stabilize Samantha.

1. What was the possible cause of Samantha's condition?
2. How could she be treated for her symptoms?

CHAPTER 19

Drug Therapy for Pediatric Respiratory Diseases

OUTLINE

OBJECTIVES

Upon completion of this chapter, the reader should be able to do the following:

1. Explain the role of surfactant in neonatal lung function.
2. Distinguish common infant respiratory disorders.
3. Explain apnea in premature infants.
4. Compare viral croup and epiglottitis in terms of incidence by age and site of infection.
5. Identify treatments for cystic fibrosis.
6. Discuss pharmacodynamics in newborns and infants.
7. Describe bronchial asthma in children.
8. Explain the factors affecting pharmacokinetics in children.
9. Define the terms *neonates*, *infants*, and *toddlers*.
10. List five drugs that cause pharmacologic effects in nursing infants.

KEY TERMS

Asphyxia
Autosomal
Cesarean section
Epiglottitis
Half-life
Hypoxemia
Incubator
Infants
Kernicterus
Lethargic
Mycoplasma pneumonia
Necrosis
Neonates
Oxygen sensor
Peristalsis
Pharmacodynamics
Pharmacokinetics
Radiant warmer
Sickle cell anemia
Stridor
Surfactant
Toddlers
Tracheotomy

INTRODUCTION

Childhood disorders may be especially threatening because children are continually changing, both physically and functionally. As a child grows, the body's immune system matures, making it better able to combat pathogens. Rapid advances in treatments and preventive medicine control many infectious diseases that previously caused serious illness, disability, and death. Pediatric pharmacology still requires special attention and knowledge, however. It is important to remember that many medications act on pediatric patients differently than adults. Research concerning neonates, infants, and children has not been as thorough as research on adults.

Common Pediatric Respiratory Disorders

Infants acquire limited natural immunity from their mothers. Still, the growing child is vulnerable to many infectious diseases and the disabilities they may cause. Common pediatric respiratory disorders include respiratory distress syndrome of newborns, acute bronchiolitis, apnea, asthma, cystic fibrosis, pneumonia, epiglottitis, and viral croup. These disorders are discussed in detail in the following sections.

Respiratory Distress Syndrome of Newborns

Respiratory distress syndrome (RDS) is also known as hyaline membrane disease. It is one of the most common causes of respiratory disease in premature infants. In these infants, pulmonary immaturity and surfactant deficiency leads to alveolar collapse. The incidence of RDS is higher among preterm male infants, white infants, infants of diabetic mothers, and those subjected to asphyxia, stress from cold temperatures, and delivery by cesarean section (if performed before the 38th week of gestation).

Surfactant synthesis is influenced by insulin and cortisol. Insulin tends to inhibit surfactant production, and cortisol can accelerate surfactant formation. When there is a deficiency of surfactant, the lungs collapse between breaths. This makes each successive breath as difficult as the first breath.

Infants with RDS show multiple signs of respiratory distress, usually within the first 24 hours after being born. Central cyanosis is an obvious sign of RDS as breathing becomes more difficult. The respiration rate increases to between 60 and 120 breaths per minute as the infant's lungs try to maintain normal ventilation. Fatigue may develop rapidly because of the increased difficulty in breathing.

To treat infants with RDS, supportive care is required, including gentle handling and a minimum of disturbances. An incubator or radiant warmer is used to prevent hypothermia and increased oxygen consumption. Oxygen levels can be assessed by using an arterial (umbilical) line or by a transcutaneous oxygen sensor. Treatment includes administration of supplemental oxygen, continuous positive airway pressure through nasal prongs, and, often, assisted mechanical ventilation.

Exogenous surfactant therapy is used to prevent and treat RDS. The two types of surfactants are as follows: natural surfactants (prepared from animal sources) and synthetic surfactants. Only the natural surfactants are currently approved for clinical use in the United States. Surfactants are suspended in saline and administered into the airways, usually through an endotracheal tube. The treatment is often initiated soon after birth in infants who are at high risk for RDS.

> **POINT TO REMEMBER**
>
> Corticosteroids may be administered to a pregnant woman to stimulate surfactant production in her fetus if it is at high risk for preterm birth.

Acute Bronchiolitis

Acute bronchiolitis is a viral infection of the lower airways. It is most commonly caused by the respiratory syncytial virus. It produces inflammatory obstruction of the small airways and necrosis of the cells that line the lower airways. Acute bronchiolitis usually occurs during the first 2 years of life, with the highest occurrence between 3 and 6 months of age.

> **POINT TO REMEMBER**
>
> Children of parents who smoke are at higher risk for respiratory tract infections, which can lead to chronic bronchitis.

Most affected infants in whom bronchiolitis develops have a history of mild upper respiratory tract infections. These symptoms usually last for several days and may be accompanied by fever as well as decreased appetite. Respiratory distress then gradually develops, with dyspnea, irritability, and a wheezing cough. The infant can usually breathe enough air in but has difficulty exhaling. The air becomes trapped in the lung distal to the site of obstruction. This interferes with gas exchange.

Infants with respiratory distress are usually hospitalized. Treatment is supportive, including administration of supplemental oxygen if the oxygen saturation consistently falls below 90%. Because the infection is viral, antibiotics are not effective. They are administered only for a secondary bacterial infection. Rapid and complete recovery usually begins after the first 48 to 72 hours of treatment.

Apnea in Premature Infants

Apnea and periodic breathing are common respiratory problems in premature infants. Apnea is defined as cessation of breathing. It is characterized by failure to breathe for 20 seconds or longer, and it is often accompanied by bradycardia or cyanosis. Because the respiratory center in the medulla oblongata is underdeveloped in premature infants, their ability for sustained normal breathing is often impaired (see Chapter 21).

In contrast to adults, infants respond to hypoxemia with only a short period of increased ventilation. This is followed by hypoventilation or apnea. About 50% of infants who weigh less than 1.5 kg often require intervention for significant spells of apnea. Periodic breathing commonly occurs in infants who weigh less than 1800 grams. This involves an intermittent failure to breathe for periods of less than 10 to 15 seconds.

The management of apnea and periodic breathing includes use of medications or ventilatory support until the central nervous system is developed and able to sustain adequate ventilatory drive. Mild episodes of apnea may be stopped by prompt tactile stimulation. Methylxanthines (such as caffeine and theophylline) are often used to treat apnea. These drugs appear to have a central stimulatory effect on brain stem respiratory neurons (see Chapter 21). They often markedly decrease how often, and how severely, apnea attacks occur.

Bronchial Asthma

Asthma is a leading cause of chronic illness in children. Many children lose school days because of different types of asthma. In children's hospitals, asthma is the most common diagnosis for admitted patients. Asthma may begin at any age, with 80% of children becoming symptomatic by 6 years of age. It affects black children more than white children and is commonly caused by either respiratory syncytial virus or parainfluenza viruses. Other factors include exposure to environmental allergens, including dust mites, cockroaches, and pet dander. Children may also exhibit asthma symptoms as a result of exposure to environmental tobacco smoke.

The signs and symptoms of asthma in infants and small children vary with the stage and severity of an attack. Many children experience acute asthma attacks at night. In these nocturnal attacks, nonproductive cough, tachypnea, dyspnea, and wheezing are common. Children with extreme respiratory distress may not exhibit wheezing. Symptoms may progress rapidly and require either emergency medical care or hospitalization.

The anti-inflammatory agents known as cromolyn and nedocromil are recommended for mild to moderate persistent asthma in infants and children. For mild intermittent symptoms (or exacerbations), inhaled short-acting beta$_2$-adrenergic agonists may be used. Severe symptoms may require the use of inhaled corticosteroids. Systemic corticosteroids may be required during an episode of severe disease.

> **POINT TO REMEMBER**
>
> Extrinsic asthma is commonly accompanied by other hereditary allergies, such as eczema and allergic rhinitis in children.

Special delivery systems for administration of inhalation medications are available for infants and small children. These include nebulizers with face masks, as well as spacers and holding chambers used with a metered dose inhaler (MDI). Nebulizer therapy is preferred for children younger than 2 years of age. MDIs with spacers and holding chambers may be used for children between 3 and 5 years of age.

Pneumonia

Pneumonia is an inflammatory condition of the lung tissue in which fluid and blood cells escape into the alveoli, impairing gas exchange. Infants and children are at risk for several forms of pneumonia, including mycoplasma pneumonia, adenovirus pneumonia, and respiratory syncytial virus pneumonia. Pneumonia may be more likely to develop if a child has a history of a recent upper respiratory infection, influenza, or a viral syndrome. Other

chronic pulmonary diseases, such as asthma, bronchitis, and tuberculosis, may also predispose a child to developing pneumonia. Additional predisposing factors include sickle cell anemia, neurological disorders that cause paralysis of the diaphragm, and malnutrition.

Cystic Fibrosis

Cystic fibrosis (CF) is the major cause of severe chronic respiratory disease in children. It is an autosomal recessive disorder that involves fluid secretion in the exocrine glands of the epithelial lining inside the respiratory, gastrointestinal, and reproductive tracts. Aside from chronic respiratory disease, CF manifests with pancreatic exocrine deficiency and elevation of sodium chloride in the sweat (also see Chapter 2). Cystic fibrosis can be diagnosed by a sweat test.

There are no currently approved treatments for correcting the genetic defects of CF. Treatment measures are therefore directed toward slowing the progression of secondary organ dysfunction, chronic lung infections, and pancreatic insufficiency. Treatment includes antibiotics to prevent and manage infections, physical therapies such as chest percussion and postural drainage, and mucolytic agents to prevent airway obstruction. Other measures include pancreatic enzyme replacement and nutritional therapy.

> **POINT TO REMEMBER**
>
> A sweat test may be inaccurate in very young infants because they may not produce enough sweat for a valid test.

Viral Croup

Croup is a childhood disease involving severe inflammation and obstruction of the upper airway, which occurs as acute laryngotracheobronchitis, laryngitis, and acute spasmodic laryngitis. Croup is characterized by inspiratory stridor, hoarseness, and a barking cough. Viral croup (also known as acute laryngotracheobronchitis) is a viral infection that affects the larynx, trachea, and bronchi. The parainfluenza viruses cause about 75% of all cases, with the remaining cases caused by other viruses. Viral croup is usually seen in children between 3 and 5 months of age. The condition may affect the entire laryngotracheal tree.

Although the respiratory manifestations of croup often appear suddenly, they are usually preceded by upper respiratory infections. Symptoms include the common cold, runny nose, low-grade fever, and hoarseness. In most children, croup only causes stridor and dyspnea before recovery begins. Symptoms usually subside when the child is exposed to moist air. Letting a shower run inside a bathroom and then bringing the child into the bathroom so the moistened air can be breathed usually provides prompt relief of croup symptoms.

Exposure to cold air also seems to relieve the airway spasms of croup. Often, severe symptoms are relieved on the way to the emergency department because the child is exposed to colder air during the trip. Treating croup is difficult because viral croup does not respond to antibiotics, and other agents (including expectorants, bronchodilating agents, and antihistamines) are not helpful. The child should be not be disturbed but should be carefully monitored for signs of respiratory distress.

Epiglottitis

Epiglottitis is an acute inflammation of the epiglottis that tends to cause airway obstruction. It is a dramatic, potentially fatal condition characterized by inflammatory edema of the supraglottic area. Epiglottitis occurs suddenly, bringing danger of airway obstruction and asphyxia. The *Haemophilus influenzae* type B bacterium was previously the most commonly identified etiologic agent, but it has been seen less commonly since the widespread use of immunizations. Therefore, other agents, such as *Streptococcus pyogenes*, *Streptococcus pneumoniae*, and *Staphylococcus aureus*, are the current common causes of pediatric epiglottitis.

Epiglottitis predominantly affects children between 2 and 6 years of age. Children with epiglottitis appear lethargic, pale, and show symptoms of toxicity. They have difficulty in swallowing, a quieter than normal voice, fever, and extreme anxiety. Epiglottitis may progress to complete airway obstruction and even death if adequate treatment is not administered. This condition is a medical emergency that requires immediate establishment of an airway by endotracheal tube or tracheotomy. If epiglottitis is suspected, the child should never be made to lie down because this position can cause the epiglottis to fall backward, leading to complete airway obstruction. The throat should not be examined with a tongue blade (tongue depressor) or other instrument except by a medical professional who has experience in intubation of small children. This is because such an examination could cause cardiopulmonary arrest. Any procedure that would increase the child's anxiety should be avoided, including drawing blood. Increased anxiety can precipitate airway spasms and cause death. Recovery from epiglottitis is usually rapid, without adverse events, after an adequate airway has been established and appropriate antibiotic therapy has been initiated.

Pharmacology in Pediatrics

The ways in which medications act on pediatric patients differ from the ways they act in adults. Pharmacokinetics and pharmacodynamics are simply not the same as in adults due to the ever-growing and developing systems of newborns, infants, and children. Research on these age groups has not been as thorough as on older children, teenagers, adults, and the

elderly. Babies are called neonates until they reach 28 days of age. Infants are babies between age 29 days and approximately 1 year. Toddlers are from 1 to 3 years of age.

Pharmacokinetics

Pharmacokinetics in children is relatively the same as in adults, with a few important differences. Soon after birth, blood flow at the site of drug administration, as well as gastrointestinal function, change rapidly. Physiologic conditions that influence pharmacokinetics include cardiovascular shock, heart failure, and vasoconstriction. Preterm infants have very little muscle mass, meaning that drugs can stay in their muscles and be absorbed much more slowly than anticipated. If the systemic blood circulation increases throughout the extremities of their bodies, the circulating medications can increase suddenly to cause potential toxicities.

Drug Absorption

Drugs have the ability to pass through barriers from the site of administration into the bloodstream. This is called drug absorption. Infants should not be given drugs that are inactivated by low pH in the gastric contents. This is because of their rapidly changing biochemical and physiologic states. The intestines' rhythmic movements (peristalsis) can be irregular or slower than anticipated. Therefore, drug absorption in neonates is very unpredictable. It is affected by the rate of gastric emptying, gestational maturity, postnatal age, and types of feeding. Gastric emptying can be delayed by conditions such as gastroesophageal reflux, congenital heart disease, and respiratory distress syndrome. Many topical agents, including hydrocortisone, laundry detergents containing pentachlorophenol, and other ingredients, can result in toxicities because of the ways neonates absorb them.

Drug Distribution

Drug distribution is the part of pharmacokinetics that deals with the movement or transport of drugs throughout the body. Although extracellular water makes up only 20% of body weight in adults, it makes up 40% of body weight in neonates. In the first 2 days after birth, most neonates experience diuresis, making it important to determine the concentration of (especially) water-soluble drugs at receptor sites. Because neonate body fat is approximately 15%, organs that accumulate lipid-soluble drugs may not be as effective as they are in older children. Drug binding to plasma proteins is below normal adult values until the infant is 10 to 12 months of age. Drugs such as local anesthetics

---

POINT TO REMEMBER

A water-soluble drug will have a higher volume of distribution in children than in adults.

POINT TO REMEMBER

Newborns have a greater percentage of weight from body water and less body fat than adults.

and ampicillin may be more concentrated in the plasma, increasing drug effects or toxicity. Drugs given to jaundiced neonates can displace bilirubin from albumin, entering the brain and causing **kernicterus**.

Drug Metabolism

The alteration or transformation of chemicals from their original form (mostly in the liver) is known as metabolism. The livers of neonates work at lower levels in the metabolizing of drugs, causing slower clearance rates and longer **half-life** elimination times. Drug doses need to be carefully calculated as a result. Lack of pediatric testing requirements by the Food and Drug Administration causes all dosages for young children to be determined based upon their body surface area, age, and weight as they compare to the systems of adults. Dose–response relationships of certain drugs can change greatly during the first weeks of life. Another consideration is that younger preterm babies (as young as 24 weeks) are now surviving, which requires even more closely scrutinized drug regimens.

Drug Excretion

Excretion is a process involving the removal of drugs, as well as active and inactive metabolites, from the body. As calculated by body surface area, the glomerular filtration rate of newborns is only 30 to 40% of adults, with premature babies having even lower rates. However, by the end of the 3rd week of life, these rates increase to 50 or even 60% of adults, with adult rates reached by 6 or 12 months of age. Drugs eliminated through the kidneys are removed from the body very slowly during the first few weeks of life. However, toddlers may have shorter elimination half-lives than older children and adults. This is most likely a result of higher renal elimination and metabolism in toddlers as compared to older children and adults.

Pharmacodynamics

The **pharmacodynamics** of newborns, infants, and children relate to the presence (or absence) of receptors, inadequate drug–receptor binding, or the inability of the developing organs and tissues to respond to a postreceptor signal. Enzyme functions are not at fully effective levels, and both biochemical and structural maturation are far from complete. Due to unique levels of distribution and elimination in younger patients, certain drugs may be unpredictable, ineffective, toxic, or able to cause unusual adverse effects. These drugs include antibiotics, digoxin, indomethacin, and methylxanthines.

POINT TO REMEMBER

Pharmacodynamics is a description of the properties of drug–receptor interaction and can be thought of as what the drug does to the body.

Drug Administration During Lactation

Although most drugs cannot pass through breast milk in sufficient quantities to harm the nursing infant, many mothers avoid breastfeeding because of medications they may be taking. More babies experience nutritional problems because of being fed baby formula in place of real breast milk than experiencing drug effects passed through breast milk. Drug concentration in breast milk is usually very low. Drugs that are safe to use during lactation should be taken by the mother 1 to 2 hours before, or 3 to 4 hours after, breastfeeding to minimize effects on the nursing infants. Most OTC medications provide information about use during lactation. Dosages should be followed strictly, and cold remedies or medications containing more than 20% alcohol should be avoided.

Drugs that are not indicated for use during lactation include many antibiotics, tetracyclines, isoniazid, sedatives, hypnotics, barbiturates, chloral hydrate, and diazepam. Narcotics such as methadone or morphine should not be used by lactating women, and alcohol should be avoided. Other drugs that should be avoided include lithium, radiopharmaceutics, chemotherapeutics, cytotoxics, and immune-modulating agents.

Patient Education

Parents should be instructed to make sure their children have all of the recommended childhood vaccinations on schedule. This can prevent many common pediatric respiratory disorders. Parents also should be aware that because children are extremely vulnerable to a variety of pulmonary disorders, signs and symptoms of such disorders should be taken seriously, and they should be treated by a physician, not simply at home. The physiology of children is completely different than that of adults. Medications must be precise and administered on a schedule provided by the physician.

SUMMARY

As a child grows, the body's systems and natural immune defense mechanisms mature and expand. Premature infants are at far more risk for infectious diseases and respiratory problems than full-term infants. Common pediatric respiratory disorders include respiratory distress syndrome of the newborn, acute bronchiolitis, apnea in premature infants, asthma, pneumonia, cystic fibrosis, viral croup, and epiglottitis.

The administration of drugs for neonates, infants, and toddlers requires special attention to prevent medication errors. Pharmacokinetics and pharmacodynamics in pediatrics are similar to adults, with several important differences. Drug absorption, drug distribution, drug metabolism, and drug excretion are influenced by the maturation and functions of various body systems. Inadequate drug–receptor binding, as well as effectiveness and insufficiency of enzymes, are important factors related to drug toxicity.

LEARNING GOALS

These learning goals correspond to the objectives at the beginning of the chapter, providing a clear summary of the chapter's most important points.

1. Surfactant is important in the very young to avoid alveolar collapse, as seen in respiratory distress syndrome (RDS). Surfactant helps the lungs to avoid collapse, and exogenous surfactant therapy may be required in certain cases. The two types of surfactants are natural surfactants (from animal sources) and synthetic surfactants. They are often administered through an endotracheal tube in infants who are at high risk of RDS.

2. Common infant respiratory disorders include respiratory distress syndrome, acute bronchiolitis, apnea, asthma, cystic fibrosis, pneumonia, epiglottitis, and viral croup.

3. Apnea (cessation of breathing) is common in premature infants. It is characterized by failure to breathe for 20 seconds or longer and is often accompanied by bradycardia or cyanosis. It may be caused as a result of an underdeveloped respiratory center in the medulla oblongata.

4. Viral croup is a viral infection of the larynx, trachea, and bronchi; it usually affects children between 3 and 5 months of age. Epiglottitis is a dramatic, potentially fatal condition characterized by inflammatory edema of the supraglottic area; it predominantly affects children between 2 and 6 years of age.

5. There are no currently approved treatments for correcting the genetic defects of cystic fibrosis. Therefore, treatment is directed toward slowing the progression of secondary organ dysfunction, chronic lung infections, and pancreatic insufficiency. Treatment includes antibiotics to prevent and manage infections, physical therapies such as chest percussion and postural drainage, and mucolytic agents to prevent airway obstruction. Other measures include pancreatic enzyme replacement and nutritional therapy.

6. The pharmacodynamics of neonates, infants, and toddlers relate to the presence or absence of receptors, inadequate drug–receptor binding, or the inability of the developing organs and tissues to respond to a postreceptor signal. Enzyme functions are not at fully effective levels. Biochemical and structural maturation are far from complete. Drug distribution and elimination are uniquely different than in adults.

7. Asthma is a leading cause of chronic illness in children. It is the most common diagnosis for children admitted into children's hospitals. Asthma may begin at any age, with 80% of children being symptomatic by 6 years of age. It is commonly caused by respiratory syncytial virus or parainfluenza viruses, as well as environmental factors. Acute asthma attacks often occur at night, and symptoms can progress rapidly until emergency medical care is required.

8. Pharmacokinetics in children is relatively the same as in adults, with a few important differences. Physiologic conditions influencing pharmacokinetics include cardiovascular shock, heart failure, and vasoconstriction. Due to very little muscle mass, drugs can stay in the muscles of preterm infants and be absorbed much more slowly than anticipated.

9. The terms *neonates*, *infants*, and *toddlers* are defined as follows:
   - Neonates: babies who are 28 days of age or younger
   - Infants: babies between age 29 days and approximately 1 year
   - Toddlers: babies between 1 and 3 years of age

10. Drugs that are not indicated for use during lactation include many antibiotics, tetracyclines, isoniazid, sedatives, hypnotics, barbiturates, chloral hydrate, diazepam, narcotics such as methadone or morphine, alcohol, lithium, radiopharmaceutics, chemotherapeutics, cytotoxics, and immune-modulating agents.

CRITICAL THINKING QUESTIONS

1. Why are premature infants more vulnerable to various diseases?
2. Why are pharmacodynamics and pharmacokinetics different in infants as compared to adults? Explain the differences.

WEB SITES

http://kidshealth.org/parent/pregnancy_newborn/medical_problems/aop.html

http://www.aafp.org/afp/20040115/325.html

http://www.jppt.org/

http://www.kidsgrowth.com/resources/articledetail.cfm?id=192

http://www.merck.com/mmhe/sec23/ch274/ch274b.html

http://www.merck.com/mmpe/sec19/ch270/ch270b.html

http://www.nlm.nih.gov/medlineplus/ency/article/001563.htm

http://www.unc.edu/courses/2008fall/nurs/721/001/pharm/pregnacyB.html

REVIEW QUESTIONS

Multiple Choice

Select the best response to each question.

1. Central cyanosis is an obvious sign of
   A. viral croup
   B. cystic fibrosis
   C. apnea and periodic breathing
   D. respiratory distress syndrome

2. Which of the following statements is true about bronchial asthma?
   A. It may begin at any age, with 80% of children being symptomatic by 6 years of age.
   B. It is an autosomal recessive disorder.
   C. It is common in children with sickle cell anemia.
   D. It is characterized by hoarseness and a barking cough.

3. Which of the following is the treatment of viral croup?
   A. bronchodilating agents
   B. antibiotics
   C. expectorants
   D. it is not easy to treat

4. What percentage of a neonate's body weight is made up of extracellular water?
   A. 20%
   B. 40%
   C. 60%
   D. 80%

5. Which of the following is a process involving removal of drugs from the body?
   A. metabolism
   B. distribution
   C. excretion
   D. absorption

6. Drugs that are *not* indicated for use during lactation include all of the following except
   A. methadone
   B. H1N1 flu vaccine
   C. isoniazid
   D. alcohol

7. Systemic corticosteroids may be required during an episode of
   A. mild asthma
   B. moderate persistent asthma
   C. mild intermittent symptoms of asthma
   D. severe asthma

8. Management of apnea and periodic breathing includes which of the following?
   A. methylxanthines
   B. corticosteroids
   C. antibiotics
   D. expectorants

9. Which of the following agents is used in premature infants to prevent alveolar collapse?
   A. theophylline
   B. penicillin G
   C. surfactant
   D. caffeine

10. Which of the following is the most common cause of viral croup?
    A. parainfluenza
    B. mumps
    C. influenza A
    D. smallpox

11. The *Haemophilus influenzae* type B bacterium was previously the most commonly identified cause of
    A. croup
    B. epiglottitis
    C. pneumonia
    D. pertussis

12. The pharmaceutical science that deals with the absorption and metabolism of drugs is called
    A. pharmacopoeia
    B. pharmacology
    C. pharmacokinetics
    D. pharmacodynamics

13. A baby between 29 days of age and approximately 1 year is referred to as a(n)
    A. toddler
    B. infant
    C. neonate
    D. newborn

14. Dose–response relationships of certain drugs can change greatly during the
    A. first weeks of life
    B. first months of life
    C. period following the first year
    D. period following the first 5 years

15. The respiration rate in respiratory distress syndrome of newborns increases to
    A. 20–40 breaths per minute
    B. 30–50 breaths per minute
    C. 40–60 breaths per minute
    D. 60–120 breaths per minute

CASE STUDY

Judy, a 4-month-old infant, took a nap around 1:00 p.m. After 1 hour, her mother went to check on her and found the infant unresponsive. She called 911, and Judy was taken to the emergency department, where she unfortunately died.

1. What was the probable cause of death for this infant?
2. Is there any prevention for this condition?

Immunization

OBJECTIVES

Upon completion of this chapter, the reader should be able to do the following:

1. Explain the role of the thymus gland in the immune system.
2. Discussion classifications of immunity.
3. Compare vaccines with gamma globulins.
4. Discuss the common vaccines recommended for children younger than 6 years of age.
5. State the type of vaccines that should not, in general, be administered to immuno-compromised patients.
6. Explain passive immunity and list three examples.
7. Compare *Haemophilus influenzae* type B with influenza A.
8. List vaccines that are administered subcutaneously and intradermally.
9. Explain the various types of immunoglobulins.
10. Compare the recommended schedules for the administration of hepatitis B and rabies.

KEY TERMS

Active immunity	Inactivated vaccine
Attenuated vaccine	Leukocytes
B lymphocytes	Mast cell
Bone marrow	Natural killer (NK) cells
Booster	Passive immunity
Cell-mediated immunity	Pathogens
Cytotoxic T cells	Phagocytic cells
Exogenous	Plasma cells
Gamma globulins	T lymphocytes
Helper T cells	Thymus gland
Immunoglobulins	Toxoid vaccine

INTRODUCTION

Widespread immunizations for major communicable diseases affecting children have been amongst the most dramatic improvements in infant health. Morbidity and mortality in infants and young children have been greatly reduced as a result. Specific immunizations are given a standard number of times to infants and children as part of the promotion of good health. Although immunization programs have lowered the prevalence of many diseases, they have not completely eradicated infectious disease. Immunization programs are only effective if adults and the elderly receive follow-up boosters for certain vaccines. These patients must follow specific recommendations concerning immunizations indicated specifically for them.

The Immune System

The immune system is able to distinguish substances that are not endogenous and then mount a targeted response to these invaders. This involves two processes known as specificity and memory. The immune system protects the body from disease-causing **pathogens**. Pathogenic microorganisms include bacteria, viruses, fungi, and protozoans. Nearly any **exogenous** molecule or cell can elicit an immune response. Pollen, chemicals, and foreign bodies are examples of substances to which the body may react. Substances that trigger the body's immune response and then react with products of that response are known as antigens.

Occasionally, the body's immune system fails to perform its normal functions. Abnormal functions of the immune system are classified as incorrect responses (autoimmune disease), lack of response (immunodeficiency disease), or overactive responses (allergies).

The immune system has two anatomical components: lymphoid tissues and the cells that are responsible for the immune response. Lymphoid tissues are located throughout the body. The two primary lymphoid tissues are the **thymus gland** and the **bone marrow**, where cells involved in the immune response form and mature. Some mature immune cells do not specialize until they are first exposed to a pathogen. Secondary lymphoid tissues are found in the spleen and the lymph nodes (see **Figure 20–1**).

The immune cells of the spleen are positioned to monitor the blood for foreign invaders. **Phagocytic cells** in the spleen also trap and then remove aging red blood cells. The lymph nodes are part of the lymphatic circulation. Inside them, clusters of immune cells intercept pathogens that have entered the interstitial fluid through breaks in the skin or through mucous membranes.

The white blood cells (WBCs), also called **leukocytes**, are the primary cells responsible for the body's immune responses. Leukocytes are divided into five basic types: neutrophils, basophils, eosinophils, monocytes, and lymphocytes. Leukocytes can be distinguished from one another in stained tissue samples by the shape and size of their nuclei (see **Figure 20–2**).

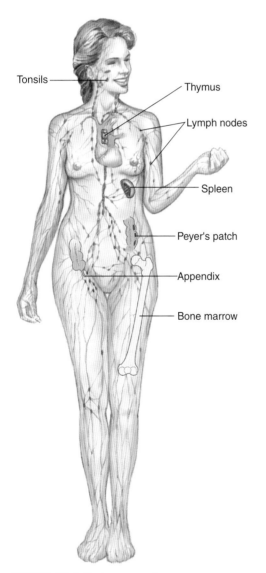

Tonsils

Thymus

Lymph nodes

Spleen

Peyer's patch

Appendix

Bone marrow

FIGURE 20–1 The immune system.

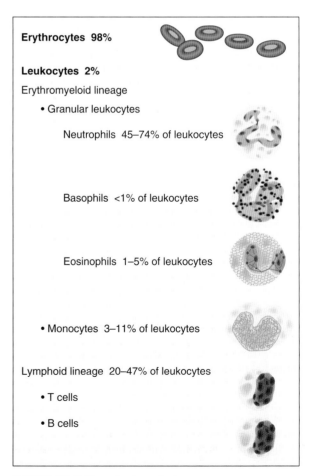

Erythrocytes 98%

Leukocytes 2%

Erythromyeloid lineage

• Granular leukocytes

Neutrophils 45–74% of leukocytes

Basophils <1% of leukocytes

Eosinophils 1–5% of leukocytes

• Monocytes 3–11% of leukocytes

Lymphoid lineage 20–47% of leukocytes

• T cells

• B cells

FIGURE 20–2 The cells of your body.

Immunity

Immunity is the state or condition of being resistant to invading microorganisms. It is normally acquired either by contracting a disease (and then developing immunity to it) or being vaccinated with proteins from the causative agent. For example, a person with a normal immune system who contracts mumps develops a lifelong immunity to the disease. Alternatively, a person may be vaccinated with live mumps viruses (weakened but not destroyed) to acquire immunity. In each case, the immune system responds to proteins in the virus and develops a memory for it.

Acquired immunity is mediated primarily by lymphocytes. There are three main types of lymphocytes: B lymphocytes, T lymphocytes, and natural killer (NK) cells. Activated B lymphocytes develop into plasma cells, which secrete antibodies. Activated T lymphocytes develop either into cells that attack and destroy virus-infected cells or into cells that regulate other immune cells. Natural killer (NK) cells attack and destroy virus-infected cells and tumor cells. All lymphocytes secrete cytokines that act on immune cells and sometimes on pathogens. T lymphocytes carry out cell-mediated immunity. In this process, T cells develop in the thymus gland from immature precursor cells that migrate there from the bone marrow (see Figure 20–3). There are several types of T lymphocytes: natural killer cells, cytotoxic T cells, helper T cells, memory T cells, and suppressor T cells.

Acquired immunity can be subdivided into active and passive immunity (see Figure 20–4). Active immunity occurs when the body is exposed to a pathogen and produces its own antibodies. Active immunity can occur naturally, when a pathogen invades the body, or artificially, when we are given vaccinations containing dead or disabled pathogens.

Passive immunity occurs when we acquire antibodies that were made in the body of another animal. Other examples of passive immunity are when a mother transfers antibodies across the placenta to her fetus or when injections containing antibodies are given. Travelers going out of the United States may be injected with gamma globulin (antibodies extracted from donated human plasma). However, this type of passive immunity only lasts for about 3 months.

Classifications of Antibodies

An antibody is a substance that develops within the immune system. It is designed to identify and destroy foreign substances. Antibodies are also called immunoglobulins and are collectively referred to as gamma globulins. Immunoglobulins (Ig) are divided into five general classes: IgG, IgA, IgE, IgM, and IgD:

- IgG: These antibodies make up 75% of the plasma antibodies in adults because they are produced in secondary immune responses. Maternal IgG crosses the placental membrane and provides the infant with immunity in the first few months of life (see Figure 20–5).
- IgA: These antibodies are found in external secretions, such as saliva, tears, intestinal and bronchial mucus, and breast milk. In these secretions, they disable pathogens before they can reach the internal environment.
- IgE: These antibodies are associated with allergic responses. When mast cell receptors bind with IgE and an antigen, the mast cells release chemical mediators, such as histamine.
- IgM: These antibodies are associated with primary immune responses and with the antibodies that react to the blood group antigen.
- IgD: These antibody proteins appear on the surfaces of B lymphocytes along with IgM. However, the physiological role of IgD is unclear.

Vaccines

Vaccines are substances administered to generate a protective immune response. They can be live (attenuated) or killed (inactivated). Vaccines are made from dead or infectious agents or those that are still living but have been rendered harmless. They trigger the body's immune response to manufacture antibodies against particular disease-causing agents. Vaccines that are available and recommended in the United States are discussed in the following sections.

An attenuated vaccine is a living but weakened microorganism that does not cause disease. Examples of attenuated vaccines are those used for polio (the injected form of the vaccine), measles, mumps, and rubella. An inactivated vaccine produces less immunity than an attenuated vaccine. Examples of inactivated vaccines are those used for flu, hepatitis A, and polio (the oral form of the vaccine). A toxoid vaccine is one that contains inactivated bacterial toxins. They retain the ability to stimulate the formation of antitoxins, which are antibodies directed against the bacterial toxin. Examples of toxoid vaccines are those used for tetanus and diphtheria. A conjugate vaccine is one that allows the immune system to recognize and attack microorganisms, exemplified by the vaccine used for *Haemophilus influenzae* type B (Hib).

Diphtheria

Diphtheria is a disease that mimics influenza, with the most significant symptom being a thick coating at the back of the throat that makes swallowing and breathing difficult. Diphtheria kills up to 10% of the people it affects. The inactivated toxin (toxoid) for diphtheria was first developed in 1921. It was later combined with the vaccines for tetanus and pertussis and was administered as the DTP vaccine. Today, the vaccines commonly available for diphtheria exist under the names DTaP and Tdap, depending on the age of the patient. The

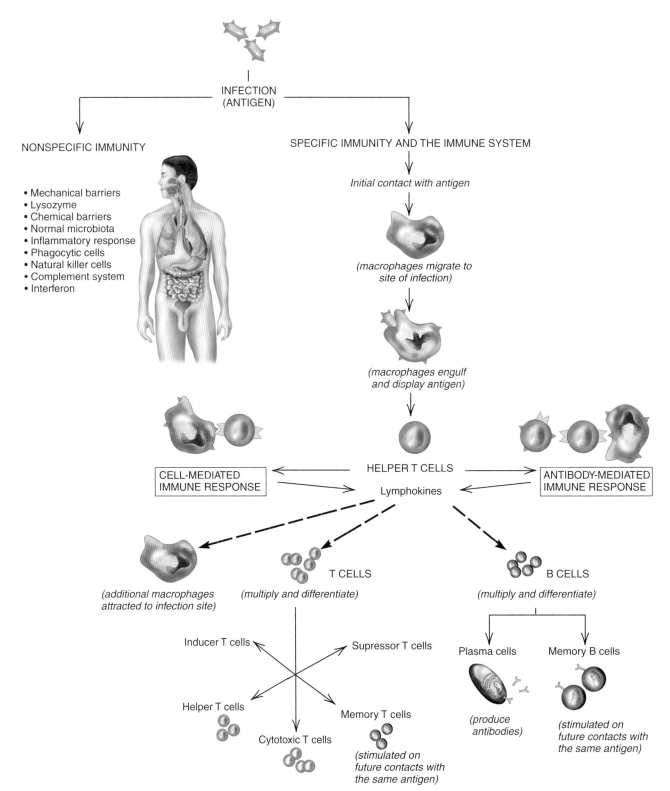

FIGURE 20-3 The process of cell-mediated immunity.

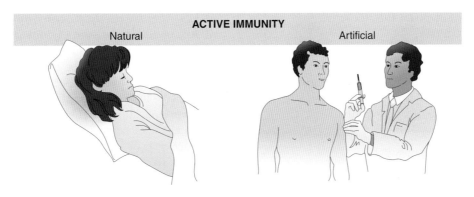

ACTIVE IMMUNITY

Natural   Artificial

(A) Naturally acquired active immunity arises from an exposure to antigens and often follows a disease.

(B) Artificially acquired active immunity results from an inoculation of toxoid or vaccine.

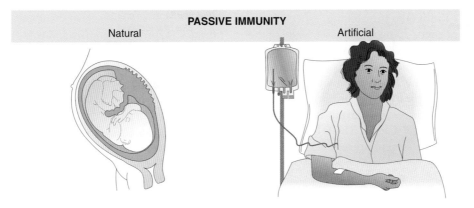

PASSIVE IMMUNITY

Natural   Artificial

(C) Naturally acquired passive immunity stems from the passage of IgG across the placenta from the maternal to the fetal circulation.

(D) Artificially acquired passive immunity is induced by an injection of antibodies taken from the circulation of an animal or another person.

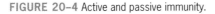

FIGURE 20–4 Active and passive immunity.

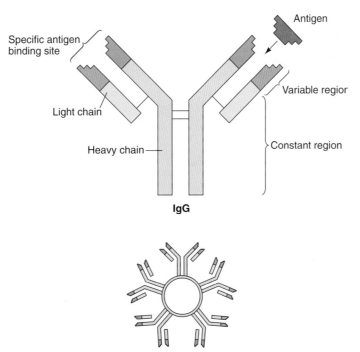

Antigen

Specific antigen binding site

Variable region

Light chain

Heavy chain

Constant region

IgG

IgM

FIGURE 20–5 Antibodies (immunoglobulins) have a characteristic "Y" shape with two antigen binding sites. The IGM isotype can exist in a pentameric (five-subunit) form.

diphtheria vaccine is given intramuscularly to people of all age groups. Infants should receive DTaP vaccine as one of their routine immunizations. Adults should receive a booster vaccine every 10 years. The vaccine is very safe, with only minor adverse effects such as pain and swelling at the injection site, agitation, tiredness, slight fever, loss of appetite, or vomiting.

Pertussis

Pertussis is a highly contagious disease that initially mimics the symptoms of influenza. Advanced cases develop an abrupt cough with a high-pitched sound upon inhaling. This sound gave the disease its commonly used name, whooping cough. The disease has the potential to appear to subside, then return and last for several months. Pertussis can be life threatening, especially for infants. One out of every 20 pertussis cases leads to the development of pneumonia. The most severe adverse effects include neuropathic conditions, including seizures and encephalopathy. The persistent coughing of this disease may cause rib fractures or hernias. Besides the vaccine for pertussis, erythromycin is effective in treating this bacteriological disease. The DTaP vaccine is most commonly administered to prevent pertussis.

Tetanus

POINT TO REMEMBER

Diphtheria and tetanus toxoids and acellular pertussis vaccine (DTaP) is not indicated for persons older than 7 years of age.

Tetanus is caused by a bacterium commonly found in soil and feces; it was first reported in the late 1940s. It usually enters the human body through a puncture wound. Tetanus targets the central nervous system, causing jaw muscle spasms, neck stiffness, difficulty swallowing, and abdominal muscle stiffness. Twenty-two percent of unvaccinated patients with tetanus will die from the disease. When tetanus causes spasm of the vocal chords, the patient may be unable to breathe normally, and convulsions can cause the spine and longer bones to break. Common risks for contracting tetanus include splinters, self-piercing, self-tattooing, and self-injection of drugs. Tetanus is the third component of the DTaP and Tdap vaccines. It is also available as the Td vaccine (which also contains the diphtheria vaccine) and as an immunoglobulin (TIG). Booster doses for tetanus should be given every 10 years. Tetanus can be contracted more than once in a person's lifetime because the toxin is so potent that only a small amount brings on the disease.

Polio

Polio is spread by a virus, usually via the fecal–oral route. Although the majority of patients with polio are asymptomatic, the disease has the potential to cause meningitis, muscle stiffness, and flaccid paralysis of the arms and legs. After the paralysis occurs, up to 5% of children and 30% of adults die from the disease. Polio vaccines have nearly eradicated the disease throughout the world. Dr. Jonas Salk developed the inactivated polio vaccine in 1955, followed by Dr. Albert Sabin's live attenuated polio vaccine in 1961. The Salk vaccine (known as IPV) is administered intramuscularly, and the Sabin vaccine (known as OPV) is given as an oral liquid. However, the OPV vaccine is no longer used in the United States. The intramuscular IPV vaccine is preferred in the United States because of the eradication of wild polio in the Western Hemisphere, but other parts of the world still report cases, which requires the live attenuated OPV vaccine for treatment.

Measles

Measles is spread by a virus and is highly contagious. It is signified by fever and a rash that begins at the hairline then moves to the face, upper neck, and downwards to the rest of the body. The rash usually lasts for 5 to 6 days. Measles is most dangerous in young children and older adults. Diarrhea is the most common complication of measles. Measles can become life threatening if it leads to pneumonia. It is most severe when contracted by immunocompromised patients. The measles vaccine was licensed in the United States in 1963. The combination measles–mumps–rubella (MMR) vaccine became available in 1971, and the measles–mumps–rubella–varicella (MMRV) vaccine became available in 2005. The vaccines are given subcutaneously, in two doses, at 12–15 months of age and then again between 4–6 years of age.

Mumps

Mumps is a viral disease that is not as contagious as measles, with the significant symptom of parotitis (swelling of the parotid glands below each ear). These are salivary glands that the disease causes to become painfully inflamed. However, patients may also have mumps and appear relatively asymptomatic. As many as 50% of males (after puberty) may experience swelling of the testicles, which has the rare potential to lead to testicular atrophy and even sterility. The vaccine for mumps was licensed in 1967. In the United States, immunization against mumps is given as part of the MMR or MMRV vaccines.

Rubella

Rubella is also known as German measles. It is a viral disease that is not as contagious as measles. It usually manifests as a rash beginning on the face and proceeding downwards over the body. Rubella is more serious when contracted by adults than by children. However, the most serious harm from rubella happens when it is contracted by pregnant women. During the first trimester of pregnancy, rubella can cause serious birth defects, premature delivery, and fetal death. The birth defects caused by congenital rubella syndrome (CRS) include deafness, defects of the eyes or heart, mental retardation, and others. The disease was first differentiated from measles in Germany in 1814. The current form of the rubella vaccine was licensed in 1979. Rubella is part of the MMR and MMRV vaccines.

Hepatitis B

Hepatitis B is a viral disease spread by contact with the infected blood of another person, commonly via sexual intercourse. Another common method of transfer is the sharing of needles used for injecting drugs. The disease is also referred to as HBV. Signs of hepatitis B include jaundice as well as yellowing of the eyes and skin. The virus attacks the liver, potentially leading to chronic liver disease that persists throughout the patient's lifetime. Most patients with hepatitis B die from cirrhosis of the liver. Worldwide, HBV is listed as the 10th leading cause of death. A person with HBV is contagious as long as the virus exists in his or her blood. The first hepatitis B vaccine became available in the United States in 1982. The vaccine is administered to all ages of patients by intramuscular injection, usually in three separate doses. Adverse effects are usually minor and not significant.

Haemophilus Influenzae Type B

Haemophilus influenzae type B is a bacterial disease that is also referred to as Hib. It is spread by direct contact or contact with respiratory droplets. The most common type of invasive Hib is meningitis. Hib is treated with antibiotics over approximately 10 days and usually requires hospitalization. The first Hib vaccine was licensed in the United States in 1985. It is administered by intramuscular injection. All infants normally receive a Hib vaccination as part of their standard regimen of immunizations. Hib is prevalent only in children age 5 years or younger, and immunization is therefore not indicated for patients older than that.

Varicella

Varicella (chickenpox) is caused by the varicella-zoster virus. It is spread by direct contact or contact with respiratory droplets. It is highly contagious and can also be spread by direct contact with someone who has shingles, which occurs as a result of the same virus. The main symptom is the development of between 250 and 500 fluid-filled blisters that spread from the scalp to the rest of the body. The symptoms last for up to 10 days. Complications from varicella can cause bacterial infections of many other parts of the body. The disease can be treated with antiviral drugs as well as acetaminophen when fever manifests. The varicella vaccine was first licensed in the

United States in 1995. The vaccine is administered by subcutaneous injection and usually causes only minor adverse effects. The first immunization should be given after the child is 12 months old, with the second dose administered between the ages of 4 and 6 years.

Hepatitis A

Hepatitis A is a viral disease caused by fecal–oral contamination. It is also transmitted sexually. Symptoms are similar to those of hepatitis B. Hepatitis A can cause nearly one-third of affected patients to be hospitalized, and it has the potential to be fatal. However, hepatitis A is an acute, not chronic, form. Travel to many countries of the world requires immunization against hepatitis A. This disease is also referred to as HAV. The first HAV vaccination became available in 1995. It is administered by intramuscular injection in two doses, 6 months apart.

Meningococcal Disease

Meningococcal disease is caused by a bacterium spread by direct contact or contact with respiratory droplets. It is not as contagious as many other diseases. It can cause very serious complications, including meningitis and septicemia. It kills as

> **POINT TO REMEMBER**
>
> Vaccination against invasive meningococcal disease is recommended for children and adolescents older than 2 years of age who have anatomic or functional asplenia; it is also recommended for certain other high-risk groups.

many as 12% of affected patients even after treatment with antibiotics. Up to 20% of recovering patients will have hearing loss, brain damage, or loss of a limb. The disease is most common in children younger than 1 year of age. It is most common in Africa and has a relatively low incidence in the United States. The first vaccination against meningococcal disease was developed in 1974. There are several different types of vaccine available, either administered subcutaneously or intramuscularly. The MCV4 vaccine is recommended for all children between 11 and 18 years of age. Adverse effects of the vaccine are minimal.

Human Papillomavirus

In 2006, the FDA licensed the human papillomavirus (HPV) vaccine to protect women from cervical cancer and other diseases caused by certain types of HPV. Females between 9 and 26 years of age should receive this vaccine. The best time to receive the vaccine is at age 10 or 11, before the onset of sexual activity. The HPV vaccine is given as three intramuscular (IM) injections, with the second dose given 2 months after the first and the final dose given 6 months after the first. The vaccine is effective for approximately 5 years.

Pneumococcal Disease

Pneumococcal disease is caused by a bacterium and is spread by respiratory droplets. It causes three major conditions: pneumonia, bacteremia, and meningitis. Pneumococcal disease kills approximately 5000 people every year in the United States. Penicillin is the drug used most commonly to treat this disease. The first vaccine for this disease was licensed in the United States in 1977. Various types of the vaccine now exist, and it is administered either intramuscularly or subcutaneously. The separate types are indicated for different age groups, ranging from infants to the elderly.

Shingles

Shingles is also known as herpes zoster, a viral disease that is related to chickenpox. Shingles is a painful skin rash that usually appears initially on one side of the face or body, following a period of pain, itching, or tingling in the same area(s). It begins as blisters, which then form scabs in 3 to 5 days. The outbreak of rash can last up to 4 weeks. Twenty percent of patients experience severe pain that lasts after the rash subsides. Shingles usually affects patients older than age 50 years and appears only once, although it can recur up to three times. Patients older than age 60 years should be vaccinated so they cannot develop shingles. Adverse effects of this subcutaneous vaccine are minimal. People with immunocompromised immune systems should not receive the shingles vaccine. The first shingles vaccine became available in the United States in 2007.

Influenza A (2009 H1N1 Flu)

Traditionally, influenza A is not common. However, the newest form of influenza A, commonly known as swine flu or H1N1 flu, was first detected in Mexico in April 2009. From then to November 2009, many countries showed outbreaks of this disease, and it was declared a global pandemic. This type of influenza is of viral origin. It is spread similarly to other forms of influenza, but diseases listed under the type A category are also likely to infect other animals besides humans.

    The incubation period for H1N1 flu is usually 1 to 4 days. This disease is usually more common in people between the ages of 5 and 24 years. Pregnant women are at high risk for 2009 H1N1 flu. Also, patients who suffer from chronic diseases, such as asthma and diabetes, are at a high risk. The clinical features of H1N1 flu include high fever, headache, extreme weakness, dry cough, sore throat, and runny nose. In children, muscle aches and stomach symptoms are common, including diarrhea and vomiting. Symptoms are similar to seasonal flu, but the more serious effects of this disease can cause respiratory problems that can lead to death.

    There are two types of vaccine for H1N1 flu, either by intramuscular injection (contains the inactivated virus) or by intranasal instillation (contains the live virus). The IM injection is more effective than the intranasal form, and it usually causes only slight soreness at the injection site. The intranasal form of this vaccine is liable to cause minor adverse effects, such as nasal congestion, sore throat, fever, headache, muscle pain, wheezing, coughing, or gastrointestinal symptoms. The primary contraindication for the nasal form of this vaccine is allergy to eggs. Pregnancy and breastfeeding are not contraindications for receiving the vaccine. This vaccine may be given concurrently with seasonal flu vaccine and other vaccines.

Influenza B (Seasonal Flu)

This type of influenza is generally less serious than influenza A, and it primarily affects only humans. Seasonal flu is also of viral origin. It is best prevented by receiving an annual flu vaccination. Approximately 36,000 people die in the United States each year due to complications from this type of flu. High-risk groups are the same for this type of flu as for influenza A.

    Serious complications of seasonal flu include bacterial pneumonia, ear infections, dehydration, sinus infections, and worsening of chronic medical conditions. The forms of the available flu vaccines are the same as for H1N1 flu vaccine, with only minimal adverse effects. It takes the body up to 2 weeks to develop antibodies against this type of flu after vaccination.

    The intramuscular form of the vaccine contains an inactivated (killed) virus, and the nasal instillation form contains a live, weakened (attenuated) virus. Neither vaccine will give patients the flu, although minor flulike symptoms may occur as the body begins to produce antibodies against the disease.

> **POINT TO REMEMBER**
>
> The minimum age for administration of influenza vaccine is 6 months for inactivated vaccine and 5 years for live (attenuated influenza) vaccine.

Tuberculosis

The first tuberculosis vaccine was administered to humans in 1921. It is known as the bacillus Calmette-Guérin (BCG) vaccine, designed to prevent the development of tuberculosis in persons who are at high risk for infection. BCG is an attenuated strain of *Mycobacterium tuberculosis bovis*. It is administered only to persons who have a negative tuberculin skin test result. This intradermal vaccine produces a local reaction that may last as long as 3 months and leave a scar at the injection site. Individuals who are vaccinated with BCG usually have a positive tuberculin skin reaction that disappears over time and is unlikely to persist beyond 10 years.

    BCG is the only tuberculosis vaccine. Worldwide, it is used as a major method of prevention for tuberculosis.

It is not generally recommended in the United States because of the low prevalence of tuberculosis infection. This is also true because of the vaccine's interference with the determination of latent tuberculosis in skin tests and its variable effectiveness against pulmonary tuberculosis. In settings where patients are infected with drug-resistant tuberculosis strains, healthcare workers may be considered for vaccination on an individual basis. BCG vaccine is contraindicated in persons who are infected with HIV.

Rabies

Rabies is a viral infection that is spread from animals to other animals or humans. If untreated, human rabies is usually fatal. When a rabid animal bites, the virus transfers from its saliva into the bite wound. Cats may transfer rabies via their claws as well as their bites. Wild animals are likely to get rabies, as are unvaccinated domesticated animals. At first, untreated bites may not result in any symptoms, but after weeks or months, a variety of indicative symptoms will occur. These include pain, fatigue, headaches, fever, and irritability. Following these symptoms, seizures, hallucinations, and paralysis result, with eventual and irreversible brain damage. The animals most likely to transmit rabies are bats, followed by skunks, raccoons, dogs, cats, coyotes, foxes, and other animals.

Bats are different from other animals in that it is possible to contract rabies by being in close contact with them and not actually receiving a bite. Rabies in humans is very rare in the United States. Humans may elect to get a series of prophylactic rabies vaccines if they work in jobs that put them in potentially high-risk situations. If a human is exposed to the rabies virus and the rabid animal cannot be located for testing, immunizations should be started. The schedule of immunizations for rabies is listed in **Table 20–1**.

Immunization

Immunization is the process of introducing an antigen into the body to induce protection against an infectious agent without causing disease. Immunization is most commonly performed by giving an injection. However, some immunizations are administered orally, such as the polio immunization. In the future, some immunizations that are currently injected will be given by means of nasal sprays or drops. Currently, the immunization for H1N1 flu is available either for nasal administration or injection. Immunizations are commonly given to all age groups, including infants, children, teenagers, adults, and the elderly.

Recommended Immunizations for Children Aged 0–6 Years

The major childhood communicable diseases include diphtheria, pertussis, tetanus, polio, measles, mumps, rubella, hepatitis B, and *Haemophilus influenzae* type B infection. According to the Advisory Committee on

TABLE 20–1 Rabies Immunization Schedule

Vaccine Type	Administration Time
Rabies immune globulin (RIG)	First day after the wound, with as much as possible (based on the size of the wound) administered around the wound and the remainder administered intramuscularly (IM) at a distant site
First rabies vaccine	Immediately following the administration of rabies immune globulin
Second rabies vaccine	On day 3 after the first administration
Third rabies vaccine	On day 7 after the first administration
Fourth rabies vaccine	On day 14 after the first administration
Fifth (final) rabies vaccine	On day 28 after the first administration

Immunization Practices (ACIP), children should be immunized against these infectious diseases. In areas of high incidence, they should also be immunized against hepatitis A. The childhood immunization schedule (from birth to 6 years) is summarized in **Table 20–2**.

Recommended Immunizations for Children Aged 7–18 Years

Annual influenza immunization is recommended for this age group if there is high risk of influenza infection. **Table 20–3** lists recommended immunizations for children between 7 and 18 years of age.

Recommended Adult Immunizations

The same vaccinations as listed previously for childhood administration are approved for adults—except for pertussis. Patients should be given only diphtheria and tetanus (DT) after age 6 years via a booster or if they did not receive any vaccines before age 6 years. This booster is approved for adults between ages 18 and 65 and can be given every 10 years. Adults should make sure that their pediatric immunizations are up to date if they travel internationally, if they become pregnant, or if they have chronic illnesses. Adults with immunosuppressed conditions (such as HIV), pulmonary or cardiovascular diseases, chronic hepatic or renal disorders, and diabetes mellitus should receive pneumococcal vaccine. Meningococcal vaccine is recommended for certain travelers and for people in areas where outbreaks can occur. International travelers may be required, depending on their travel itinerary, to receive immunizations against yellow fever, hepatitis A, cholera, typhoid, or plague. Healthcare workers may be required to receive hepatitis B vaccine due to higher risks of exposure in their workplaces. Other vaccines that are recommended for adults are summarized in **Table 20–4**.

TABLE 20-2 Childhood Immunization Schedule (From Birth to Six Years)

Recommended Immunization Schedule for Persons Aged 0 Through 6 Years—United States • 2010
For those who fall behind or start late, see the catch-up schedule

Vaccine ▼ Age ►	Birth	1 month	2 months	4 months	6 months	12 months	15 months	18 months	19–23 months	2–3 years	4–6 years
Hepatitis B[1]	HepB	HepB				HepB					
Rotavirus[2]			RV	RV	RV[2]						
Diphtheria, Tetanus, Pertussis[3]			DTaP	DTaP	DTaP	see footnote[3]	DTaP				DTaP
Haemophilus influenzae type b[4]			Hib	Hib	Hib[4]	Hib					
Pneumococcal[5]			PCV	PCV	PCV	PCV				PPSV	
Inactivated Poliovirus[6]			IPV	IPV		IPV					IPV
Influenza[7]						Influenza (Yearly)					
Measles, Mumps, Rubella[8]						MMR		see footnote[8]			MMR
Varicella[9]						Varicella		see footnote[9]			Varicella
Hepatitis A[10]						HepA (2 doses)				HepA Series	
Meningococcal[11]										MCV	

Range of recommended ages for all children except certain high-risk groups

Range of recommended ages for certain high-risk groups

This schedule includes recommendations in effect as of December 15, 2009. Any dose not administered at the recommended age should be administered at a subsequent visit, when indicated and feasible. The use of a combination vaccine generally is preferred over separate injections of its equivalent component vaccines. Considerations should include provider assessment, patient preference, and the potential for adverse events. Providers should consult the relevant Advisory Committee on Immunization Practices statement for detailed recommendations: **http://www.cdc.gov/vaccines/pubs/acip-list.htm**. Clinically significant adverse events that follow immunization should be reported to the Vaccine Adverse Event Reporting System (VAERS) at **http://www.vaers.hhs.gov** or by telephone, **800-822-7967.**

1. **Hepatitis B vaccine (HepB).** (Minimum age: birth)
   At birth:
   - Administer monovalent HepB to all newborns before hospital discharge.
   - If mother is hepatitis B surface antigen (HBsAg)-positive, administer HepB and 0.5 mL of hepatitis B immune globulin (HBIG) within 12 hours of birth.
   - If mother's HBsAg status is unknown, administer HepB within 12 hours of birth. Determine mother's HBsAg status as soon as possible and, if HBsAg-positive, administer HBIG (no later than age 1 week).
   After the birth dose:
   - The HepB series should be completed with either monovalent HepB or a combination vaccine containing HepB. The second dose should be administered at age 1 or 2 months. Monovalent HepB vaccine should be used for doses administered before age 6 weeks. The final dose should be administered no earlier than age 24 weeks.
   - Infants born to HBsAg-positive mothers should be tested for HBsAg and antibody to HBsAg 1 to 2 months after completion of at least 3 doses of the HepB series, at age 9 through 18 months (generally at the next well-child visit).
   - Administration of 4 doses of HepB to infants is permissible when a combination vaccine containing HepB is administered after the birth dose. The fourth dose should be administered no earlier than age 24 weeks.
2. **Rotavirus vaccine (RV).** (Minimum age: 6 weeks)
   - Administer the first dose at age 6 through 14 weeks (maximum age: 14 weeks 6 days). Vaccination should not be initiated for infants aged 15 weeks 0 days or older.
   - The maximum age for the final dose in the series is 8 months 0 days
   - If Rotarix is administered at ages 2 and 4 months, a dose at 6 months is not indicated.
3. **Diphtheria and tetanus toxoids and acellular pertussis vaccine (DTaP).** (Minimum age: 6 weeks)
   - The fourth dose may be administered as early as age 12 months, provided at least 6 months have elapsed since the third dose.
   - Administer the final dose in the series at age 4 through 6 years.
4. ***Haemophilus influenzae* type b conjugate vaccine (Hib).** (Minimum age: 6 weeks)
   - If PRP-OMP (PedvaxHIB or Comvax [HepB-Hib]) is administered at ages 2 and 4 months, a dose at age 6 months is not indicated.
   - TriHiBit (DTaP/Hib) and Hiberix (PRP-T) should not be used for doses at ages 2, 4, or 6 months for the primary series but can be used as the final dose in children aged 12 months through 4 years.
5. **Pneumococcal vaccine.** (Minimum age: 6 weeks for pneumococcal conjugate vaccine [PCV]; 2 years for pneumococcal polysaccharide vaccine [PPSV])
   - PCV is recommended for all children aged younger than 5 years. Administer 1 dose of PCV to all healthy children aged 24 through 59 months who are not completely vaccinated for their age.
   - Administer PPSV 2 or more months after last dose of PCV to children aged 2 years or older with certain underlying medical conditions, including a cochlear implant. See *MMWR* 1997;46(No. RR-8).

6. **Inactivated poliovirus vaccine (IPV)** (Minimum age: 6 weeks)
   - The final dose in the series should be administered on or after the fourth birthday and at least 6 months following the previous dose.
   - If 4 doses are administered prior to age 4 years a fifth dose should be administered at age 4 through 6 years. See *MMWR* 2009;58(30):829–30.
7. **Influenza vaccine (seasonal).** (Minimum age: 6 months for trivalent inactivated influenza vaccine [TIV]; 2 years for live, attenuated influenza vaccine [LAIV])
   - Administer annually to children aged 6 months through 18 years.
   - For healthy children aged 2 through 6 years (i.e., those who do not have underlying medical conditions that predispose them to influenza complications), either LAIV or TIV may be used, except LAIV should not be given to children aged 2 through 4 years who have had wheezing in the past 12 months.
   - Children receiving TIV should receive 0.25 mL if aged 6 through 35 months or 0.5 mL if aged 3 years or older.
   - Administer 2 doses (separated by at least 4 weeks) to children aged younger than 9 years who are receiving influenza vaccine for the first time or who were vaccinated for the first time during the previous influenza season but only received 1 dose.
   - For recommendations for use of influenza A (H1N1) 2009 monovalent vaccine see *MMWR* 2009;58(No. RR-10).
8. **Measles, mumps, and rubella vaccine (MMR).** (Minimum age: 12 months)
   - Administer the second dose routinely at age 4 through 6 years. However, the second dose may be administered before age 4, provided at least 28 days have elapsed since the first dose.
9. **Varicella vaccine.** (Minimum age: 12 months)
   - Administer the second dose routinely at age 4 through 6 years. However, the second dose may be administered before age 4, provided at least 3 months have elapsed since the first dose.
   - For children aged 12 months through 12 years the minimum interval between doses is 3 months. However, if the second dose was administered at least 28 days after the first dose, it can be accepted as valid.
10. **Hepatitis A vaccine (HepA).** (Minimum age: 12 months)
    - Administer to all children aged 1 year (i.e., aged 12 through 23 months). Administer 2 doses at least 6 months apart.
    - Children not fully vaccinated by age 2 years can be vaccinated at subsequent visits
    - HepA also is recommended for older children who live in areas where vaccination programs target older children, who are at increased risk for infection, or for whom immunity against hepatitis A is desired.
11. **Meningococcal vaccine.** (Minimum age: 2 years for meningococcal conjugate vaccine [MCV4] and for meningococcal polysaccharide vaccine [MPSV4])
    - Administer MCV4 to children aged 2 through 10 years with persistent complement component deficiency, anatomic or functional asplenia, and certain other conditions placing them at high risk.
    - Administer MCV4 to children previously vaccinated with MCV4 or MPSV4 after 3 years if first dose administered at age 2 through 6 years. See *MMWR* 2009;58:1042–3.

The Recommended Immunization Schedules for Persons Aged 0 through 18 Years are approved by the Advisory Committee on Immunization Practices (**http://www.cdc.gov/vaccines/recs/acip**), the American Academy of Pediatrics (**http://www.aap.org**), and the American Academy of Family Physicians (**http://www.aafp.org**).

CS207330-A

TABLE 20-2 Recommended Immunizations for Children Between 7 and 18 Years of Age

Recommended Immunization Schedule for Persons Aged 7 Through 18 Years—United States • 2010
For those who fall behind or start late, see the schedule below and the catch-up schedule

Vaccine ▼ Age ▶	7–10 years	11–12 years	13–18 years
Tetanus, Diphtheria, Pertussis[1]		Tdap	Tdap
Human Papillomavirus[2]	see footnote 2	HPV (3 doses)	HPV series
Meningococcal[3]	MCV	MCV	MCV
Influenza[4]	Influenza (Yearly)		
Pneumococcal[5]	PPSV		
Hepatitis A[6]	HepA Series		
Hepatitis B[7]	Hep B Series		
Inactivated Poliovirus[8]	IPV Series		
Measles, Mumps, Rubella[9]	MMR Series		
Varicella[10]	Varicella Series		

Legend:
- Range of recommended ages for all children except certain high-risk groups
- Range of recommended ages for catch-up immunization
- Range of recommended ages for certain high-risk groups

This schedule includes recommendations in effect as of December 15, 2009. Any dose not administered at the recommended age should be administered at a subsequent visit, when indicated and feasible. The use of a combination vaccine generally is preferred over separate injections of its equivalent component vaccines. Considerations should include provider assessment, patient preference, and the potential for adverse events. Providers should consult the relevant Advisory Committee on Immunization Practices statement for detailed recommendations: http://www.cdc.gov/vaccines/pubs/acip-list.htm. Clinically significant adverse events that follow immunization should be reported to the Vaccine Adverse Event Reporting System (VAERS) at http://www.vaers.hhs.gov or by telephone, 800-822-7967.

1. **Tetanus and diphtheria toxoids and acellular pertussis vaccine (Tdap).** (Minimum age: 10 years for Boostrix and 11 years for Adacel)
   - Administer at age 11 or 12 years for those who have completed the recommended childhood DTP/DTaP vaccination series and have not received a tetanus and diphtheria toxoid (Td) booster dose.
   - Persons aged 13 through 18 years who have not received Tdap should receive a dose.
   - A 5-year interval from the last Td dose is encouraged when Tdap is used as a booster dose; however, a shorter interval may be used if pertussis immunity is needed.
2. **Human papillomavirus vaccine (HPV).** (Minimum age: 9 years)
   - Two HPV vaccines are licensed: a quadrivalent vaccine (HPV4) for the prevention of cervical, vaginal and vulvar cancers (in females) and genital warts (in females and males), and a bivalent vaccine (HPV2) for the prevention of cervical cancers in females.
   - HPV vaccines are most effective for both males and females when given before exposure to HPV through sexual contact.
   - HPV4 or HPV2 is recommended for the prevention of cervical precancers and cancers in females.
   - HPV4 is recommended for the prevention of cervical, vaginal and vulvar precancers and cancers and genital warts in females.
   - Administer the first dose to females at age 11 or 12 years.
   - Administer the second dose 1 to 2 months after the first dose and the third dose 6 months after the first dose (at least 24 weeks after the first dose).
   - Administer the series to females at age 13 through 18 years if not previously vaccinated.
   - HPV4 may be administered in a 3-dose series to males aged 9 through 18 years to reduce their likelihood of acquiring genital warts.
3. **Meningococcal conjugate vaccine (MCV4).**
   - Administer at age 11 or 12 years, or at age 13 through 18 years if not previously vaccinated.
   - Administer to previously unvaccinated college freshmen living in a dormitory.
   - Administer MCV4 to children aged 2 through 10 years with persistent complement component deficiency, anatomic or functional asplenia, or certain other conditions placing them at high risk.
   - Administer to children previously vaccinated with MCV4 or MPSV4 who remain at increased risk after 3 years (if first dose administered at age 2 through 6 years) or after 5 years (if first dose administered at age 7 years or older). Persons whose only risk factor is living in on-campus housing are not recommended to receive an additional dose. See MMWR 2009;58:1042–3.

4. **Influenza vaccine (seasonal).**
   - Administer annually to children aged 6 months through 18 years.
   - For healthy nonpregnant persons aged 7 through 18 years (i.e., those who do not have underlying medical conditions that predispose them to influenza complications), either LAIV or TIV may be used.
   - Administer 2 doses (separated by at least 4 weeks) to children aged younger than 9 years who are receiving influenza vaccine for the first time or who were vaccinated for the first time during the previous influenza season but only received 1 dose.
   - For recommendations for use of influenza A (H1N1) 2009 monovalent vaccine. See MMWR 2009;58(No. RR-10).
5. **Pneumococcal polysaccharide vaccine (PPSV).**
   - Administer to children with certain underlying medical conditions, including a cochlear implant. A single revaccination should be administered after 5 years to children with functional or anatomic asplenia or an immunocompromising condition. See MMWR 1997;46(No. RR-8).
6. **Hepatitis A vaccine (HepA).**
   - Administer 2 doses at least 6 months apart.
   - HepA is recommended for children aged older than 23 months who live in areas where vaccination programs target older children, who are at increased risk for infection, or for whom immunity against hepatitis A is desired.
7. **Hepatitis B vaccine (HepB).**
   - Administer the 3-dose series to those not previously vaccinated.
   - A 2-dose series (separated by at least 4 months) of adult formulation Recombivax HB is licensed for children aged 11 through 15 years.
8. **Inactivated poliovirus vaccine (IPV).**
   - The final dose in the series should be administered on or after the fourth birthday and at least 6 months following the previous dose.
   - If both OPV and IPV were administered as part of a series, a total of 4 doses should be administered, regardless of the child's current age.
9. **Measles, mumps, and rubella vaccine (MMR).**
   - If not previously vaccinated, administer 2 doses or the second dose for those who have received only 1 dose, with at least 28 days between doses.
10. **Varicella vaccine.**
   - For persons aged 7 through 18 years without evidence of immunity (see MMWR 2007;56[No. RR-4]), administer 2 doses if not previously vaccinated or the second dose if only 1 dose has been administered.
   - For persons aged 7 through 12 years, the minimum interval between doses is 3 months. However, if the second dose was administered at least 28 days after the first dose, it can be accepted as valid.
   - For persons aged 13 years and older, the minimum interval between doses is 28 days.

TABLE 20-4 Adult Immunization Schedule

Recommended Adult Immunization Schedule
UNITED STATES - 2010

Note: These recommendations *must* be read with the footnotes that follow containing number of doses, intervals between doses, and other important information.

Figure 1. Recommended adult immunization schedule, by vaccine and age group

VACCINE ▼ AGE GROUP ▶	19–26 years	27–49 years	50–59 years	60–64 years	≥65 years
Tetanus, diphtheria, pertussis (Td/Tdap)[1],*	Substitute 1-time dose of Tdap for Td booster; then boost with Td every 10 yrs				Td booster every 10 yrs
Human papillomavirus (HPV)[2],*	3 doses (females)				
Varicella[3],*	2 doses				
Zoster[4]				1 dose	
Measles, mumps, rubella (MMR)[5],*	1 or 2 doses		1 dose		
Influenza[6],*	1 dose annually				
Pneumococcal (polysaccharide)[7,8]	1 or 2 doses				1 dose
Hepatitis A[9],*	2 doses				
Hepatitis B[10],*	3 doses				
Meningococcal[11],*	1 or more doses				

*Covered by the Vaccine Injury Compensation Program.

For all persons in this category who meet the age requirements and who lack evidence of immunity (e.g., lack documentation of vaccination or have no evidence of prior infection)

Recommended if some other risk factor is present (e.g., on the basis of medical, occupational, lifestyle, or other indications)

No recommendation

Report all clinically significant postvaccination reactions to the Vaccine Adverse Event Reporting System (VAERS). Reporting forms and instructions on filing a VAERS report are available at www.vaers.hhs.gov or by telephone, 800-822-7967.

Information on how to file a Vaccine Injury Compensation Program claim is available at www.hrsa.gov/vaccinecompensation or by telephone, 800-338-2382. To file a claim for vaccine injury, contact the U.S. Court of Federal Claims, 717 Madison Place, N.W., Washington, D.C. 20005; telephone, 202-357-6400.

Additional information about the vaccines in this schedule, extent of available data, and contraindications for vaccination is also available at www.cdc.gov/vaccines or from the CDC-INFO Contact Center at 800-CDC-INFO (800-232-4636) in English and Spanish, 24 hours a day, 7 days a week.

Use of trade names and commercial sources is for identification only and does not imply endorsement by the U.S. Department of Health and Human Services.

Figure 2. Vaccines that might be indicated for adults based on medical and other indications

VACCINE ▼ / INDICATION ▶	Pregnancy	Immuno-compromising conditions (excluding human immunodeficiency virus [HIV])[3-5,13]	HIV infection[3-5,12,13] CD4+ T lymphocyte count <200 cells/µL	HIV infection CD4+ T lymphocyte count ≥200 cells/µL	Diabetes, heart disease, chronic lung disease, chronic alcoholism	Asplenia[12] (including elective splenectomy and persistent complement component deficiencies)	Chronic liver disease	Kidney failure, end-stage renal disease, receipt of hemodialysis	Health-care personnel
Tetanus, diphtheria, pertussis (Td/Tdap)[1,*]	Td	Substitute 1-time dose of Tdap for Td booster; then boost with Td every 10 yrs							
Human papillomavirus (HPV)[2,*]		3 doses for females through age 26 yrs							
Varicella[3,*]	Contraindicated	Contraindicated		2 doses					
Zoster[4]	Contraindicated	Contraindicated		1 dose					
Measles, mumps, rubella (MMR)[5,*]	Contraindicated	Contraindicated		1 or 2 doses					
Influenza[6,*]		1 dose TIV annually								1 dose TIV or LAIV annually
Pneumococcal (polysaccharide)[7,8]		1 or 2 doses							
Hepatitis A[9,*]		2 doses							
Hepatitis B[10,*]		3 doses							
Meningococcal[11,*]		1 or more doses							

* Covered by the Vaccine Injury Compensation Program.

Recommended if some other risk factor is present (e.g., on the basis of medical, occupational, lifestyle, or other indications)

For all persons in this category who meet the age requirements and who lack evidence of immunity (e.g., lack documentation of vaccination or have no evidence of prior infection)

No recommendation

These schedules indicate the recommended age groups and medical indications for which administration of currently licensed vaccines is commonly indicated for adults ages 19 years and older, as of January 1, 2010. Licensed combination vaccines may be used whenever any components of the combination are indicated and when the vaccine's other components are not contraindicated. For detailed recommendations on all vaccines, including those used primarily for travelers or that are issued during the year, consult the manufacturers' package inserts and the complete statements from the Advisory Committee on Immunization Practices (www.cdc.gov/vaccines/pubs/acip-list.htm).

The recommendations in this schedule were approved by the Centers for Disease Control and Prevention's (CDC) Advisory Committee on Immunization Practices (ACIP), the American Academy of Family Physicians (AAFP), the American College of Obstetricians and Gynecologists (ACOG), and the American College of Physicians (ACP).

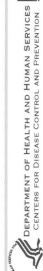

DEPARTMENT OF HEALTH AND HUMAN SERVICES
CENTERS FOR DISEASE CONTROL AND PREVENTION

CS209938-A

TABLE 20-4 (continued)

Footnotes

Recommended Adult Immunization Schedule—UNITED STATES · 2010

For complete statements by the Advisory Committee on Immunization Practices (ACIP), visit www.cdc.gov/vaccines/pubs/ACIP-list.htm.

1. Tetanus, diphtheria, and acellular pertussis (Td/Tdap) vaccination

Tdap should replace a single dose of Td for adults aged 19 through 64 years who have not received a dose of Tdap previously.

Adults with uncertain or incomplete history of primary vaccination series with tetanus and diphtheria toxoid-containing vaccines should begin or complete a primary vaccination series. A primary series for adults is 3 doses of tetanus and diphtheria toxoid-containing vaccines; administer the first 2 doses at least 4 weeks apart and the third dose 6–12 months after the second; Tdap can substitute for any one of the doses of Td in the 3-dose primary series. The booster dose of tetanus and diphtheria toxoid-containing vaccine should be administered to adults who have completed a primary series and if the last vaccination was received ≥10 years previously. Tdap or Td vaccine may be used, as indicated.

If a woman is pregnant and received the last Td vaccination ≥10 years previously, administer Tdap during the second or third trimester. If the woman received the last Td vaccination <10 years previously, administer Tdap during the immediate postpartum period. A dose of Tdap is recommended for postpartum women, close contacts of infants aged <12 months, and all health-care personnel with direct patient contact if they have not previously received Tdap. An interval as short as 2 years from the last Td is suggested; shorter intervals can be used. Td may be deferred during pregnancy and Tdap substituted in the immediate postpartum period, or Tdap can be administered instead of Td to a pregnant woman. Consult the ACIP statement for recommendations for giving Td as prophylaxis in wound management.

2. Human papillomavirus (HPV) vaccination

HPV vaccination is recommended at age 11 or 12 years with catch-up vaccination at ages 13 through 26 years.

Ideally, vaccine should be administered before potential exposure to HPV through sexual activity; however, females who are sexually active should still be vaccinated consistent with age-based recommendations. Sexually active females who have not been infected with any of the four HPV vaccine types (types 6, 11, 16, 18 all of which HPV4 prevents) or any of the two HPV vaccine types (types 16 and 18 both of which HPV2 prevents) receive the full benefit of the vaccination. Vaccination is less beneficial for females who have already been infected with one or more of the HPV vaccine types. HPV4 or HPV2 can be administered to persons with a history of genital warts, abnormal Papanicolaou test, or positive HPV DNA test, because these conditions are not evidence of prior infection with all vaccine HPV types.

HPV4 may be administered to males aged 9 through 26 years to reduce their likelihood of acquiring genital warts. HPV4 would be most effective when administered before exposure to HPV through sexual contact.

A complete series for either HPV4 or HPV2 consists of 3 doses. The second dose should be administered 1–2 months after the first dose; the third dose should be administered 6 months after the first dose.

Although HPV vaccination is not specifically recommended for persons with the medical indications described in Figure 2, "Vaccines that might be indicated for adults based on medical and other indications," it may be administered to these persons because the HPV vaccine is not a live-virus vaccine. However, the immune response and vaccine efficacy might be less for persons with the medical indications described in Figure 2 than in persons who do not have the medical indications described or who are immunocompetent. Health-care personnel are not at increased risk because of occupational exposure, and should be vaccinated consistent with age-based recommendations.

3. Varicella vaccination

All adults without evidence of immunity to varicella should receive 2 doses of single-antigen varicella vaccine if not previously vaccinated or the second dose if they have received only 1 dose, unless they have a medical contraindication. Special consideration should be given to those who 1) have close contact with persons at high risk for severe disease (e.g., health-care personnel and family contacts of persons with immunocompromising conditions) or 2) are at high risk for exposure or transmission (e.g., teachers; child-care employees; residents and staff members of institutional settings, including correctional institutions; college students; military personnel; adolescents and adults living in households with children; nonpregnant women of childbearing age; and international travelers).

Evidence of immunity to varicella in adults includes any of the following: 1) documentation of 2 doses of varicella vaccine at least 4 weeks apart; 2) U.S.-born before 1980 (although for health-care personnel and pregnant women, birth before 1980 should not be considered evidence of immunity); 3) history of varicella based on diagnosis or verification of varicella by a health-care provider (for a patient reporting a history of or presenting with an atypical case, a mild case, or both, health-care providers should seek either an epidemiologic link with a typical varicella case or evidence of laboratory confirmation, if it was performed at the time of acute disease); 4) history of herpes zoster based on diagnosis or verification of herpes zoster by a health-care provider; or 5) laboratory evidence of immunity or laboratory confirmation of disease.

Pregnant women should be assessed for evidence of varicella immunity. Women who do not have evidence of immunity should receive the first dose of varicella vaccine upon completion or termination of pregnancy and before discharge from the health-care facility. The second dose should be administered 4–8 weeks after the first dose.

4. Herpes zoster vaccination

A single dose of zoster vaccine is recommended for adults aged ≥60 years regardless of whether they report a prior episode of herpes zoster. Persons with chronic medical conditions may be vaccinated unless their condition constitutes a contraindication.

5. Measles, mumps, rubella (MMR) vaccination

Adults born before 1957 generally are considered immune to measles and mumps.

Measles component: Adults born during or after 1957 should receive 1 or more doses of MMR vaccine unless they have 1) a medical contraindication; 2) documentation of vaccination with 1 or more doses of MMR vaccine; 3) laboratory evidence of immunity; or 4) documentation of physician-diagnosed measles.

A second dose of MMR vaccine, administered 4 weeks after the first dose, is recommended for adults who 1) have been recently exposed to measles or are in an outbreak setting; 2) have been vaccinated previously with killed measles vaccine; 3) have been vaccinated with an unknown type of measles vaccine during 1963–1967; 4) are students in postsecondary educational institutions; 5) work in a health-care facility; or 6) plan to travel internationally.

Mumps component: Adults born during or after 1957 should receive 1 dose of MMR vaccine unless they have 1) a medical contraindication; 2) documentation of vaccination with 1 or more doses of MMR vaccine; 3) laboratory evidence of immunity; or 4) documentation of physician-diagnosed mumps.

A second dose of MMR vaccine, administered 4 weeks after the first dose, is recommended for adults who 1) live in a community experiencing a mumps outbreak and are in an affected age group; 2) are students in postsecondary educational institutions; 3) work in a health-care facility; or 4) plan to travel internationally.

Rubella component: 1 dose of MMR vaccine is recommended for women who do not have documentation of rubella vaccination, or who lack laboratory evidence of immunity. For women of childbearing age, regardless of birth year, rubella immunity should be determined and women should be counseled regarding congenital rubella syndrome. Women who do not have evidence of immunity should receive MMR vaccine upon completion or termination of pregnancy and before discharge from the health-care facility.

Health-care personnel born before 1957: For unvaccinated health-care personnel born before 1957 who lack laboratory evidence of measles, mumps, and/or rubella immunity or laboratory confirmation of disease, health-care facilities should consider vaccinating personnel with 2 doses of MMR vaccine at the appropriate interval (for measles and mumps) and 1 dose of MMR vaccine (for rubella), respectively.

During outbreaks, health-care facilities should recommend that unvaccinated health-care personnel born before 1957, who lack laboratory evidence of measles, mumps, and/or rubella immunity or laboratory confirmation of disease, receive 2 doses of MMR vaccine during an outbreak of measles or mumps, and 1 dose during an outbreak of rubella.

Complete information about evidence of immunity is available at www.cdc.gov/vaccines/recs/provisional/default.htm.

6. Seasonal Influenza vaccination

Vaccinate all persons aged ≥50 years and any younger persons who would like to decrease their risk of getting influenza. Vaccinate persons aged 19 through 49 years with any of the following indications.

Medical: Chronic disorders of the cardiovascular or pulmonary systems, including asthma; chronic metabolic diseases, including diabetes mellitus; renal or hepatic dysfunction, hemoglobinopathies, or immunocompromising conditions (including immunocompromising conditions caused by medications or HIV); cognitive, neurologic or neuromuscular disorders; and pregnancy during the influenza season. No data exist on the risk for severe or complicated influenza disease among persons with asplenia; however, influenza is a risk factor for secondary bacterial infections that can cause severe disease among persons with asplenia.

Occupational: All health-care personnel, including those employed by long-term care and assisted-living facilities, and caregivers of children aged <5 years.

Other: Residents of nursing homes and other long-term care and assisted-living facilities; persons likely to transmit influenza to persons at high risk (e.g., in-home household contacts and caregivers of children aged <5 years, persons aged ≥50 years, and persons of all ages with high-risk conditions).

Healthy, nonpregnant adults aged <50 years without high-risk medical conditions who are not contacts of severely immunocompromised persons in special-care units may receive either intranasally administered live, attenuated influenza vaccine (FluMist) or inactivated vaccine. Other persons should receive the inactivated vaccine.

7. Pneumococcal polysaccharide (PPSV) vaccination

Vaccinate all persons with the following indications.

Medical: Chronic lung disease (including asthma); chronic cardiovascular diseases; diabetes mellitus; chronic liver diseases, cirrhosis, chronic alcoholism; functional or anatomic asplenia (e.g., sickle cell disease or splenectomy [if elective splenectomy is planned, vaccinate at least 2 weeks before surgery]); immunocompromising conditions including chronic renal failure or nephrotic syndrome; and cochlear implants and cerebrospinal fluid leaks. Vaccinate as close to HIV diagnosis as possible.

Other: Residents of nursing homes or long-term care facilities and persons who smoke cigarettes. Routine use of PPSV is not recommended for American Indians/Alaska Natives or persons aged <65 years unless they have underlying medical conditions that are PPSV indications. However, public health authorities may consider recommending PPSV for American Indians/Alaska Natives and persons aged 50 through 64 years who are living in areas where the risk for invasive pneumococcal disease is increased.

8. Revaccination with PPSV

One-time revaccination after 5 years is recommended for persons with chronic renal failure or nephrotic syndrome; functional or anatomic asplenia (e.g., sickle cell disease or splenectomy); and for persons with immunocompromising conditions. For persons aged ≥65 years, one-time revaccination is recommended if they were vaccinated ≥5 years previously and were younger than aged <65 years at the time of primary vaccination.

9. Hepatitis A vaccination

Vaccinate persons with any of the following indications and any person seeking protection from hepatitis A virus (HAV) infection.

Behavioral: Men who have sex with men and persons who use injection drugs.

Occupational: Persons working with HAV-infected primates or with HAV in a research laboratory setting.

Medical: Persons with chronic liver disease and persons who receive clotting factor concentrates.

Other: Persons traveling to or working in countries that have high or intermediate endemicity of hepatitis A (a list of countries is available at www.cdc.gov/travel/contentdiseases.aspx).

Unvaccinated persons who anticipate close personal contact (e.g., household contact or regular babysitting) with an international adoptee from a country of high or intermediate endemicity during the first 60 days after arrival of the adoptee in the United States should consider vaccination. The first dose of the 2-dose hepatitis A vaccine series should be administered as soon as adoption is planned, ideally ≥2 weeks before the arrival of the adoptee.

Single-antigen vaccine formulations should be administered in a 2-dose schedule at either 0 and 6–12 months (Havrix), or 0 and 6–18 months (Vaqta). If the combined hepatitis A and hepatitis B vaccine (Twinrix) is used, administer 3 doses at 0, 1, and 6 months; alternatively, a 4-dose schedule, administered on days 0, 7, and 21–30 followed by a booster dose at month 12 may be used.

10. Hepatitis B vaccination

Vaccinate persons with any of the following indications and any person seeking protection from hepatitis B virus (HBV) infection.

Behavioral: Sexually active persons who are not in a long-term, mutually monogamous relationship (e.g., persons with more than one sex partner during the previous 6 months); persons seeking evaluation or treatment for a sexually transmitted disease (STD); current or recent injection-drug users; and men who have sex with men.

Occupational: Health-care personnel and public-safety workers who are exposed to blood or other potentially infectious body fluids.

Medical: Persons with end-stage renal disease, including patients receiving hemodialysis; persons with HIV infection; and persons with chronic liver disease.

Other: Household contacts and sex partners of persons with chronic HBV infection; clients and staff members of institutions for persons with developmental disabilities; and international travelers to countries with high or intermediate prevalence of chronic HBV infection (a list of countries is available at www.cdc.gov/travel/contentdiseases.aspx).

Hepatitis B vaccination is recommended for all adults in the following settings: STD treatment facilities; HIV testing and treatment facilities; facilities providing drug-abuse treatment and prevention services; health-care settings targeting services to injection-drug users or men who have sex with men; correctional facilities; end-stage renal disease programs and facilities for chronic hemodialysis patients; and institutions and nonresidential daycare facilities for persons with developmental disabilities.

Administer or complete a 3-dose series of HepB to those persons not previously vaccinated. The second dose should be administered 1 month after the first dose; the third dose should be administered at least 2 months after the second dose (and at least 4 months after the first dose). If the combined hepatitis A and hepatitis B vaccine (Twinrix) is used, administer 3 doses at 0, 1, and 6 months; alternatively, a 4-dose schedule, administered on days 0, 7, and 21–30 followed by a booster dose at month 12 may be used.

Adult patients receiving hemodialysis or with other immunocompromising conditions should receive 1 dose of 40 μg/mL (Recombivax HB) administered on a 3-dose schedule or 2 doses of 20 μg/mL (Engerix-B) administered simultaneously on a 4-dose schedule at 0, 1, 2 and 6 months.

TABLE 20-4 (continued)

11. Meningococcal vaccination

Meningococcal vaccine should be administered to persons with the following indications.

Medical: Adults with anatomic or functional asplenia, or persistent complement component deficiencies.

Other: First-year college students living in dormitories; microbiologists routinely exposed to isolates of *Neisseria meningitidis*; military recruits; and persons who travel to or live in countries in which meningococcal disease is hyperendemic or epidemic (e.g., the "meningitis belt" of sub-Saharan Africa during the dry season [December through June]), particularly if their contact with local populations will be prolonged. Vaccination is required by the government of Saudi Arabia for all travelers to Mecca during the annual Hajj.

Meningococcal conjugate vaccine (MCV4) is preferred for adults with any of the preceding indications who are aged ≤55 years; meningococcal polysaccharide vaccine (MPSV4) is preferred for adults aged ≥56 years. Revaccination with MCV4 after 5 years is recommended for adults previously vaccinated with MCV4 or MPSV4 who remain at increased risk for infection (e.g., adults with anatomic or functional asplenia). Persons whose only risk factor is living in on-campus housing are not recommended to receive an additional dose.

12. Selected conditions for which *Haemophilus influenzae* type b (Hib) vaccine may be used

Hib vaccine generally is not recommended for persons aged ≥5 years. No efficacy data are available on which to base a recommendation concerning use of Hib vaccine for older children and adults. However, studies suggest good immunogenicity in patients who have sickle cell disease, leukemia, or HIV infection or who have had a splenectomy. Administering 1 dose of Hib vaccine to these high-risk persons who have not previously received Hib vaccine is not contraindicated.

13. Immunocompromising conditions

Inactivated vaccines generally are acceptable (e.g., pneumococcal, meningococcal, influenza [inactivated influenza vaccine]) and live vaccines generally are avoided in persons with immune deficiencies or immunocompromising conditions. Information on specific conditions is available at www.cdc.gov/vaccines/pubs/acip-list.htm.

Vaccines Recommended for Special Conditions

Vaccination of pregnant women is generally avoided until after delivery due to the concern about potential risk to the fetus. Administration of live attenuated vaccines should not be done during pregnancy, and inactivated vaccines may be administered to pregnant women if the benefits outweigh the risks. Hepatitis A, hepatitis B, meningococcal, inactivated polio, and pneumococcal polysaccharide vaccines should be administered to pregnant women who are at risk for contracting these infections.

In general, severely immunocompromised individuals should not receive live vaccines, such as patients with chronic conditions that cause limited immune deficiency. These conditions include renal disease, diabetes, liver disease, and asplenia (lack of a functioning spleen). These patients, when not receiving immunosuppressants, may receive live attenuated and killed vaccines, as well as toxoid vaccines. Patients with active malignant disease may receive killed vaccines or toxoids, but they should not be given live vaccines. Live virus vaccines may be administered to persons with leukemia who have not received chemotherapy for at least 3 months. Those receiving high-dose corticosteroids, or those who have had a course of drug therapy lasting longer than 2 weeks, should wait 1 month before being immunized with live virus vaccines.

Patient Education

Patients must understand the importance of immunization. In history, millions of people died from various infectious diseases that are no longer serious health threats. This is due to the discovery of vaccines for a wide variety of diseases. Patients should make sure that their own immunization records, as well as those of their children, are on hand. Because most vaccines require booster doses, it is important to know when these doses are due. All vaccines used today are safe for administration, although there is a possibility of allergic reactions or nonserious adverse effects.

SUMMARY

The immune system protects the body from disease-causing pathogens, including bacteria, viruses, fungi, and protozoans. The two anatomical components of the immune system are the lymphoid tissues (primarily the thymus gland and bone marrow) and the cells responsible for the immune response. The white blood cells (WBCs), or leukocytes, are the primary cells responsible for the body's immune responses. Immunity is the state or condition of being resistant to invading microorganisms. Acquired immunity occurs either by contracting a disease and becoming immune to it or by being vaccinated with proteins from the causative agent. Acquired immunity is subdivided into active and passive immunity. Antibodies are also called immunoglobulins, and they are collectively referred to as gamma globulins. Vaccines are administered to generate a protective immune response, and they may be live (attenuated) or killed (inactivated). Examples of diseases that are commonly vaccinated against include diphtheria, pertussis, tetanus, polio, measles, mumps, rubella, hepatitis B, *Haemophilus influenzae* type B, varicella, hepatitis A, meningococcal disease, human papillomavirus, pneumococcal disease, shingles, influenza A, influenza B, tuberculosis, and rabies. Immunizations are commonly administered by injection or by oral or nasal instillation.

LEARNING GOALS

These learning goals correspond to the objectives at the beginning of the chapter, providing a clear summary of the chapter's most important points.

1. The thymus gland is one of the two primary lymphoid tissues. It is a major part of the immune system, along with the bone marrow and cells responsible for the immune response. It is located in the upper chest cavity, just under the sternum.
2. Acquired immunity is obtained by contracting a disease and developing immunity to it or by being vaccinated with proteins from the causative agent. Acquired immunity is primarily mediated by lymphocytes, and it is subdivided into active and passive immunity:
   - Active immunity occurs when the body is exposed to a pathogen and produces its own antibodies.
   - Passive immunity occurs when antibodies made in the body of another animal are acquired or when a mother transfers antibodies across the placenta to her fetus.
3. Vaccines are substances administered to generate a protective immune response, and they can be live (attenuated) or killed (inactivated). They are made from infectious (causative) agents of the specific disease being vaccinated against. The term *gamma globulins* collectively refers to antibodies, which are substances that develop within the immune system to identify and destroy foreign substances.
4. Children younger than 6 years of age should be vaccinated against diphtheria, pertussis, tetanus, polio, measles, mumps, rubella, hepatitis B, and *Haemophilus influenzae* type B. In areas of high incidence, they should also be immunized against hepatitis A.
5. In general, severely immunocompromised individuals, such as patients with chronic conditions that cause limited immune deficiency, should not receive live vaccines.

6. Passive immunity occurs when we acquire antibodies that were made in the body of another animal. Other examples are when a mother transfers antibodies across the placenta to her fetus or when injections containing antibodies are given. Gamma globulin injections only last for about 3 months.

7. *Haemophilus influenzae* type B is a bacterial disease (Hib) that is spread by direct contact or contact with respiratory droplets. Its most common type is meningitis. Hib is treated with antibiotics and usually requires hospitalization. Hib vaccination is administered intramuscularly. Influenza A is a viral disease and includes the H1N1 or swine flu. It is spread in a similar fashion, but it can also infect other animals besides humans. Its vaccination is administered either intramuscularly or by intranasal instillation.

8. Subcutaneous vaccines include those given for measles, mumps, rubella, varicella, meningococcal disease, pneumococcal disease, and shingles. The only intradermal vaccine discussed in this chapter is the vaccine for tuberculosis.

9. The five general classes of immunoglobulins are as follows:
   - IgG: These antibodies make up 75% of the plasma antibodies in adults because they are produced in secondary immune responses.
   - IgA: These antibodies are found in external secretions.
   - IgE: These antibodies are associated with allergic responses.
   - IgM: These antibodies are associated with primary immune responses and with the antibodies that react to the blood group antigen.
   - IgD: These antibody proteins appear on the surfaces of B lymphocytes along with IgM. However, the physiological role of IgD is unclear.

10. Immunization for hepatitis B is given to all ages of patients by intramuscular injection, usually in three separate doses. Immunization for rabies begins with rabies immune globulin (RIG) on the first day after the wound, followed immediately by the first of five rabies vaccines. The second vaccine is given 3 days later; the third vaccine is given on the 7th day; the fourth vaccine is given on the 14th day; and the fifth (final) vaccine is given on the 28th day.

CRITICAL THINKING QUESTIONS

1. Why is a yearly flu shot needed to prevent the contraction of seasonal influenza?
2. List two examples of infectious diseases that have been used by bioterrorists against the general public.

WEB SITES

http://uhaweb.hartford.edu/BUGL/immune.htm
http://www.aafp.org/afp/20000215/1089.html
http://www.biology-online.org/1/11_cell_defense_2.htm
http://www.cdc.gov/vaccines/recs/schedules/adult-schedule.htm
http://www.cdc.gov/vaccines/recs/schedules/child-schedule.htm
http://www.cellsalive.com/antibody.htm

REVIEW QUESTIONS

Multiple Choice

Select the best response to each question.

1. Pneumococcal polysaccharide vaccine is administered to children or adolescents in one dose of 0.5 mL by which of the following routes?
   A. intramuscular
   B. intradermal
   C. subcutaneous
   D. A and B

2. Annual vaccinations may be indicated in some adolescents for which of the following diseases?
   A. rabies
   B. chickenpox
   C. hepatitis A
   D. influenza

3. BCG vaccination is *not* recommended for children who are
   A. infected with HIV
   B. infected with hepatitis A virus
   C. malnourished
   D. anemic

4. Treatment for which of the following diseases requires a series of six injections over a 4-week period?
   A. influenza
   B. viral meningitis
   C. rabies
   D. hepatitis B

5. Which of the following vaccines can be administered at birth?
   A. H1N1 flu
   B. polio
   C. hepatitis A
   D. hepatitis B

6. Which of the following immunoglobulins crosses the placental membrane and provides infants with immunity in the first few months of life?
   A. IgG
   B. IgA
   C. IgM
   D. IgE

7. Which of the following lymphocytes attack and destroy virus-infected cells and tumor cells?
   A. memory B cells
   B. cytotoxic T cells
   C. natural killer cells
   D. helper T cells

8. The HPV vaccine is effective for approximately
   A. 1 year
   B. 3 years
   C. 5 years
   D. 15 years

9. The BCG vaccine is given
   A. intramuscularly
   B. intradermally
   C. intranasally
   D. orally

10. Which of the following vaccines is recommended as a booster every 10 years?
    A. HPV
    B. DTP
    C. TDaP
    D. MMR

11. MMRV is the abbreviation of
    A. measles–mumps–rubella vaccine
    B. measles–mumps–rubella–varicella
    C. measles–mumps–rubella–variola
    D. measles–mumps–rubella–viruses

12. Which of the following is the best time to give human papillomavirus vaccine to protect women from cervical cancer?
    A. at age 3 to 5 years
    B. at age 10 to 11 years
    C. at age 15 to 18 years
    D. at age 30 to 40 years

13. H1N1 flu is caused by which of the following types of flu viruses?
    A. type C
    B. type D
    C. type A
    D. type B

14. Which of the following vaccines is a live vaccine?
    A. tetanus
    B. polio
    C. diphtheria
    D. *Haemophilus influenzae* type B

15. An example of a conjugate vaccine is
    A. mumps
    B. diphtheria
    C. rubella
    D. *Haemophilus influenzae* type B

CASE STUDY

A 67-year-old man developed a painful skin rash on one side of his face after first experiencing pain and itching in the same place. The rash began as blisters, which then formed scabs in 3 to 5 days.

1. What is the likely diagnosis of his condition?
2. Is his skin disorder preventable by any vaccine?

Treatment of Nervous System Disorders

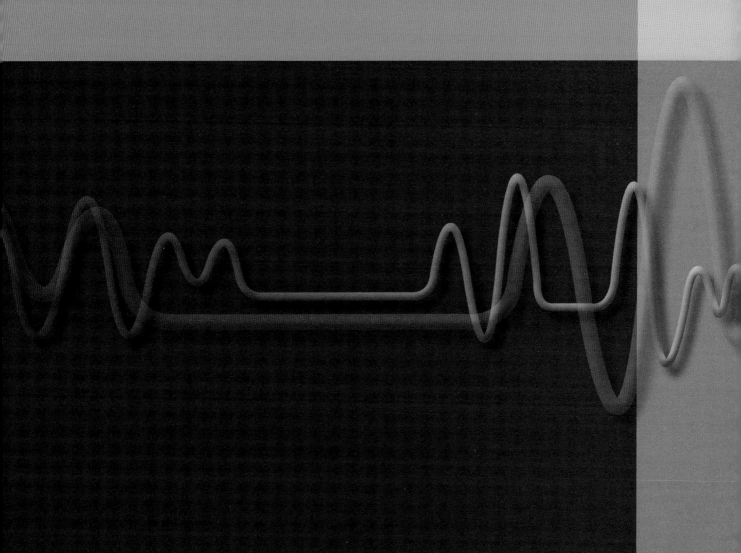

Effects of Drugs on the Central Nervous System

OBJECTIVES

Upon completion of this chapter, the reader should be able to do the following:
1. List the neurotransmitters that are most involved in anxiety.
2. Explain the structure of a neuron.
3. Name the major parts and functions of the brain.

4. Explain the newest drugs for the treatment of depression.
5. Classify medications used to treat anxiety.
6. Describe the methods of action for each class of drugs used to treat depression.
7. Name the four stages of anesthesia and explain which of them is the most dangerous.
8. Classify the different types of painkillers.
9. Describe the cause of pain.
10. Classify medications used in the treatment of sleep disorders.

KEY TERMS

Ataxia	Foramen magnum
Axons	Glial cells
Brain	Medulla oblongata
Central nervous system (CNS)	Neurons
Cerebellum	Peripheral nervous system (PNS)
Dendrites	Thalamus
Dysthymia	

INTRODUCTION

Various agents are prescribed for different disorders of both the central nervous system and the autonomic nervous system. These agents may be used for the treatment of anxiety, insomnia, depression, pain management, seizures, other conditions, and for anesthesia. The discussion of drugs used to treat these disorders will focus on agents that commonly affect cardiopulmonary systems.

Structures and Functions

The nervous system is divided into the central nervous system (CNS), which includes the brain and spinal cord, and the peripheral nervous system (PNS), which includes the cranial nerves arising from the brain and the spinal nerves arising from the spinal cord. Although this chapter focuses on the CNS, the structures and functions of the PNS will be summarized in Chapter 22.

The nervous system is composed of two main types of cells: neurons and supporting cells. Neurons are the basic structural and functional units of the nervous system. They are specialized and respond to physical and chemical stimuli. They also conduct electrochemical impulses and release chemical regulators. These activities enable neurons to perceive sensory stimuli, learn, remember, and control muscles and glands. Neurons are made up of three parts: dendrites, cell bodies, and axons.

Supporting cells aid the functions of neurons. In the CNS, supporting cells are collectively called neuroglia or glial cells. This chapter will focus on a brief discussion of the structure and functions of the central nervous system.

The Brain

The brain can be divided into four major portions: cerebrum, diencephalon, brainstem, and cerebellum (see Figure 21–1). The cerebrum is the largest part of the brain, including nerve centers associated with sensory and motor functions. It provides higher mental functions, including memory and reasoning. The diencephalon also processes sensory information. Nerve pathways in the brainstem connect various parts of the nervous system and regulate certain visceral activities. The cerebellum includes centers that coordinate voluntary muscle movements.

> **POINT TO REMEMBER**
>
> Conscious thought and intelligence are provided by the neural cortex of the cerebral hemispheres.

Cerebrum

The lobes of the cerebral hemispheres are named after the skull bones (see Figure 21–2). These include the

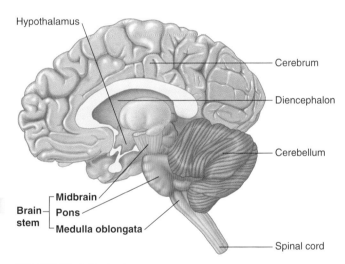

FIGURE 21–1 The brain.

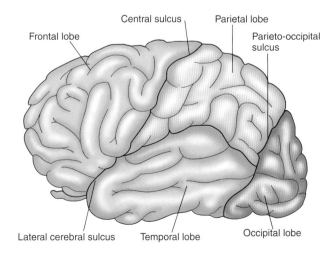

FIGURE 21–2 The lobes of the cerebrum.

frontal, parietal, temporal, and occipital lobes. The cerebrum has centers for interpreting sensory impulses arriving from sense organs and centers for initiating voluntary muscular movements.

Diencephalon

The diencephalon is located between the cerebral hemispheres and above the midbrain. The two main parts of the diencephalon are the thalamus and the hypothalamus (see **Figure 21–3**). The thalamus is a central relay station for sensory impulses that ascend from other parts of the nervous system to the cerebral cortex. The thalamus produces a general awareness of certain sensations, including pain, temperature, and touch. The hypothalamus maintains homeostasis by regulating a variety of activities. It also connects the nervous and endocrine systems. The hypothalamus regulates the following functions:

- body temperature
- control of hunger and body weight
- heart rate and arterial blood pressure
- movement and glandular secretions of the stomach and intestines
- sleep and wakefulness
- stimulation of the pituitary gland to secrete hormones
- water and electrolyte balance

Brainstem

The brainstem is a bundle of nervous tissue that connects the cerebrum to the spinal cord. The three parts of the brainstem include the midbrain, pons, and medulla oblongata, which are also shown in Figure 21–1. The midbrain is a short section of the brainstem between the diencephalon and the pons. The pons is a part of the brainstem above the medulla oblongata and below the midbrain. The pons, along with the center of the medulla oblongata, maintains basic breathing rhythm.

The medulla oblongata extends from the pons to the foramen magnum of the skull. The medulla oblongata controls vital visceral activities. These include altering the heart rate, stimulating blood vessels to contract, elevating blood pressure, and dilating blood vessels (which results in reducing blood pressure). The medulla oblongata also is the center of the respiratory system; it adjusts the rate and depth of breathing. There are also some nuclei within the medulla oblongata associated with the reflexes needed for coughing, sneezing, swallowing, and vomiting.

Cerebellum

The cerebellum is a large mass of tissue located below the occipital lobes of the cerebrum. It is situated posterior to the pons and medulla oblongata (as shown in Figure 21–1). The cerebellum is a center for coordinating skeletal muscle movements. It also helps to maintain posture. Damage to the cerebellum may cause tremors, loss of muscle tone, and loss of equilibrium.

The Spinal Cord

The spinal cord is the major pathway for information between the brain and the skin, joints, and muscles of the body. In addition, the spinal cord contains neural networks responsible for locomotion. The spinal cord is divided into the following four regions: cervical, thoracic, lumbar, and sacral. These regions are named to correspond to adjacent vertebrae (see **Figure 21–4**).

Anxiety Disorders and Treatments

Anxiety disorders involve intense fearfulness, which arises without the occurrence of a precipitating and potentially dangerous event. Anxiety may be accompanied by subjective and objective manifestations. Although grief is a normal response to personal loss, anxiety is a normal response to a threatening situation. Anxiety disorders are the most common of the various psychiatric disorders. They affect more

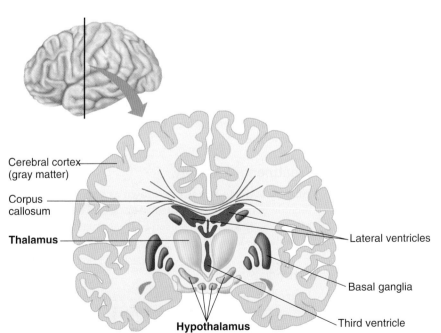

Cerebral cortex (gray matter)

Corpus callosum

Thalamus

Hypothalamus

Lateral ventricles

Basal ganglia

Third ventricle

FIGURE 21–3 The thalamus, hypothalamus, and associated structures in a coronal section of the brain.

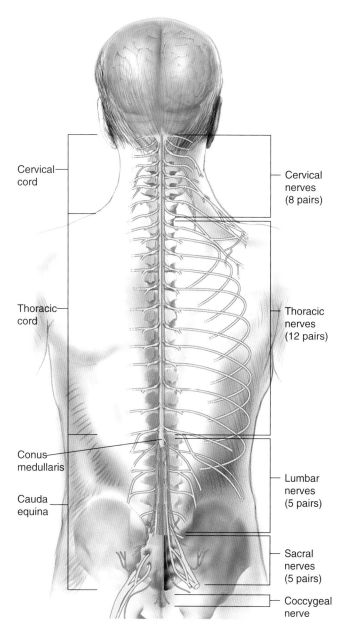

Cervical cord

Cervical nerves (8 pairs)

Thoracic cord

Thoracic nerves (12 pairs)

Conus medullaris

Cauda equina

Lumbar nerves (5 pairs)

Sacral nerves (5 pairs)

Coccygeal nerve

FIGURE 21–4 The spinal cord.

TABLE 21–1 Drugs Used to Treat Anxiety		
Generic Name	**Trade Name**	**Average Adult Dosage**
Benzodiazepines		
• alprazolam	Xanax, etc.	PO: 0.25–2 mg
• clonazepam	Klonopin	PO: 0.5–2 mg
• clorazepate	Tranxene, etc.	PO: 3.75–15 mg
• diazepam	Valium, etc.	PO: 2–10 mg
• lorazepam	Ativan, etc.	PO: 0.5–2 mg
• midazolam	Generic only	PO: 2 mg/mL
• oxazepam	Serax, et	PO: 10–30 mg
Azapirones		
• buspirone	BuSpar	PO: 5–30 mg
Miscellaneous anxiolytics		
• hydroxyzine HCl	Atarax, etc.	PO: 10–50 mg
• hydroxyzine pamoate	Generic only	PO: 25–100 mg

stress disorder is characterized by a variety of symptoms experienced as states of intrusion, avoidance, and hyperarousal. Intrusion refers to flashbacks that occur during waking hours or nightmares in which a past traumatic event is relived. Posttraumatic stress disorder may occur after having experienced a terrifying event such as war, sexual abuse, rape, an accident, or a natural disaster.

Neurotransmitters and Anxiety

A neurotransmitter is a biochemical that is formed in and released from a neuron to stimulate or inhibit the action of another cell. The neurotransmitters most involved in anxiety include gamma-aminobutyric acid (GABA), serotonin, and norepinephrine (NE). GABA is the major nervous system neurotransmitter with inhibitory actions. It acts to reduce neuronal excitability and decrease nerve impulse transmission. Serotonin plays a minor role in the treatment of anxiety. Norepinephrine mediates certain adrenergic-related symptoms of anxiety. It is very effective in the treatment of depression but not as effective in treating anxiety. Other examples of neurotransmitters include dopamine, acetylcholine, and epinephrine.

Treatment of Anxiety

Anxiety is treated by drugs known as **anxiolytics**. These include benzodiazepines, azapirones, and miscellaneous anxiolytic agents. Drugs used to treat anxiety are shown in **Table 21–1**.

Benzodiazepines

Benzodiazepines are the most commonly used agents in the treatment of short-term anxiety. Benzodiazepines are rapidly and completely absorbed and can cross the blood–brain barrier. These drugs are capable of producing tolerance as well as dependence, and they are classified as Schedule IV controlled substances.

than 40 million adults in the United States, with women being affected more often than men. Anxiety disorders have a high occurrence rate among members of the same family. Common symptoms of anxiety include increased heart rate, palpitations, rapid breathing, shortness of breath, nausea, dry mouth, and sweating.

There are five major types of anxiety disorders: generalized anxiety disorder, panic disorder, obsessive-compulsive disorder (OCD), social phobia, and posttraumatic stress disorder (PTSD). Generalized anxiety disorder is characterized by excessive, uncontrollable worrying. Panic disorder is characterized by intense fear, with neurologic, cardiac, respiratory, and psychological symptoms. Obsessive-compulsive disorder is characterized by repetitive thoughts and actions. Social phobia is an intense fear reaction to social interaction. Posttraumatic

Azapirones differ from benzodiazepines because they do not produce tolerance or dependence. Currently, the only drug in this class is buspirone, which has a slow onset of action. Unlike the benzodiazepines, buspirone produces only slight sedation. Miscellaneous anxiolytic agents include various types of hydroxyzine, which does not produce tolerance or dependence but causes a small amount of sedation.

Method of Action
Antianxiety drugs affect the CNS in a manner that appears to be closely related to how they increase the action of the neurotransmitter known as GABA.

Clinical Implications
Benzodiazepines are also used for panic attacks, insomnia, seizure disorders, status epilepticus, and muscle relaxation.

Adverse Effects

POINT TO REMEMBER

The withdrawal syndrome of benzodiazepines is very long in duration (lasting from weeks to months). Seizures can occur and can result in status epilepticus and death.

Antianxiety drugs, in general, produce sedation as a common adverse effect. Other adverse effects include ataxia, drowsiness, fatigue, impaired judgment, development of tolerance, and rebound insomnia. Benzodiazepine overdosage may cause CNS and respiratory depression, hypotension, cardiovascular collapse, or coma.

Contraindications
Benzodiazepines, particularly flurazepam, should be avoided during pregnancy because they are able to cause abnormalities in the developing fetus. They are also contraindicated in severe kidney disease, severe liver disease, and in hyperactive children. They should be used carefully due to many different drug interactions.

Precautions
To avoid serious adverse effects, gradual withdrawal of benzodiazepines is recommended. Benzodiazepines and other antianxiety drugs should not be taken with alcohol or other CNS depressants. Patients should not drive or operate machinery while taking these agents. These agents may cause moderate to severe renal or hepatic impairment.

The Concept of Sleep, Sleep Disorders, and Treatments

Sleep is defined as a period of inactivity as well as restoration of mental and physical function. Sufficient sleep is vital for body growth and maintenance, as well as healthy immune and nervous system function. There are two types of sleep: rapid eye movement (REM) and non-REM sleep. REM sleep is associated with rapid eye movements, loss of muscle movement, and vivid dreaming.

Non-REM sleep is a quiet type of sleep characterized by a relatively inactive state while the brain remains fully regulated and the body remains fully movable. It is divided into five stages that reflect an increasing depth of sleep:

- Stage I: a brief transitional stage that occurs at the onset of sleep, during which a person is easily aroused
- Stage II: a deeper sleep, lasting approximately 10 to 25 minutes
- Stages III and IV: deep sleep in which the muscles of the body relax, the heart rate and blood pressure decrease, and gastrointestinal activity is increased
- Stage V: rapid eye movement (REM) sleep, which lasts about 2 hours per night

Normally, sleep and wakefulness occur in a cyclic manner that is integrated into the 24-hour solar day, with its standard periods of light and dark. These 24-hour diurnal periods include rhythms referred to as circadian. This term comes from the Latin word *circa* (about) and *dies* (day). The function of the circadian time system is to provide organization of physiologic processes and behaviors. This organization promotes effective adaptation to the environment. Behaviorally, this is expressed in regular sleep and waking cycles. It is also expressed in body functions, including temperature regulation and hormone secretion. These functional changes are based on the 24-hour light–dark solar day.

Sleep disorders include a variety of symptoms, such as the inability to fall sleep and stay asleep, circadian rhythm and sleep–wake transition disorders, sleep-related breathing, movement disorders, and excessive sleepiness. Sleep disorders have existed for centuries. However, only within the last 3 or 4 decades has attention been focused on the diagnosis and classification of sleep disorders. These classifications include circadian rhythm disorders, insomnias, hypersomnias (narcolepsy), sleep-related movement disorders, and sleep-related breathing disorders.

In the United States, millions of people experience sleep disorders. Insomnia, restless leg syndrome, sleep apnea, and narcolepsy are among the most common forms. Insomnia is the inability to sleep or to remain asleep. Restless leg syndrome is more common in elderly patients and can also be caused by anemia, diabetes, and pregnancy. Sleep apnea involves interruption of the oxygen supply while sleeping, causing the patient to awaken; in extreme cases, it may cause respiratory arrest and be fatal. Narcolepsy is the least common sleep disorder of the four; it is characterized by falling asleep suddenly for a few seconds to 30 minutes. It may be due to heredity or brain trauma.

Sleep disorders may be treated with a variety of prescription or OTC medications, as well as natural remedies. Prescription drugs used for insomnia include barbiturates, benzodiazepines, and other sedative–hypnotics. **Table 21–2** lists various types of agents used for sleep disorders.

TABLE 21-2 Agents Used to Treat Sleep Disorders

Generic Name	Trade Name	Average Adult Dosage
Barbiturates		
• amobarbital	Amytal	Injection: 500 mg
• pentobarbital	Nembutal	Injection: 50 mg/mL
• secobarbital	Seconal	PO: 100 mg
Benzodiazepines		
• flurazepam	Dalmane	PO: 15–30 mg
• temazepam	Restoril	PO: 15–30 mg
• triazolam	Halcion	PO: 0.125–0.25 mg
Miscellaneous agents		
• eszopiclone	Lunesta	PO: 1–3 mg
• zaleplon	Sonata	PO: 5–10 mg
• zolpidem	Ambien, etc.	PO: 5–10 mg

Barbiturates

Barbiturates are sedative–hypnotics that greatly affect GABA binding, promoting relaxation and sleep. In low doses, they decrease anxiety. Higher doses cause sedation, then somnolence or hypnosis. They can produce tolerance and dependence and are usually considered Schedule II or Schedule IV controlled substances. Barbiturates are listed in **Table 21–2**.

Method of Action

Barbiturates enhance GABA binding and appear to have a direct action on chloride ion channels.

Clinical Implications

Barbiturates are used to decrease anxiety and promote relaxation and sleep, with dose-dependent effects. These drugs are also used for partial epilepsy and tonic-clonic seizures.

Adverse Effects

POINT TO REMEMBER

Barbiturates may cause the development of cross-tolerance to alcohol, general anesthetics, benzodiazepines, and other sedative–hypnotics.

Increased doses of barbiturates may cause general anesthesia, and toxic doses produce coma and death. Other adverse effects of barbiturates include ataxia, confusion, hypotension, and reduced motor performance. They can produce tolerance and dependence. The toxic effects of barbiturates include respiratory depression, circulatory collapse, and renal or hepatic impairment.

Contraindications

Barbiturates are contraindicated in known hypersensitivity and in patients with history of manifest or latent porphyria (a group of disorders involving purple

discoloration of feces and urine). Barbiturates are also contraindicated in cases of severe respiratory or renal disease.

Precautions

Barbiturates should be used with caution by patients with chronic obstructive pulmonary disease (COPD), heart failure, mental status changes, sleep apnea, major depression, renal impairment or failure, if suicidal thoughts persist, and in neonates.

POINT TO REMEMBER

Barbiturate withdrawal can be severe and life threatening, with prolonged delirium and grand mal convulsions.

Benzodiazepines

Benzodiazepines have replaced many barbiturates in the treatment of a variety of sleep disorders. Benzodiazepines used to treat sleep disorders are listed in Table 21–2.

Method of Action

Benzodiazepines enhance the GABA–benzodiazepine receptor complex to produce sedation, skeletal muscle relaxation, and anticonvulsant effects.

Clinical Implications

In the treatment of sleep disorders, benzodiazepines are used for insomnia and to treat patients with poor sleeping habits.

Adverse Effects

Benzodiazepines may cause coma if an overdosage occurs. Other adverse effects include dizziness or lightheadedness, ataxia, headache, apprehension, nervousness, irritability, depression, hallucinations, confusion, nightmares, excitement, euphoria, disorientation, and hyperactivity. Additional adverse effects include blurred vision, burning of the eyes, heartburn, nausea or vomiting, abdominal pain, diarrhea, allergic reactions, and hypotension. Rare effects include granulocytopenia and jaundice.

Contraindications

Benzodiazepines are contraindicated for long-term use, in hypersensitive patients, and in sleep apnea, COPD, ethanol intoxication, major depression, intermittent porphyria, acute narrow-angle glaucoma, and psychosis. They should not be used in children younger than 15 years of age or during pregnancy and lactation.

Precautions

Benzodiazepines should be used with caution in impaired kidney or liver function, mental depression, history of suicidal tendencies, bipolar disorder, and in addiction-prone individuals, as well as elderly or debilitated patients.

Miscellaneous Agents

Miscellaneous agents used to treat sleep disorders include eszopiclone, zaleplon, and zolpidem, which are listed in Table 21–2.

Method of Action

The actions of these agents are similar to those of barbiturates and benzodiazepines.

Clinical Implications

These agents are primarily used to treat insomnia.

Adverse Effects

Adverse effects of these miscellaneous agents include anxiety, confusion, depression, dizziness, hallucinations, headache, decreased libido, irritability, nervousness, and somnolence. Additional adverse effects may include pericardial infusion, tachycardia, left ventricular systolic dysfunction, dry mouth, dyspepsia, nausea, and vomiting. Other adverse effects may include dysmenorrhea, gynecomastia, respiratory infections, skin rash, pruritus, or unpleasant tastes.

Contraindications

These agents are contraindicated in hypersensitive patients, with certain inhibitory agents, with alcohol, in patients with suicidal tendencies or ideation, in children younger than age 18 years, and during pregnancy.

Precautions

Miscellaneous agents used for sleep disorders should be used cautiously in elderly or debilitated patients, with hepatic impairment, during use of CNS depressants, in depressed patients, with COPD, and during lactation.

Depression and Treatments

Depression is among the leading causes of disability worldwide. In the United States, the lifetime incidence of depression is 20% of women and 12% of men. Nearly 20 million people in the United States are affected by depression. This condition affects most aspects of the patient's life, including mood, self-esteem, eating, sleeping, and thought patterns. It reduces their ability to think and concentrate.

The three primary types of depressive disorders include major depression, bipolar disorder, and **dysthymia**. Major depression is characterized by feelings of worthlessness and guilt, decreased concentration, alterations in sleep and appetite, and possible suicidal ideation. Bipolar depression is characterized by alternating periods of depression and mania. During the manic phase, there is a decreased need for food and sleep, racing thoughts, irritability, and high distractibility. Dysthymia is characterized by the same symptoms as major depression but in a milder form. These include low self-esteem, sleep and energy problems, and appetite disturbances. Persons with dysthymia are at risk for the development of major depression and other psychiatric disorders, including substance abuse disorders. Although the root cause of depression is unknown, neurotransmitter deficiency is involved. Treatment with medications for depression is designed to restore normal levels of various neurotransmitters. Major depression may be treated with medications, psychotherapy, or electroconvulsive therapy.

There are three classes of drugs available today for the treatment of depression. The oldest types are the tricyclic antidepressants (TCIs), with the other two types being the selective serotonin reuptake inhibitors (SSRIs) and monoamine oxidase inhibitors (MAOIs). Drugs used to treat depression are shown in **Table 21–3**.

> **POINT TO REMEMBER**
>
> The primary clinical indication for antidepressants is major depression (unipolar disorder).

Tricyclic Antidepressants

The tricyclic antidepressants (TCAs) are used for depression as well as other conditions (see Clinical Implications). Tricyclic antidepressants include imipramine, nortriptyline, clomipramine, and amitriptyline. TCAs are readily absorbed via oral administration (see Table 21–3).

Method of Action

Tricyclic antidepressants increase the effects of both norepinephrine and serotonin into presynaptic nerve terminals by blocking their neuronal uptake.

Clinical Implications

TCAs are used for endogenous (of internal origin) depression and sometimes for reactive (as a result of external stimuli) depression. They are also used for bedwetting (enuresis), obsessive-compulsive disorder, and chronic pain.

Adverse Effects

Adverse effects of TCAs vary among specific drugs and include blurred vision, constipation, dry mouth, tachycardia, and urine retention. Other effects include mental confusion, postural hypotension, sedation, weight gain, erectile dysfunction, and orthostatic hypotension.

Contraindications

TCAs are contraindicated in hypersensitive patients, those recovering from a heart attack, and in severe kidney or liver impairment.

TABLE 21-3 Drugs Used to Treat Depression

Generic Name	Trade Name	Average Adult Dosage
Tricyclic antidepressants (TCAs)		
• amitriptyline	Elavil	PO: Up to 300 mg/day in divided doses
• amoxapine	Asendin	PO: Start at 50 mg b.i.d.–t.i.d., up to 100 mg t.i.d. on day 3
• clomipramine	Anafranil	PO: 50–150 mg/day in single or divided doses
• desipramine	Norpramin	PO: 100–300 mg/day
• doxepin	Sinequan	PO: 25–30 mg/day in divided doses
• imipramine	Tofranil	PO: 75–300 mg/day in divided doses
• nortriptyline	Aventyl, etc.	PO: 25 mg t.i.d.–q.i.d.
• protriptyline	Vivactil	PO: 15–40 mg/day in 3–4 divided doses, up to 60 mg/day
• trimipramine	Surmontil	PO: 100–300 mg/day in divided doses
Selective serotonin reuptake inhibitors (SSRIs)		
• citalopram	Celexa	PO: 20–40 mg/day
• escitalopram	Lexapro	PO: 10–20 mg/day
• fluoxetine	Prozac, etc.	PO: 20 mg/day (in morning); may increase by 40–80 mg/day in divided doses; or 1 capsule/week
• fluvoxamine	Luvox	PO: 50–300 mg/day in divided doses
• paroxetine	Paxil	PO: 25–50 mg/day
• sertraline	Zoloft	PO: 50–200 mg/day
Monoamine oxidase inhibitors (MAOIs)		
• isocarboxazid	Marplan	PO: 10–30 mg/day
• phenelzine	Nardil	PO: 15 mg t.i.d. increased rapidly to 60 mg/day; up to 90 mg/day
• tranylcypromine	Parnate	PO: 30–60 mg/day in divided doses at 3-week intervals
Second- and third-generation antidepressants		
• bupropion	Wellbutrin, Zyban	PO: 75–300 mg in various tablet forms
• mirtazapine	Remeron	PO: 15–45 mg in various tablet forms
• nefazodone	Generic only	PO: 50–250 mg
• trazodone	Desyrel	PO: 50–300 mg
• venlafaxine	Effexor	PO: 25–150 mg in various tablet forms

Precautions

Patients should be warned not to stop taking TCAs abruptly and that they should be taken at bedtime. They should also be advised to report severe postural hypotension to their physician. These drugs take approximately 2 weeks to become effective.

Selective Serotonin Reuptake Inhibitors

Lack of adequate serotonin in the CNS can lead to depression. Selective serotonin reuptake inhibitors (SSRIs) are the newest and most widely prescribed type of antidepressants used today. They are as effective as TCAs but do not have the cardiotoxic effects of the TCAs. Therefore, SSRIs can be used in patients with heart disease. Common SSRIs include fluoxetine, paroxetine, and sertraline (see Table 21–3).

Method of Action

Selective serotonin reuptake inhibitors selectively target serotonin by blocking the effects of serotonin reuptake. They are comparable in effectiveness to the TCAs.

Clinical Implications

SSRIs are commonly used for depression, bulimia nervosa, obsessive-compulsive disorder, posttraumatic stress disorder, social anxiety disorder, and premenstrual dysphoric disorder.

> **POINT TO REMEMBER**
>
> The main advantage of SSRIs is that they are much safer due to a lack of sedation, orthostatic hypotension, and anticholinergic effects.

Adverse Effects

SSRIs usually offer relatively mild adverse effects that are usually of short duration. A common adverse effect of SSRIs is insomnia, therefore they are commonly administered in the morning. The most serious adverse effects of SSRIs include serotonin syndrome (confusion, agitation, diarrhea, tremors, increased blood pressure, and seizures) and suicide ideation (persistent thoughts of suicide).

Contraindications

SSRIs are contraindicated in hypersensitive patients, during pregnancy, and in children younger than age 7 years.

Precautions

There is an important warning concerning SSRIs: they may cause an increased risk of suicide. To avoid serotonin syndrome or suicide ideation, doses should be increased or decreased gradually. They should be used with caution in kidney or liver impairment, kidney failure, cardiac disease, diabetes mellitus, or during lactation.

Monoamine Oxidase Inhibitors

These agents are also known as MAO inhibitors or MAOIs, and they are eliminated very slowly from the body. They are as effective as TCAs and SSRIs in treating depression. However, there are numerous interactions with other medications as well as certain foods and beverages. MAOIs are shown in Table 21–3.

Method of Action

MAOIs block the enzyme known as MAO, but their actual method of action is believed to only prevent the natural breakdown of neurotransmitters. This inhibition increases the concentration of norepinephrine, dopamine, and serotonin. They may prolong and intensify the effects of many other drugs.

Clinical Implications

MAOIs are used to treat major endogenous depression, depressive psychosis, severe reactive depression not responsive to other therapies, and Parkinson disease. MAOIs are now reserved for patients who are not responsive to other classes of antidepressants.

Adverse Effects

A primary concern is that MAOIs interact with a large number of medications and foods, causing serious adverse effects. This includes hypertensive crisis caused by interactions with other drugs or foods that contain tyramine, such as fruits (avocados, bananas, canned figs, and raisins); dairy products (cheese, sour cream, and yogurt); alcohol (beer and red wine); and meats (beef and chicken liver, salami, sausage, and hot dogs).

Common adverse effects of MAOIs include dry mouth, sedation, constipation, orthostatic hypotension, impotence, urinary retention, nausea, diarrhea, dizziness, vertigo, headache, and weight gain. Severe adverse effects include hepatotoxicity, CNS stimulation, hypertensive crisis, and stroke when taken with food containing tyramine. Combining an MAOI with an SSRI may cause serotonin syndrome. Other antidepressants or sympathomimetic drugs are discussed in Chapter 22.

Contraindications

MAOIs are contraindicated in hypersensitive patients and in patients with epilepsy, liver disease, or severe cardiovascular disease.

Precautions

Patients should use MAOIs with caution and avoid foods that contain tyramine, including red wine, beer, caffeine, cheese, sauerkraut, yogurt, certain fruits, soy sauce, liver, chocolate, and others. Patients should be instructed that the effectiveness of these drugs occurs after about 2 weeks.

Second- and Third-Generation Antidepressants

Second- and third-generation antidepressants were developed to offer patients treatments that do not have as many adverse effects as TCAs or MAOIs. These agents include serotonin–noradrenaline reuptake inhibitors (SNRIs) and noradrenaline–dopamine reuptake inhibitors (NADRIs). Second- and third-generation antidepressants include bupropion, mirtazapine, trazodone, venlafaxine, and others.

Method of Action

These antidepressants appear to work by selectively inhibiting neuronal uptake of dopamine and other neurotransmitters.

Clinical Implications

Second- and third-generation antidepressants are indicated for mental depression, as adjunct therapy for smoking cessation, and for seasonal affective disorder.

Adverse Effects

Common adverse effects of these agents include sedation, dry mouth, and nausea. Other adverse effects include somnolence, increased appetite, constipation, flulike symptoms, hypertension, sinusitis, rash, and urinary frequency.

Contraindications

These agents are contraindicated in hypersensitive patients, seizure disorders, eating disorders, suicidal ideation, head trauma, CNS tumors, recent myocardial infarction, in children younger than 18 years of age, and during lactation.

Precautions

These agents should not be discontinued abruptly. They should be used with caution in kidney or liver impairment, patients who abuse drugs, cardiac diseases, hypertension, bipolar disorder, diabetes mellitus, elderly patients, and during pregnancy.

Anesthesia and Anesthetics

Anesthesia is a medical procedure performed by administering drugs that cause a loss of sensation. Anesthesia can be limited to a small area (local anesthesia) or can cause loss of sensation and consciousness through the whole body (general anesthesia). This chapter examines drugs used only for general anesthesia. For local anesthesia, refer to other textbooks.

Patients who are about to undergo operations often receive preoperative agents and/or general anesthetics before, during, and after surgery. Most other medication orders are withheld when the patient goes to surgery. General anesthetics are usually used to produce loss of consciousness before and during surgery.

Anesthetic agents should, ideally, have the following characteristics:

- analgesia to relieve pain but not cause unconsciousness
- a wide therapeutic index
- chemical inertness
- high potency
- noninflammability
- rapid, pleasant induction and withdrawal from anesthesia
- skeletal muscle relaxation

The four stages of general anesthesia are analgesia, excitement (delirium), surgical anesthesia, and medullary paralysis. Analgesia abolishes pain but allows the patient to remain conscious. The excitement stage may cause the patient to become violent or afraid of what is occurring, so it is important that this second stage be managed so that the next stage is achieved as quickly as possible. Surgical anesthesia (stage 3) is characterized by progressive muscle relaxation but must be monitored closely so that respiratory paralysis does not occur. Stage 4 is medullary paralysis, which can lead to circulatory collapse. Obviously, this stage must be avoided at all costs.

Preoperative agents, also known as preanesthetics, are usually given about 45 to 70 minutes before surgery. Common preoperative agents include benzodiazepines, opioid analgesics, antacids, H_2-receptor antagonists, gastric acid pump inhibitors, antiemetics, and anticholinergics.

General anesthetics are usually given by inhalation or by intravenous injection. Inhaled general anesthetics include volatile liquids (desflurane, enflurane, halothane, isoflurane, methoxyflurane, and sevoflurane) and gases (nitrous oxide). **Table 21–4** shows volatile liquids and gases used for general anesthesia.

Intravenous general anesthetics include

TABLE 21–4 General Anesthetics for Inhalation

Generic Name	Trade Name	Average Adult Dosage
Gases		
• nitrous oxide	Generic only	The anesthesiologist determines the dosage.
Volatile liquids		
• desflurane	Suprane	
• enflurane	Ethrane	The anesthesiologist determines the dosage for these agents.
• halothane	Fluothane	
• isoflurane	Forane	
• methoxyflurane	Penthrane	
• sevoflurane	Ultane	

barbiturates and barbiturate-like agents, benzodiazepines, opioids, and miscellaneous anesthetics (see **Table 21–5**). Dosages must be individualized for each patient, but the table shows the average adult dosages for each drug.

Method of Action

General anesthetics work by blocking neuronal pain impulses, primarily in the CNS. This is accomplished by blocking sodium channels inside neuronal membranes. General anesthetics must cross the blood–brain barrier to be effective. All general anesthetics are lipophilic (able to dissolve easily in lipids rather than in water).

Clinical Implications

General anesthesia is indicated for all types of surgery that cannot be accomplished simply with a local anesthetic. It is also indicated for various nonsurgical procedures wherein the patient should not be conscious. Often, inhaled and intravenous general anesthetics are used in combination.

Adverse Effects

Common adverse effects of inhaled and intravenous general anesthetics include drowsiness, tiredness that lasts for several days, and overall weakness. Other adverse effects include blurred vision, problems with coordination, and fuzzy thoughts. Patients should not drive, operate machinery, or perform other potentially dangerous activities while general anesthetics are still in their systems. Adverse effects that may occur after general anesthesia include headache, muscle pain, mental or mood changes, nausea or vomiting, shivering, nightmares, and sore throat.

Contraindications

IV anesthetics are contraindicated in patients who have taken monoamine oxidase inhibitors (MAOIs) within the last 14 days. Other contraindications include

TABLE 21-5 General Anesthetics for Intravenous Injection

Generic Name	Trade Name	Average Adult Dosage
Barbiturates and barbiturate-like agents		
• etomidate	Amidate	200–600 mcg/kg given over 30–60 seconds
• methohexital sodium	Brevital	50–120 mg at 5 mg every 5 minutes, then 20–40 mg every 4–6 minutes p.r.n.
• propofol	Diprivan	Induction: 2–2.5 mg/kg every 10 seconds until onset; maintenance: 100–200 mcg/kg/min
Benzodiazepines		
• diazepam	Valium	5–15 mg 5–10 minutes before procedure
• lorazepam	Ativan	0.044 mg/kg up to 2 mg 15–20 minutes before procedure
• midazolam hydrochloride	Versed	Premedicated: 0.15–0.25 mg/kg over 20–30 seconds, allowing 2 minutes for effect; non-pre-medicated: 0.3–0.35 mg/kg over 20–30 seconds, allowing 2 minutes for effect
Opioids		
• alfentanil hydrochloride	Alfenta	3–8 mcg/kg; maintenance of monitored anesthesia care (MAC); 3–5 mcg/kg q5–20 minutes or 0.25–1 mcg/kg/min; total dose: 3–40 mcg/kg
• fentanyl citrate	Sublimaze, etc.	2–20 mcg/kg, additional doses of 25–100 mcg as required
• remifentanil hydrochloride	Ultiva	0.5–1 mcg/kg/min or 1 mcg/kg bolus
• sufentanil citrate	Sufenta	1–30 mcg/kg with 100% oxygen and a muscle relaxant; may give additional doses of 10–50 mcg if needed
Miscellaneous agents		
• ketamine	Ketalar	2 mg/kg with additional doses after 5–10 minutes as needed

hypersensitive patients, acute narrow-angle glaucoma, increased intracranial pressure, impaired cerebral circulation, acute alcohol intoxication, intra-arterial injection, history of paradoxic excitation, myasthenia gravis, porphyrias, and status asthmaticus. General anesthetics are also contraindicated in shock, coma, obstetric procedures, labor, delivery, and during lactation. Drug regimens should be monitored closely due to many potential interactions.

Precautions

General anesthetics should be used with caution during pregnancy and in children younger than age 12 years. Patients should be questioned about OTC medications they may be taking due to potential interactions. This is also true for herbal supplements. Patients should be encouraged to breathe and cough deeply to clear anesthetics from the respiratory system.

Pain Management

Acute pain occurs because of injuries, burns, infections, or other causes and is considered self-limiting. Chronic pain often originates from neuropathic origins. It may persist for months or even years and requires pain management therapies. Patient-controlled analgesia (PCA) is a method of pain management wherein the patient uses a device with a button that is connected to an intravenous line; the patient can push the button to deliver a specific dose of pain medication. Conditions that produce pain include those from nociceptive origins, including inflammation, arthritis, lower back pain, headache, burns, and trauma. Conditions that produce pain from neuropathic origins include diabetic neuropathy, phantom limb, shingles, and trigeminal neuralgia.

Histamine and bradykinin are substances that produce inflammation, vasodilation, and pain. Prostaglandins trigger pain responses from peripheral nociceptors. Serotonin causes pain when released by mast cells as part of the inflammatory response. Glutamate is a neurotransmitter that carries pain messages to higher brain centers. A peptide known as substance P controls pain perception by acting as a neurotransmitter at junctions between nociceptors in the spinal cord. Endorphins, enkephalin, and dynorphin are peptides released when painful stimuli occur—they are the body's natural painkillers. GABA also helps to control pain by reducing the release of glutamate and substance P.

Opioids

Opioids are natural or synthetic substances extracted from the poppy plant that exert their effects through interaction with mu and kappa receptors in the brain. Natural opioids have been used for thousands of years to relieve pain. Opiates include morphine and heroin. The term *opioid* describes a drug that acts like morphine. Opiates and opioid agents produce analgesia. Opioids are classified as agonists and antagonists. A complete list of opioid agonists and antagonists is shown in **Table 21-6**.

TABLE 21–6 Opioid Agonists and Antagonists

Generic Name	Trade Name	Average Adult Dosage
Agonists		
• alfentanil	Alfenta	Injection: 8–20 mcg/kg
• codeine	Generic only	Injection: 15–30 mg/mL; PO: 15–200 mg
• codeine with acetaminophen (APAP)	Tylenol with Codeine No. 2, etc.	PO: 8–60 mg codeine with 120–300 mg APAP
• fentanyl	Actiq, Duragesic, Sublimaze	Injection: 0.05 mg/mL; PO: 200–1600 mcg; transdermal: 25–100 mcg
• hydrocodone with acetaminophen	Lortab, etc.	PO: 2.5–10 mg hydrocodone with 400–660 mg APAP
• hydrocodone with ibuprofen	Vicoprofen	PO: 5–7.5 mg hydrocodone with 200 mg ibuprofen
• hydromorphone	Dilaudid, etc.	Injection: 1–10 mg/mL; PO: 2–32 mg; suppository: 3 mg
• levorphanol	Levo-Dromoran	Injection: 2 mg/mL; PO: 2 mg
• meperidine	Demerol, etc.	Injection: 10–100 mg/mL; PO: 50–100 mg
• methadone	Dolophine, etc.	Injection: 10 mg/mL; PO: 5–40 mg
• morphine	Duramorph, etc.	Injection: 0.5–25 mg/mL; PO: 15–200 mg
• oxycodone	OxyContin, etc.	PO: 5–160 mg
• oxycodone with acetaminophen	Percocet, etc.	PO: 2.5–10 mg oxycodone with 325–650 mg APAP
• oxymorphone	Numorphan	Injection: 1–1.5 mg/mL; suppository: 5 mg
• sufentanil	Sufenta	Injection: 1–2 mcg/kg
Antagonists		
• naloxone	Narcan	Injection: 0.4–1 mg/mL
• naltrexone	ReVia	PO: 50 mg

Opioid Agonists

Opioid agonists produce analgesia. There are many different opioid agonists available, with the most common including codeine, hydrocodone, and morphine.

Method of Action
Opioid agonists work by reducing nociceptive stimulation to decrease pain sensation and raise the pain threshold.

Clinical Implications
Opioid agonists are used for symptomatic relief of serious acute and chronic pain after nonnarcotic analgesics have failed. Morphine is also used as a preanesthetic medication, to relieve shortness of breath associated with heart failure, and for pulmonary edema. Another indication of morphine is for acute chest pain connected with myocardial infarction. Opioids are used to decrease the cough reflex and slow the motility of the GI tract. Methadone is used for the treatment of addiction to narcotics.

Adverse Effects
Opioid agonists may cause euphoria, pupil constriction, hallucinations, nausea, constipation, dizziness, itching sensations, and physical dependence. Overdose may result in severe respiratory depression or cardiac arrest. Tolerance to opioid agonists and sedatives is a common development. Cross-tolerance also develops between morphine and other opioids, such as meperidine, methadone, and heroin.

Contraindications
Opioid agonists are contraindicated in asthmatics (especially before surgery). They are also contraindicated in GI obstruction and severe hepatic or renal impairment. Morphine may intensify or mask the pain of gallbladder disease.

Precautions
Opioid agonists must be used with caution in patients because of their potential to produce tolerance and dependence.

Opioid Antagonists

Opioid antagonists interfere with agonist binding. They bind to opioid receptors but do not activate them. They are used for reversal of respiratory depression that may be caused by opioid use. Opioid antagonists include naltrexone and naloxone. Naloxone is a pure opioid antagonist.

Method of Action
Opioid antagonists work by blocking the actions of both mu and kappa opioid receptors. They can also prevent receptors from being activated by opioid agonists.

Clinical Implications
Opioid antagonists are used for complete or partial reversal of opioid effects in emergency situations when acute opioid overdose is suspected. They are also used to treat postoperative opioid depression. Naltrexone is also used for treating opioid overdose and to manage alcohol and drug dependence.

Adverse Effects
Naloxone itself has minimal toxicity. However, reversal of the effects of opioids may result in rapid loss of analgesia, drowsiness, increased blood pressure, hyperventilation, nausea, and vomiting. Drowsiness may impair the ability of the patient to drive or operate machinery.

Contraindications

Opioid antagonists should not be taken with alcohol. They should not be used for respiratory depression that is caused by nonopioid drugs.

Precautions

Opioid antagonists should be used with caution in opioid-dependent patients because they can precipitate withdrawal symptoms.

Nonopioid Analgesics

Nonopioid analgesics include acetaminophen, aspirin, and the selective COX-2 inhibitors. They are effective in treating mild to moderate pain, inflammation, and fever.

Method of Action

Nonopioid analgesics decrease prostaglandin synthesis by inhibiting the action of cyclooxygenase (COX). When cyclooxygenase is inhibited, inflammation and pain are reduced. There are two forms of this substance, known as COX-1 and COX-2. These agents work similarly to aspirin but have greater potency. The only COX-2 inhibitor still on the market is celecoxib.

Clinical Implications

Nonopioid analgesics are used to treat mild to moderate pain, with or without inflammation, and when fever conditions exist because these agents can also reduce fever.

Adverse Effects

Nonopioid analgesics can cause headache, GI bleeding, ulceration, nausea, abdominal pain, and dizziness. Serious adverse effects include salicylism, agranulocytosis, and hepatic toxicity. Hepatotoxicity with alcohol is one of the serious adverse effects of acetaminophen.

Contraindications

Nonopioid analgesics are contraindicated primarily in hypersensitive patients, and celecoxib is also contraindicated after coronary artery bypass graft surgery. Aspirin should not be given to patients receiving anticoagulant therapy, such as warfarin, heparin, or plicamycin.

Precautions

Patients taking nonopioid analgesics must be instructed to contact their physician immediately if they have trouble breathing or experience chest pain, weakness in body parts, slurred speech, or swelling of the face or throat.

Patient Education

Respiratory therapists should instruct patients taking medications that affect the CNS not to drink alcohol, take other similar medications, take antihistamines, alter the prescribed dosage in any way, or drive cars or operate heavy machinery. They should report extreme lethargy, slurred speech, disorientation, or ataxia to their physician.

SUMMARY

There are many disorders that affect the central nervous system. The most common disorders of the central nervous system include anxiety, depression, and sleep disorders. Anxiety may be classified as generalized anxiety, phobias, obsessive-compulsive disorder, panic attacks, and posttraumatic stress disorder. Anxiety can be managed with a variety of medications. Insomnia is a sleep disorder that may be caused by anxiety. CNS agents, including anxiolytics, sedatives, and hypnotics, are used to treat anxiety and insomnia. Benzodiazepines are the drugs of choice for generalized anxiety and insomnia.

Depression has many causes and types. Major depression may be treated with medications, psychotherapy, or electroconvulsive therapy. Antidepressants act by correcting neurotransmitter imbalances in the brain and can reduce symptoms of depression. Common antidepressants include the tricyclic antidepressants (TCAs), monoamine oxidase inhibitors (MAOIs), and selective serotonin reuptake inhibitors (SSRIs).

General anesthesia produces a complete loss of sensation accompanied by loss of consciousness. This state is usually achieved through the use of several medications. Inhaled general anesthetics are used to maintain surgical anesthesia. Some types, such as nitrous oxide, have low efficacy, and the anesthetic known as halothane can induce deep anesthesia. IV anesthetics are used either alone for short procedures or in combination with inhaled anesthetics. Numerous nonanesthetic medications, including opioids, antianxiety agents, barbiturates, and neuromuscular blockers, are administered as adjuncts to surgery.

Opioids are natural or synthetic substances extracted from the poppy plant. They exert their effects through interaction with mu and kappa receptors. Opioids are the drugs of choice for severe pain, and they also have other important therapeutic effects. Opioid antagonists may be used to reverse the symptoms of opioid toxicity or overdose, including sedation or respiratory depression. Nonopioid analgesics, such as acetaminophen, aspirin, and the selective COX-2 inhibitors, are effective in treating mild or moderate pain, inflammation, and fever.

LEARNING GOALS

These learning goals correspond to the objectives at the beginning of the chapter, providing a clear summary of the chapter's most important points.

1. The neurotransmitters most involved in anxiety include gamma-aminobutyric acid (GABA), serotonin, and norepinephrine (NE).
2. Neurons are made up of three parts: dendrites, cell bodies, and axons. Dendrites are nerve cell processes that carry nervous impulses toward cell

bodies. Axons are nerve cell structures that carry impulses away from cell bodies to the dendrites.

3. The brain can be divided into four major portions: cerebrum, diencephalon, brainstem, and cerebellum. The cerebrum is the largest part of the brain, including nerve centers associated with sensory and motor functions. It provides higher mental functions, including memory and reasoning. The diencephalon also processes sensory information. Nerve pathways in the brainstem connect various parts of the nervous system and regulate certain visceral activities. The cerebellum includes centers that coordinate voluntary muscle movements.

4. Selective serotonin reuptake inhibitors (SSRIs) are the newest drugs for the treatment of depression. They are also the most widely prescribed antidepressants used today.

5. Anxiety is treated by drugs known as anxiolytics. These include benzodiazepines, azapirones, and miscellaneous anxiolytic agents.

6. The methods of action for each class of drugs used to treat depression are as follows:
    - Tricyclic antidepressants (TCAs) increase the effects of both norepinephrine and serotonin in presynaptic nerve terminals by blocking their neuronal uptake.
    - Selective serotonin reuptake inhibitors (SSRIs) selectively target serotonin by blocking the effects of serotonin reuptake.
    - Monoamine oxidase inhibitors (MAOIs) block the enzyme known as MAO, but their actual method of action is believed to only prevent the natural breakdown of neurotransmitters.
    - Second- and third-generation antidepressants appear to work by selectively inhibiting neuronal uptake of dopamine and other neurotransmitters.

7. The four stages of general anesthesia are analgesia, excitement (delirium), surgical anesthesia, and medullary paralysis. Analgesia abolishes pain but allows the patient to remain conscious. The excitement stage may cause the patient to become violent or afraid of what is occurring, so it is important that this second stage be managed so that the next stage is achieved as quickly as possible. Surgical anesthesia (stage 3) is characterized by progressive muscle relaxation but must be monitored closely so that respiratory paralysis does not occur. Stage 4 is medullary paralysis, which can lead to circulatory collapse. Obviously, this stage must be avoided at all costs.

8. Opioids are natural or synthetic substances extracted from the poppy plant that exert their effects through interaction with mu and kappa receptors in the brain. Opiates and opioid agents produce analgesia. Opioids are classified as agonists and antagonists. Nonopioid analgesics include acetaminophen, aspirin, and the selective COX-2 inhibitors.

9. Acute pain occurs because of injuries, burns, infections, or other causes, and it is considered self-limiting. Chronic pain often originates from neuropathic origins.

10. Sleep disorders may be treated with a variety of prescription or OTC medications, as well as with natural remedies. Prescription drugs used for insomnia include barbiturates, benzodiazepines, and other sedative–hypnotics.

CRITICAL THINKING QUESTIONS

1. Explain why antianxiety agents and drugs used for insomnia may cause cardiac collapse and respiratory depression.
2. Describe overdose and toxicity of morphine and its treatment.

WEB SITES

http://users.rcn.com/jkimball.ma.ultranet/
    BiologyPages/C/CNS.html
http://www.aapainmanage.org/
http://www.adaa.org/
http://www.depression.com/
http://www.depression-screening.org/
http://www.nimh.nih.gov/health/topics/anxiety-
    disorders/index.shtml
http://www.nlm.nih.gov/medlineplus/anesthesia.html
http://www.sleepforscience.org/study/
http://www.webmd.com/sleep-disorders/default.htm

REVIEW QUESTIONS

Multiple Choice

Select the best response to each question.

1. Which of the following is the greatest threat from morphine poisoning?
    A. cardiovascular collapse
    B. renal shutdown
    C. respiratory depression
    D. paralysis of the spinal cord
2. Which of the following is *not* a toxic effect of barbiturates?
    A. circulatory collapse
    B. renal impairment
    C. respiratory depression
    D. hypertension
3. Which of the following drugs is used to treat postoperative opioid depression?
    A. methadone
    B. meperidine
    C. naloxone
    D. atropine

4. Lorazepam is classified as an
   A. antianxiety agent
   B. anticholinergic
   C. antipyretic
   D. analgesic

5. Which of the following is a specific narcotic antagonist?
   A. meprobamate
   B. naltrexone
   C. propranolol
   D. phenytoin

6. Celecoxib is used as a(n)
   A. cardiotonic
   B. antihistamine
   C. analgesic
   D. antispasmodic

7. Which of the following is *not* an adverse effect of codeine?
   A. nausea
   B. diarrhea
   C. addiction
   D. respiratory depression

8. Combining an MAOI with an SSRI may cause
   A. serotonin syndrome
   B. Cushing syndrome
   C. pulmonary hypertension
   D. chronic obstructive pulmonary disease

9. Which of the following is classified as a monoamine oxidase inhibitor?
   A. fluvoxamine
   B. isocarboxazid
   C. trimipramine
   D. citalopram

10. Which of the following antidepressants also has an indication for smoking cessation?
    A. paroxetine
    B. citalopram
    C. bupropion
    D. mirtazapine

11. Which of the following drugs may increase the risk of suicide?
    A. benzodiazepines
    B. tricyclic antidepressants
    C. selective serotonin reuptake inhibitors
    D. opioids

12. Which of the following parts of the brainstem maintain basic breathing rhythm?
    A. medulla oblongata and pons
    B. cerebellum and midbrain
    C. midbrain and thalamus
    D. pons and hypothalamus

13. Which of the following stages of general anesthesia is called surgical anesthesia?
    A. stage 1
    B. stage 2
    C. stage 3
    D. stage 4

14. Hepatotoxicity is a serious adverse effect that may occur if alcohol is used with
    A. naloxone
    B. aspirin
    C. acetaminophen
    D. oxycodone

15. Which of the following is the main part of the diencephalon?
    A. pons
    B. hypothalamus
    C. midbrain
    D. cerebrum

CASE STUDY

An 80-year-old woman complains that she cannot sleep normally through the night. She has not altered her lifestyle in any way and is frustrated at the change in her sleep habits. She says that she wakes up suddenly many times during the night.

1. What possible condition could this patient have developed?
2. Has her age affected her sleeping habits in some way?

Effects of Drugs on the Autonomic Nervous System

OBJECTIVES

Upon completion of this chapter, the reader should be able to do the following:

1. Describe the structure and function of the autonomic nervous system.
2. Explain the roles of adrenergic and cholinergic agonists and antagonists.
3. Compare the anatomical components of the sympathetic and parasympathetic divisions of the autonomic nervous system.
4. Compare the fight-or-flight response to the rest-and-digest response.
5. List the neurotransmitters that are important to the autonomic nervous system.
6. Classify adrenergic agonists and antagonists.
7. List the contraindications of beta$_2$-receptor agonists.
8. Explain the clinical implications of alpha$_1$-rceptor agonists.
9. Describe the method of action of alpha$_2$-receptor agonists.
10. Explain the clinical implications of cholinergic agonists.

KEY TERMS

Acetylcholine (ACh)	Muscarinic receptor
Adrenal medulla	Nicotinic receptor
Adrenergic fibers	Norepinephrine (NE)
Adrenergic receptors	Pheochromocytoma
Cholinergic fiber	Sympathetic division
Cholinergic receptor	Synapses

INTRODUCTION

In the preceding chapter, the activities of the human nervous system of which we are consciously aware were discussed. These include the general and special senses, cognitive processes, emotions, and voluntary movements. In this chapter, the branch of the nervous system that primarily operates unconsciously will be discussed—the autonomic nervous system (ANS). The ANS operates almost entirely without any ability to control it, think about it, modify it, or suppress it.

The ANS is self-governed and almost completely independent of our will. It regulates fundamental life processes and states, including blood pressure, heart rate, body temperature, respiration, diameter of the pupils of the eyes, energy metabolism, digestion, defecation, and urination. The ANS quietly controls many unconscious processes of homeostasis. It is essential to understand the anatomy and physiology of the ANS to understand the effects of various medications that may increase (excite) or decrease (inhibit) its activities.

Structures and Functions of the Autonomic Nervous System

The peripheral nervous system (PNS) is the part of the nervous system that is located outside of the brain and spinal cord. The autonomic nervous system (ANS) is a division of the PNS. The ANS can itself be divided into two sections: motor and sensory neurons. The motor neurons of the ANS are divided into two subsystems: the sympathetic and parasympathetic divisions (see **Figure 22–1**). These divisions differ in structure and function. However, they often innervate the same target organs. They may have cooperative or contrasting effects on these organs.

Sympathetic Nervous System

The sympathetic division adapts the body for many types of physical activity. It increases alertness, blood pressure, heart rate, pulmonary airflow, blood glucose concentration, and blood flow to cardiac and skeletal muscles. At the same time, it reduces blood flow to the skin and digestive tract.

The sympathetic division is also called the thoracolumbar division because it arises from the thoracic and lumbar regions of the spinal cord. It has relatively short preganglionic and long postganglionic fibers

> **POINT TO REMEMBER**
>
> Cells that produce epinephrine have methyltransferase (an enzyme), which converts norepinephrine to epinephrine.

(see **Figure 22–2**). Preganglionic sympathetic neurons release acetylcholine (ACh). Postganglionic sympathetic neurons release norepinephrine. This is true throughout the body except in the sweat glands, where the postganglionic neurons release acetylcholine. The sympathetic division prepares the body for situations that expend energy, are stressful, or are emergency situations. This is part of the fight-or-flight response.

The sympathetic nervous system and adrenal medulla are very closely related in development and function. They are referred to collectively as the sympathoadrenal system. When stimulated, the adrenal medulla secretes a mixture of hormones into the bloodstream. These include approximately 85% epinephrine (adrenaline), 15% norepinephrine (noradrenaline), and a trace of dopamine.

Parasympathetic Nervous System

The parasympathetic division of the nervous system, in comparison, has a calming effect on many body systems. It is associated with reduced expenditure of energy and normal bodily maintenance. These include such functions as digestion and elimination of wastes. The effects of this division can be expressed as resting and digesting. The parasympathetic division decreases the heart rate, constricts breathing and the pupils, stimulates salivation

and digestion, stimulates the gallbladder, contracts the urinary bladder, and stimulates the sex organs.

The parasympathetic division is also called the craniosacral division because it arises from the brain and sacral region of the spinal cord. Its fibers travel through certain cranial and sacral nerves. The parasympathetic division has long preganglionic fibers that reach nearly all the way to the target cells. It also has short postganglionic fibers that cover the rest of the distance (see Figure 22–2).

Parasympathetic preganglionic neurons release acetylcholine at

> **POINT TO REMEMBER**
>
> Parasympathetic and sympathetic responses are coordinated. When one is generally decreased, the other is increased.

> **POINT TO REMEMBER**
>
> The effects of all parasympathetic actions are similar to the effects of parasympathomimetic nerve stimulations.

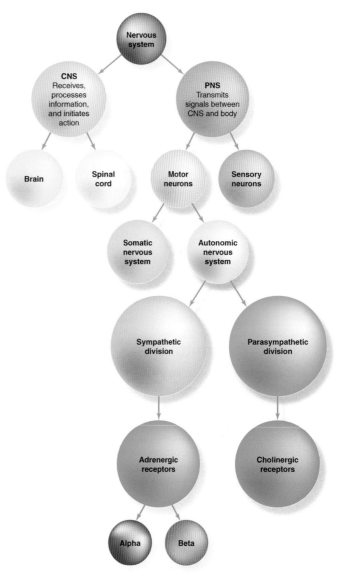

FIGURE 22–1 Divisions of the nervous system.

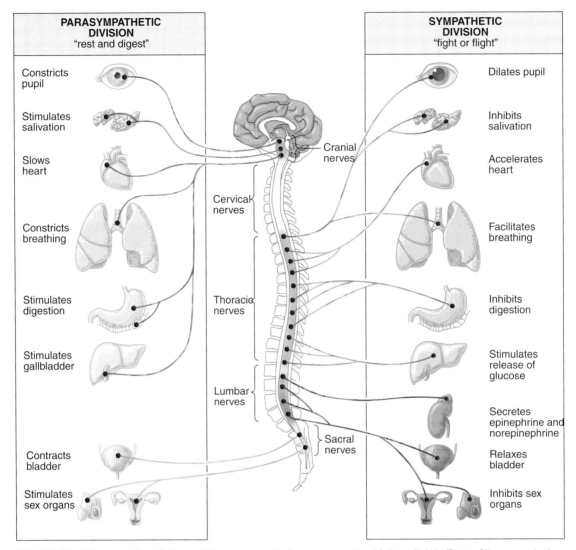

FIGURE 22–2 "Rest and digest" effects of the parasympathetic nervous system; "fight or flight" effects of the sympathetic nervous system.

the ganglia. The parasympathetic postganglionic neurons also release acetylcholine, which binds to the target tissue.

Neurotransmitters

Different autonomic neurons can have contrasting effects. This is because sympathetic and parasympathetic neurons secrete different neurotransmitters. It is also because cells respond in varying ways to the same neurotransmitter, depending upon which receptors they have for that neurotransmitter. **Figure 22–3** shows basic categories of autonomic neurotransmitters and receptors.

A nerve fiber that secretes acetylcholine (ACh) is called a cholinergic fiber. Any receptor that binds it is called a cholinergic receptor, which may be either a muscarinic receptor or a nicotinic receptor. All cardiac muscle, smooth muscle, and gland cells that receive cholinergic innervation have muscarinic receptors. Nicotinic receptors are found at synapses where autonomic

preganglionic neurons stimulate postganglionic cells, including the cells of the adrenal medulla and the neuromuscular junctions of skeletal muscle fibers. ACh excites all cells that have nicotinic receptors.

Norepinephrine (NE) is secreted by most sympathetic postganglionic neurons. Nerve fibers that secrete NE are called adrenergic fibers, and the receptors for it are called adrenergic receptors. NE is also called noradrenaline. The origin of the term *adrenergic* is from *adrenaline*. Adrenergic receptors include α-adrenergic receptors (which usually have excitatory effects) and β-adrenergic receptors (which usually have inhibitory effects).

Drugs and the Autonomic Nervous System

Autonomic nervous system drugs are categorized by which receptors they stimulate or block. They include adrenergic agonists (sympathomimetics), adrenergic

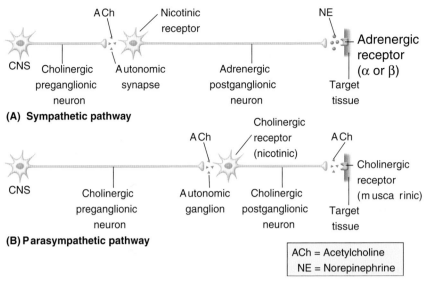

FIGURE 22–3 Receptors in the autonomic nervous system: (A) sympathetic pathways (acetylcholine [Ach] and norepinephrine [NE]); (B) parasympathetic pathway (acetylcholine [Ach]).

antagonists (blockers), cholinergic agonists (parasympathomimetics), and cholinergic antagonists (blockers).

Adrenergic Agonists

Adrenergic agonists (sympathomimetics) are either catecholamines or noncatecholamines. These agonists mimic the actions of the sympathetic nervous system. Catecholamines include norepinephrine, epinephrine, and dopamine. These naturally secreted neurotransmitters can also be manufactured synthetically. Noncatecholamines are more selective of receptor sites, slower acting, and have a longer duration. **Table 22–1** summarizes the classifications of adrenergic agonists.

TABLE 22–1 Classifications of Adrenergic Agonists

Generic name	Trade name	Indications
Alpha$_1$ agonists		
• methoxamine	Vasoxyl	Maintenance of blood pressure during anesthesia
• midodrine	Pro Amatine	Orthostatic hypotension
• oxymetazoline	Afrin	Nasal congestion
• phenylephrine	Neo-Synephrine	Nasal congestion
• xylometazoline	Otrivin, et	Nasal congestion
Alpha$_2$ agonists		
• apraclonidine	Iopidine	Operative eye pressure, glaucoma
• clonidine	Catapres (in CNS)	Hypertension
• guanabenz	Wytensin	Hypertension
• guanfacine	Tenex	Hypertension
• methyldopa	AdoMet (in CNS)	Hypertension
Beta$_1$ agonists		
• dobutamine	Dobutrex	Cardiac stimulant
Beta$_2$ agonists		
• albuterol	Ventolin	Asthma
• metaproterenol	Alupent	Asthma
• ritodrine	Yutopar	Slow uterine contractions
• salmeterol	Serevent	Decongestant
• terbutaline	Brethine	Asthma
Catecholamines		
• dopamine	Intropin (α_1 and β_1)	Shock
• epinephrine	Adrenalin, Primatene (α and β)	Asthma and cardiac arrest
• isoproterenol	Isuprel (β_1 and β_2)	Asthma, dysrhythmias, and heart failure
• norepinephrine	Levarterenol, Levophed (α and β)	Shock
Miscellaneous adrenergic agonists		
• amphetamine	Generic only	Attention-deficit/hyperactivity disorder, narcolepsy, and obesity
• ephedrine	Generic only	Allergies, asthma, and narcolepsy
• methylphenidate	Ritalin	Attention-deficit/hyperactivity disorder and obesity
• pemoline	Cylert	Attention-deficit/hyperactivity disorder
• pseudoephedrine	Sudafed (α and β)	Coryza, rhinitis, and sinusitis

Alpha₁-Receptor Agonists

Alpha₁-receptors are found on blood vessels. They affect blood pressure and blood flow into tissues (tissue perfusion). They are also found on muscles of the iris in each eye, smooth gastrointestinal (GI) tract muscles, smooth reproductive tract muscles, and in liver cells, urinary bladder sphincters, and sweat glands. These agonists affect alpha₁ receptors to cause vasoconstriction, some dilation, and other actions.

Method of Action

Alpha₁-receptor agonists cause blood vessel constriction, pupil dilation (mydriasis), decreased GI motility, external bladder sphincter contraction, decreased secretion of bile, and sweat gland stimulation.

Clinical Implications

Alpha₁-receptor agonists are used for hypotension, nasal congestion, and red eye (subconjunctival hemorrhage).

Adverse Effects

Alpha₁-receptor agonists may cause blurred vision, constipation, hypertension, gooseflesh, sweating, or urine retention.

Contraindications

Alpha₁-receptor agonists are contraindicated in severe cardiovascular or coronary disease, glaucoma, acute kidney disease, hypovolemia (within 2 weeks of taking MAOIs), adrenal tumor, hyperthyroidism or Graves disease, urine retention, hypersensitivity to these types of agents, supine hypertension, and ventricular tachycardia. They should not be used during pregnancy or lactation or in very young patients.

Precautions

Patients taking alpha₁-receptor agonists should be instructed to inform their physician if they have high blood pressure, enlarged prostate, glaucoma, thyroid disease, or if they are breastfeeding. There are many interactions with other medications, so a complete drug regimen review should be undertaken before taking these agonists. Dosages must be administered exactly as prescribed.

Alpha₂-Receptor Agonists

Alpha₂-receptor agonists are located primarily on the presynaptic neurons. They appear to control the release of neurotransmitters by these neurons, usually to reduce blood pressure.

Method of Action

Alpha₂-receptor agonists stimulate alpha₂-receptors to inhibit sympathetic vasomotor centers. This reduces plasma concentrations of norepinephrine, decreases systolic blood pressure and heart rate, and inhibits the kidneys from releasing renin.

Clinical Implications

Alpha₂-receptor agonists are used for hypertension either with other hypertensive agents or alone. They are also used as adjunct therapy for severe pain via epidural injection.

Adverse Effects

Alpha₂-receptor agonists may cause hypotension, dry mouth, dry eyes, peripheral edema, constipation, dizziness, drowsiness, pruritus, impotence, nausea, vomiting, rash, hallucinations, depression, hepatitis, and recurrent herpes simplex.

Contraindications

Alpha₂-receptor agonists are contraindicated in hypertension related to pregnancy toxemia, swollen or damaged arteries, scleroderma (skin hardening), cirrhosis, hepatitis, **pheochromocytoma**, blood dyscrasias, and in pregnancy or lactation. They are also contraindicated in pediatric patients.

Precautions

Alpha₂-receptor agonists should be used with caution in hypertension with excessive sodium that can lead to fluid retention. Patients should avoid foods high in sodium, including certain types of soup, processed cheese, potato chips, pretzels, and salted crackers.

Beta₁-Receptor Agonists

These agonists are found on the myocardium, fat cells, GI sphincters and smooth muscle, and the renal arterioles.

Method of Action

Beta₁-receptor agonists work by increasing the heart's rate and force of contraction. This increases lipolysis in fatty (adipose) tissue, decreases digestion and GI motility, and increases glomerular filtration.

Clinical Implications

These agonists are used for circulatory shock, cardiac arrest, and hypotension.

Adverse Effects

Beta₁-receptor agonists may cause hypertension, constipation, and tachycardia.

Contraindications

These agonists are contraindicated in hypersensitive patients, after an acute myocardial infarction, and in ventricular tachycardia. They should not be used in pediatric, pregnant, or lactating patients.

Precautions

Isoproterenol may turn sputum and saliva pink after it is inhaled. Women should not breastfeed while taking beta₁-receptor agonists. Patients should be cautioned about any anginal pain, which should be reported to their physician immediately. Doses should not be increased, decreased, or omitted, and intervals between doses should not be changed.

Beta₂-Receptor Agonists

Beta₂-adrenoreceptors are found on bronchiole smooth muscle and in liver cells, skeletal muscles, and the blood vessels that supply the brain, heart, kidneys, and skeletal muscles.

Method of Action

These agonists stimulate the beta₂ receptors, causing bronchodilation, increased skeletal muscle excitability, relaxation of the uterus during pregnancy, and vasodilation of the blood vessels to the brain, heart, kidneys, and skeletal muscles.

Clinical Implications

Beta₂-receptor agonists are used for chronic obstructive pulmonary disease, circulatory shock, peripheral vascular disease, and premature labor.

Adverse Effects

These agonists may cause increased muscle tension, feelings of warmth, muscle tremor in the hands, and increased blood glucose. Other adverse effects include dizziness, tremor, and postural hypotension.

Contraindications

Beta₂-receptor agonists are contraindicated in hypersensitive patients, patients with cardiac arrhythmias (associated with tachycardia or digitalis intoxication), hyperthyroidism, hypertension during pregnancy (preeclampsia), coma and convulsions related to pregnancy (eclampsia), hypertension, diabetes mellitus, hypovolemia, intrauterine infection, asthma (treated with beta-mimetics), coronary artery disease (within 14 days of MAOI therapy), angle-closure glaucoma, and thyrotoxicosis. They should not be used in pediatric, pregnant, or lactating patients.

Precautions

Patients should be instructed on the correct use of the inhaler required for these agonists, and the technique should be demonstrated to them. Doses and the frequency of doses should not be changed. Other OTC drugs should be avoided, and patients should report any failure of symptom reduction to their physician.

Adrenergic Antagonists

These antagonists can show specificity for blocking a certain receptor or subtype. They are subdivided as alpha-receptor antagonists and beta-receptor antagonists.

Alpha-Receptor Antagonists

These antagonists can be reversible or irreversible, and they may be nonselective or highly selective. They all antagonize the effects of endogenous catecholamines.

Method of Action

Adrenergic antagonists work by selectively inhibiting alpha adrenoreceptors. This produces arteriole and venal vasodilation, reducing peripheral vascular resistance and blood pressure.

> **POINT TO REMEMBER**
>
> Adrenergic antagonists have no affects on adrenergic receptors. Instead, they reduce the release of norepinephrine from the postganglionic adrenergic neurons.

Clinical Implications

These antagonists are used for controlling hypertension and to treat adrenal medulla tumor, peripheral vascular disease, and urinary retention.

Adverse Effects

Adrenergic antagonists may cause nasal congestion, inhibited ejaculation, lack of energy, and postural hypotension.

Contraindications

These antagonists should be avoided with known hypersensitivity, and they may have interactions with many different types of drugs, including diuretics, various neurotransmitters, other hypotensive agents, and NSAIDs.

Precautions

Because of their ability to cause dizziness (from postural hypotension), patients should be advised to change positions slowly and avoid driving for at least 12 hours after taking the first dose. They should avoid OTC drugs for respiratory conditions unless approved by their physician. Women should not breastfeed while taking adrenergic antagonists.

Beta-Receptor Antagonists

These antagonists reduce receptor occupancy by beta agonists and are usually pure antagonists that cause no activation of beta receptors.

Method of Action

Beta-receptor antagonists block beta receptors to cause decreased peripheral resistance, orthostatic hypotension, and vasodilation. They primarily target cardiac muscles.

Clinical Implications

These antagonists are used for management of hypertension when patients have not responded to diet, exercise, and weight reduction. They are also used for cardiac arrhythmias, myocardial infarction, hypertrophic sub-aortic stenosis, tachyarrhythmias, angina pectoris, hereditary essential tremor, and pheochromocytoma.

Adverse Effects

Beta-receptor antagonists may cause dizziness, insomnia, diarrhea, and lethargy.

Contraindications

These agonists are contraindicated in heart block, cardiogenic shock, severe heart failure, and other severe circulatory disorders. They should be avoided if there is a history of asthma or chronic obstructive pulmonary disease. They may interact with many other drugs and hypotensive agents.

Precautions

Patients must be instructed on how to monitor their own heart rate and blood pressure, and they should report decreases in either of them during therapy with beta-receptor antagonists. Patients should change positions slowly and avoid driving for at least 12 hours after taking the first dose. Breastfeeding should be avoided. OTC drugs for respiratory conditions should not be taken concurrently unless approved by a physician.

Cholinergic Agonists

These agents (also known as parasympathomimetics or cholinomimetics) mimic the effects of acetylcholine to stimulate the parasympathetic nervous system. Cholinergic agonists contain two types of receptors: muscarinic receptors and nicotinic receptors. Muscarinic receptors innervate smooth muscle and slow the heart rate, and nicotinic receptors affect skeletal muscles. Because most of these agonists are nonselective, they can innervate both types of receptors. Some of these agonists are selective only for muscarinic receptors.

Method of Action

Cholinergic agonists work either directly or indirectly to stimulate smooth and skeletal muscle and slow the heart rate.

POINT TO REMEMBER

Congenital megacolon is a disorder of the large intestine, characterized by the absence or marked reduction of parasympathetic ganglion cells in the colorectal wall.

Clinical Implications

These agonists are used to reduce elevated intraocular pressure (in glaucoma) and to treat constipation, congenital megacolon, postoperative

and postpartum obstruction of the bowel, reflux esophagitis, nonobstructive urine retention, neurogenic urinary bladder with retention, diagnosis of atrial tachycardia, diagnosis of asthma, and dry mouth (see **Table 22–2**).

Adverse Effects

Cholinergic agonists may cause bronchospasm, excessive salivation, flushing, abdominal cramps, difficulty in visual accommodation, sweating, convulsions, nausea, vomiting, diarrhea, urinary frequency, and headache.

Contraindications

These agonists are contraindicated with atrioventricular arrhythmias, coronary insufficiency, asthma, hyperthyroidism, and peptic ulcer. They may interact with many other types of drugs.

Precautions

Patients should be cautioned that many other types of drugs may cause interactions and that they must report all drugs they are currently using before beginning cholinergic agonist therapy. They should change positions slowly to avoid dizziness. Women should not breastfeed while taking these agonists.

Cholinergic Antagonists

Cholinergic antagonists (blockers) are also known as anticholinergics or parasympatholytics. They inhibit the actions of acetylcholine by occupying the acetylcholine receptors. These antagonists primarily affect the heart, respiratory tract, eyes, GI tract, sweat glands, and urinary bladder.

Method of Action

These agents act primarily on muscarinic receptors, with little effect on nicotinic receptors.

Clinical Implications

Cholinergic antagonists are primarily used for GI disorders, ophthalmic disorders, bronchial conditions,

TABLE 22–2   Common Cholinergic Agonists

Generic Name	Trade Name	Average Adult Dosage
Direct acting		
• bethanechol	Duvoid, Urabeth	PO: 2.5–5 mg, repeat at 15–30 minute intervals p.r.n.
• carbachol	Miostat	Intraocular (topical): 1–2 drops q4–8h; (approximately 0.5 mL)
• cevimeline	Evoxac	PO: 30 mg t.i.d.
• pilocarpine	Pilocar	Intraocular: 1–2 gtt in eye 1–6 times/day
Indirect acting		
• ambenonium	Mytelase	PO: 5–75 mg q.i.d.
• edrophonium	Enlon, Tensilon	V: 2 mg injected over 15–30 seconds; if needed inject another 8 mg after 45 seconds
• neostigmine	Prostigmin	PO: 15–375 mg/day in 3–6 divided doses
• pyridostigmine	Mestinon	PO: 60 mg–1.5 g/day; 180–540 mg 1–2 times/day sustained release
• tacrine	Cognex	PO: 10–40 mg/day (max: 160 mg/day)

various cardiac conditions, chronic obstructive pulmonary disease, upper respiratory infections, preoperative situations, and to counteract mushroom poisoning.

Adverse Effects

Common adverse effects of these antagonists include decreased perspiration, dry mouth, blurred vision, tachycardia, constipation, and urine retention. Other adverse effects may include headache, nausea, abdominal distention, dry skin, hypotension or hypertension, impotence, photophobia, and coma.

Contraindications

Cholinergic antagonists are contraindicated in hypersensitive patients, angle-closure glaucoma, inflammation of the saliva glands, weakness of intestinal muscles, obstructive uropathy, GI obstructions, paralytic ileus, severe ulcerative colitis, toxic megacolon, acute hemorrhage, tachycardia, myasthenia gravis, and in pregnant or lactating patients.

Precautions

Patients taking these antagonists should be cautioned to use frequent mouth rinses or to chew gum or suck on candy to relieve dry mouth. Their dental hygiene should be increased to counteract the effects of these agents. Patients should avoid driving and breastfeeding while taking cholinergic antagonists. Any tachycardia or palpitations should be reported to a physician immediately.

Patient Education

Respiratory therapists should instruct patients to use sympathomimetic drugs exactly as prescribed and not to double their dose. These medications should be taken early in the day to prevent insomnia. Patients must immediately report shortness of breath, palpitations, dizziness, or chest pain to their physician. They should be told to avoid driving and other activities that require visual acuity until blurring subsides (in the case of ophthalmic sympathomimetics).

Patients should report nausea, vomiting, diarrhea, jaundice, and changes in color of stool when they use parasympathomimetics. They must also be instructed to take the drug as directed on a regular schedule to maintain serum levels and control symptoms. Oral parasympathomimetics should be taken on an empty stomach to lessen the incidence of nausea and vomiting and to increase absorption.

SUMMARY

The peripheral nervous system is divided into a somatic portion and an autonomic portion. The somatic portion is under voluntary control; the autonomic portion is involuntary and controls smooth muscle, cardiac muscle, and glandular secretions. Stimulation of the sympathetic division of the autonomic nervous system causes symptoms of the fight-or-flight response, and stimulation of the parasympathetic branch induces rest-and-digest responses.

Drugs can prevent the synthesis, storage, or release of neurotransmitters. They can also prevent the destruction of neurotransmitters or bind neurotransmitters to receptors. Norepinephrine is the primary neurotransmitter released at adrenergic receptors, which are divided into alpha and beta subtypes. Acetylcholine is the other primary neurotransmitter of the autonomic nervous system. Acetylcholine is the primary neurotransmitter released at cholinergic receptors (nicotinic and muscarinic) in both the sympathetic and parasympathetic nervous systems.

Autonomic drugs are classified by the receptors they stimulate or block. Sympathomimetics stimulate sympathetic nerves, and parasympathomimetics stimulate parasympathetic nerves. Adrenergic antagonists inhibit the sympathetic division, whereas anticholinergics inhibit the parasympathetic branch.

LEARNING GOALS

These learning goals correspond to the objectives at the beginning of the chapter, providing a clear summary of the chapter's most important points.

1. The autonomic nervous system is a division of the peripheral nervous system. The ANS can be divided into motor and sensory neurons. The motor neurons of the ANS can be divided into the sympathetic and parasympathetic divisions that may have cooperative or contrasting effects when innervating target organs.

2. The roles of adrenergic and cholinergic agonists and antagonists are as follows:
    -   Adrenergic agonists (sympathomimetics) mimic the actions of the sympathetic nervous system.
    -   Adrenergic antagonists (blockers) can show specificity for blocking a certain receptor or subtype. They are subdivided as alpha-receptor antagonists and beta-receptor antagonists.
    -   Cholinergic agonists (also known as parasympathomimetics or cholinomimetics) mimic the effects of acetylcholine to stimulate the parasympathetic nervous system.
    -   Cholinergic antagonists (blockers) are also known as anticholinergics or parasympatholytics. They inhibit the actions of acetylcholine by occupying the acetylcholine receptors.

3. The sympathetic division of the ANS adapts the body for many types of physical activities and reduces blood flow to the skin and digestive tract. It arises from the thoracic and lumbar regions of the spinal cord. This is the fight-or-flight division.

The parasympathetic division has a calming effect on many body systems, including digestion and elimination of wastes. It is the rest-and-digest division. It arises from the brain and sacral region of the spinal cord.

4. The fight-or-flight response increases alertness, blood pressure, heart rate, pulmonary airflow, blood glucose concentration, and blood flow to cardiac and skeletal muscles. The rest-and-digest response decreases the heart rate, constricts breathing and the pupils, stimulates salivation and digestion, stimulates the gallbladder, contracts the urinary bladder, and stimulates the sex organs.

5. Neurotransmitters that are important to the autonomic nervous system include acetylcholine, adrenaline (epinephrine), noradrenaline (norepinephrine), serotonin, dopamine, and GABA.

6. Adrenergic agonists (sympathomimetics) are either catecholamines (norepinephrine, epinephrine, and dopamine) or noncatecholamines. They are naturally selected neurotransmitters that can also be manufactured synthetically. Adrenergic antagonists are subdivided as alpha-receptor antagonists and beta-receptor antagonists. Alpha-receptor antagonists antagonize the effects of endogenous catecholamines. Beta-receptor antagonists reduce receptor occupancy by beta agonists and are usually pure antagonists that cause no activation of beta receptors.

7. Beta$_2$-receptor agonists are contraindicated in hypersensitive patients, patients with cardiac arrhythmias, hyperthyroidism, preeclampsia, eclampsia, hypertension, diabetes mellitus, hypovolemia, intrauterine infection, asthma (treated with beta-mimetics), coronary artery disease (within 14 days of MAOI therapy), angle-closure glaucoma, and thyrotoxicosis. They should not be used in pediatric, pregnant, or lactating patients.

8. Alpha$_1$-receptor agonists are used for hypotension, nasal congestion, and subconjunctival hemorrhage.

9. Alpha$_2$-receptor agonists work by inhibiting sympathetic vasomotor centers to reduce norepinephrine in the plasma, decrease systolic blood pressure and heart rate, and inhibit renal release of renin.

10. Cholinergic agonists are indicated for GI disorders, ophthalmic disorders, bronchial conditions, cardiac conditions, chronic obstructive pulmonary disease, upper respiratory infections, preoperative situations, and to counteract mushroom poisoning.

CRITICAL THINKING QUESTIONS

1. Explain neurotransmitters that are released from preganglionic and postganglionic neurons of both the sympathetic and parasympathetic nervous systems.
2. Explain the clinical implications of alpha$_1$- and beta$_1$- receptor agonists.

WEB SITES

http://ni.cvm.umn.edu/pdfs/AutonomicPharmacology .pdf

http://www.becomehealthynow.com/article/ bodynervousadvanced/821/

http://www.benbest.com/science/anatmind/anatmd10 .html

http://www.mediglyphics.com/public/Pharmacology/ cholinergic_agonists_and_overview

http://www.sciencedaily.com/articles/s/sympathetic_ nervous_system.htm

http://www.studystack.com/flashcard-197463

http://www.uic.edu/classes/phar/phar402/katz/ adragonist/

REVIEW QUESTIONS

Multiple Choice

Select the best response to each question.

1. Which of the following is secreted by most sympathetic postganglionic neurons?
   A. dopamine and acetylcholine
   B. norepinephrine and acetylcholine
   C. only norepinephrine
   D. only acetylcholine

2. Muscarine is a parasympathetic substance that mimics the effect of
   A. epinephrine
   B. norepinephrine
   C. acetylcholine
   D. serotonin

3. Which is the major neurotransmitter secreted from the adrenal medulla?
   A. epinephrine
   B. norepinephrine
   C. dopamine
   D. acetylcholine

4. Beta$_1$-receptor agonists are used for all of the following conditions except
   A. hypotension
   B. cardiac arrest
   C. shock
   D. hypertension

5. Beta$_2$-receptor agonists are contraindicated in
   A. premature labor
   B. hypersensitive patients
   C. circulatory shock
   D. chronic obstructive pulmonary disease
6. Cholinergic antagonists are also known as
   A. sympathomimetics
   B. catecholamines
   C. adrenergic antagonists
   D. anticholinergics
7. Which of the following is an example of an alpha$_1$ agonist?
   A. phenylephrine (Neo-Synephrine)
   B. dopamine (Intropin)
   C. albuterol (Ventolin)
   D. salmeterol (Serevent)
8. Brethine is the trade name of
   A. methyldopa
   B. terbutaline
   C. amphetamine
   D. norepinephrine
9. Which of the following is an indication of phenylephrine (Neo-Synephrine)?
   A. nasal congestion
   B. hypertension
   C. shock
   D. asthma
10. Which of the following are the clinical implications of epinephrine?
   A. sinusitis and attention-deficit/hyperactivity disorder
   B. hypertension and glaucoma
   C. asthma and cardiac arrest
   D. obesity and narcolepsy
11. All of the following are adverse effects of beta$_1$-receptor agonists except
   A. hypertension
   B. constipation
   C. bradycardia
   D. tachycardia
12. Pheochromocytoma is a malignant tumor of the adrenal medulla that secretes
   A. serotonin
   B. catecholamine
   C. acetylcholine
   D. all of the above
13. Cholinergic antagonists act primarily on which of the following receptors?
   A. muscarinic
   B. nicotinic
   C. both A and B
   D. none of the above
14. Ventolin is the trade name of
   A. metaproterenol
   B. terbutaline
   C. albuterol
   D. salmeterol
15. The parasympathetic division of the nervous system can be expressed as
   A. the fight-or-flight division
   B. the rest-and-digest division
   C. either A or B
   D. none of the above

CASE STUDY

A 53-year-old male patient was diagnosed with Parkinson disease 2 years ago. He is being treated with benztropine (Cogentin), an anticholinergic agent.

1. How does this medication work in treating Parkinson disease?
2. Discuss the potential adverse effects of benztropine.

100 Commonly Prescribed Drugs for Cardiopulmonary Care

Certain drugs have multiple uses, but these are the most common uses for each.

Type	Generic Name	Trade Name
Angiotensin acting drugs	captopril	Capoten
	trandolapril	Mavik
Antianginals		
• Nitrates	isosorbide	Imdur
• Others	clonidine	Catapres
	methyldopa	Aldomet
	prazosin	Minipress
Antiarrhythmics	amiodarone	Cordarone
	digoxin	Digitek
	disopyramide	Norpace
	mexiletine	Mexitil
	procainamide	Procanbid
	propafenone	Rythmol
	propranolol	Inderal
	quinidine	Quinidex
	tocainide	Tonocard
Antiasthmatics	albuterol	ProAir HFA
	fluticasone/salmeterol	Advair Diskus
	montelukast	Singulair
Anticoagulants	enoxaparin	Lovenox
	heparin	Hep-Lock
	warfarin	Coumadin
Antidiabetics	glipizide	Glucotrol
	glyburide	Micronase
	metformin	Glucophage
	pioglitazone	Actos
	rosiglitazone	Avandia
Antihistamines	astemizole	Hismanal
	brompheniramine	Dimetane
	cetirizine	Zyrtec
	chlorpheniramine	Chlor-Trimeton
	clemastine	Tavist
	cyproheptadine	Periactin
	desloratadine	Clarinex
	diphenhydramine	Benadryl
	fexofenadine	Allegra
	loratadine	Claritin
	promethazine	Phenergan
	terfenadine	Seldane

Type	Generic Name	Trade Name
Antihypertensives	amlodipine	Norvasc
	amlodipine/benazepril	Lotrel
	carvedilol	Coreg
	diltiazem	Cartia XL
	losartan	Cozaar
	metoprolol	Toprol XL
	quinapril	Prinivil
	ramipril	Altace
	valsartan	Diovan
Antilipidemics	atorvastatin	Lipitor
	ezetimibe	Zetia
	ezetimibe/simvastatin	Vytorin
	fenofibrate	TriCor
	gemfibrozil	Lopid
	rosuvastatin	Crestor
Antitussives	codeine	Codeine Sulfate
	codeine/chlorpheniramine	Codeprex
Beta-blockers	atenolol	Tenormin
	nadolol	Corgard
	pindolol	Visken
	sotalol	Betapace AF
Bronchodilators	albuterol	Proventil
	epinephrine	Epinephrine Mist
	metaproterenol	Alupent
	pirbuterol	Maxair
	salmeterol	Serevent
	terbutaline	Brethine
	theopylline	Theo-Dur
Calcium channel blockers	amlodipine/olmesartan	Azor
	isradipine	DynaCirc
	nifedipine	Procardia
	verapamil	Calan
Decongestants	l-desoxyephedrine	Vicks Inhaler
	oxymetazoline	Afrin
	phenylephrine	Neo-Synephrine
	pseudoephedrine	Sudafed
Diuretics	amiloride	Midamor
	bumetanide	Bumex
	chlorothiazide	Diuril
	furosemide	Lasix
	hydrochlorothiazide	Hydrodiuril
	indapamide	Lozol
	mannitol	Mannitol IV
	methyclothiazide	Enduron
	metolazone	Dialo
	spironolactone	Aldactone
	spironolactone/amiloride	Alazide
	triamterene	Dyrenium
	triamterene/hydrochlorothiazide	Dyazide
Expectorants	guaifenesin	Robitussin
Intranasal agents	budesonide	Rhinocort

Type	Generic Name	Trade Name
Respiratory inhalants	beclomethasone cromolyn flunisolide fluticasone ipratropium triamcinolone	Beclovent Intal AeroBid Flovent Atrovent Azmacort
Vasoconstrictors	dopamine norepinephrine	Intropin Levophed
Vasodilators	enalapril lisinopril nitroglycerin	Vasotec Prinivil Nitrostat

Commonly Confused Drug Names

Generic Names	Brand Names	Potential Confusion
amiodarone amantadine	Cordarone (generic only)	Easily confused generic names. Amiodarone is an antiarrhythmic, whereas amantadine is an antiviral.
amlodipine amiloride	Norvasc Midamor	Easily confused generic names. Amlodipine is a calcium channel blocker, whereas amiloride is a potassium-sparing diuretic.
benazepril diphenhydramine	Lotensin Benadryl	Generic name benazepril may be confused with brand name Benadryl. Benazepril is an ACE inhibitor, whereas diphenhydramine is an antihistamine.
captopril carvedilol	Capoten Coreg	Easily confused generic names. Captopril is an ACE inhibitor, whereas carvedilol is a beta-blocker.
cetirizine sertraline olanzapine	Zyrtec Zoloft Zyprexa IM	Generic names may be confused with each other, and brand names may also be confused with each other. Cetirizine is an antihistamine, sertraline is an antidepressant, and olanzapine is an antipsychotic.
clonidine clonazepam	Catapres Klonopin	Easily confused generic or trade names. Clonidine is an antihypertensive, whereas clonazepam is a benzodiazepine.
codeine etodolac	Codeine Sulfate Lodine	Generic name codeine may be confused with brand name Lodine. Codeine is a narcotic analgesic, whereas etodolac is a non-steroidal anti-inflammatory drug (NSAID).
diphenhydramine dimenhydrinate	Benadryl Dramamine	Easily confused generic names. Diphenhydramine is an antihistamine, whereas dimenhydrinate is used to treat dizziness, vertigo, nausea, and vomiting.
disopyramide desipramine	Norpace Norpramin	Generic names may be confused with each other, and brand names may also be confused with each other. Disopyramide is an antiarrhythmic, whereas desipramine is an antidepressant.
dopamine dobutamine	Intropin (generic only)	Easily confused generic names. Dopamine is a vasopressor and inotropic agent, whereas dobutamine is a direct-acting inotropic agent. Dopamine is from a natural catecholamine source; dobutamine is synthetic. Any combination of these drugs requires diligent monitoring.
ephedrine epinephrine	(generic only) Epinephrine Mist	Since these drugs have similar names and uses, they may be stored close to each other. They are also packaged somewhat similarly. Ephedrine is a decongestant, whereas epinephrine is often used as an antiasthmatic.
glipizide glyburide	Glucotrol Micronase	Easily confused generic names. They are both antidiabetic medications used to treat type 2 diabetes mellitus. Glipizide may be taken in higher doses than glyburide; therefore, confusion between the two has the potential to be harmful to the patient.
guaifenesin guanfacine	Robitussin Tenex	Easily confused generic names. Guaifenesin is an expectorant, whereas guanfacine is an alpha agonist used for high blood pressure.

Generic Names	Brand Names	Potential Confusion
heparin hetastarch in sodium chloride	Hep-Lock Hespan	Generic name heparin may be confused with the brand name Hespan. Heparin is an anticoagulant, whereas hetastarch is a plasma volume expander.
Insulin glargine Insulin zinc suspension Human insulin Insulin lispro Human insulin aspart	Lantus Lente Humulin Humalog Novolog	Similar names, strengths, and concentrations can lead to medication errors. Confusion between 100 units per mL and 500 units per mL may occur.
metformin metronidazole	Glucophage Flagyl	Easily confused generic names. Metformin is an antidiabetic, whereas metronidazole is an antibiotic.
metolazone methimazole	Dialo Tapazole	Easily confused generic names. Metolazone is a diuretic, whereas methimazole is an antithyroid agent.
metoprolol succinate metoprolol tartrate	Toprol XL Lopressor	Different types of the drug "metoprolol." They are both beta-blockers, but the succinate formulation is stronger than the tartrate formulation. Therefore, caution must be used based on dosage.
nifedipine nicardipine nimodipine	Procardia Cardene IV (generic only)	Easily confused generic names. They are also calcium channel blockers. Nifedipine has a shorter half-life than nicardipine, and nimodipine should only be taken orally due to life-threatening complications when injected.
quinidine quinine	Quinidex Qualaquin	Easily confused generic names, which also may be confused with the trade name Quinidex. Quinidine is an antiarrhythmic that is also an antimalarial, whereas quinine has been banned in the United States by the FDA except for the formulation known as Qualaquin, an antimalarial.
sotalol pseudoephedrine	Betapace AF Sudafed	Generic name sotalol may be confused with the trade name Sudafed. Sotalol is a beta-blocker, whereas pseudoephedrine is a decongestant.

Reporting of Medical Errors

Thousands of people are harmed each year in the United States by medical errors. Hundreds die as a result of these errors. Recent studies have shown that 10 to 25 percent of all medical errors are caused by medication errors. This form is used by the FDA for the documentation of adverse events that are related to medications, medical devices, and other medical products. All respiratory therapists should fall under the FDA's MedWatch reporting program.

U.S. Department of Health and Human Services

Form Approved: OMB No. 0910-0291, Expires: 12/31/2011
See OMB statement on reverse.

MEDWATCH

For VOLUNTARY reporting of
adverse events, product problems and
product use errors

The FDA Safety Information and
Adverse Event Reporting Program

FDA USE ONLY

Triage unit
sequence #

PLEASE TYPE OR USE BLACK INK

A. PATIENT INFORMATION

1. Patient Identifier	2. Age at Time of Event or Date of Birth:	3. Sex	4. Weight
In confidence		☐ Female ☐ Male	_____ lb or _____ kg

B. ADVERSE EVENT, PRODUCT PROBLEM OR ERROR

Check all that apply:

1. ☐ Adverse Event ☐ Product Problem (e.g., defects/malfunctions)
☐ Product Use Error ☐ Problem with Different Manufacturer of Same Medicine

2. Outcomes Attributed to Adverse Event
(Check all that apply)

☐ Death: _____ (mm/dd/yyyy)   ☐ Disability or Permanent Damage
☐ Life-threatening   ☐ Congenital Anomaly/Birth Defect
☐ Hospitalization - initial or prolonged ☐ Other Serious (Important Medical Events)
☐ Required Intervention to Prevent Permanent Impairment/Damage (Devices)

3. Date of Event (mm/dd/yyyy)	4. Date of this Report (mm/dd/yyyy)

5. Describe Event, Problem or Product Use Error

6. Relevant Tests/Laboratory Data, Including Dates

7. Other Relevant History, Including Preexisting Medical Conditions (e.g.,
allergies, race, pregnancy, smoking and alcohol use, liver/kidney problems, etc.)

C. PRODUCT AVAILABILITY

Product Available for Evaluation? (Do not send product to FDA)

☐ Yes ☐ No ☐ Returned to Manufacturer on: _____ (mm/dd/yyyy)

D. SUSPECT PRODUCT(S)

1. **Name, Strength, Manufacturer** (from product label)
#1 Name:
  Strength:
  Manufacturer:
#2 Name:
  Strength:
  Manufacturer:

2. Dose or Amount	Frequency	Route
#1		
#2		

3. Dates of Use (If unknown, give duration) from/to (or best estimate)	5. Event Abated After Use Stopped or Dose Reduced?
#1	#1 ☐ Yes ☐ No ☐ Doesn't Apply
#2	#2 ☐ Yes ☐ No ☐ Doesn't Apply

4. Diagnosis or Reason for Use (Indication)	8. Event Reappeared After Reintroduction?
#1	#1 ☐ Yes ☐ No ☐ Doesn't Apply
#2	#2 ☐ Yes ☐ No ☐ Doesn't Apply

6. Lot #	7. Expiration Date	9. NDC # or Unique ID
#1	#1	
#2	#2	

E. SUSPECT MEDICAL DEVICE

1. Brand Name

2. Common Device Name

3. Manufacturer Name, City and State

4. Model #	Lot #	5. Operator of Device
		☐ Health Professional
Catalog #	Expiration Date (mm/dd/yyyy)	☐ Lay User/Patient
		☐ Other:
Serial #	Other #	_____

6. If Implanted, Give Date (mm/dd/yyyy)	7. If Explanted, Give Date (mm/dd/yyyy)

8. Is this a Single-use Device that was Reprocessed and Reused on a Patient?
☐ Yes ☐ No

9. If Yes to Item No. 8, Enter Name and Address of Reprocessor

F. OTHER (CONCOMITANT) MEDICAL PRODUCTS

Product names and therapy dates (exclude treatment of event)

G. REPORTER (See confidentiality section on back)

1. **Name and Address**
  Name:
  Address:

  City: State: ZIP:

Phone #	E-mail

2. Health Professional?	3. Occupation	4. Also Reported to:
☐ Yes ☐ No		☐ Manufacturer
5. If you do NOT want your identity disclosed to the manufacturer, place an "X" in this box: ☐		☐ User Facility ☐ Distributor/Importer

FORM FDA 3500 (1/09)   Submission of a report does not constitute an admission that medical personnel or the product caused or contributed to the event.

ADVICE ABOUT VOLUNTARY REPORTING

Detailed instructions available at: http://www.fda.gov/medwatch/report/consumer/instruct.htm

Report adverse events, product problems or product use errors with:

- Medications *(drugs or biologics)*
- Medical devices *(including in-vitro diagnostics)*
- Combination products *(medication & medical devices)*
- Human cells, tissues, and cellular and tissue-based products
- Special nutritional products *(dietary supplements, medical foods, infant formulas)*
- Cosmetics

Report product problems - quality, performance or safety concerns such as:

- Suspected counterfeit product
- Suspected contamination
- Questionable stability
- Defective components
- Poor packaging or labeling
- Therapeutic failures (product didn't work)

Report SERIOUS adverse events. An event is serious when the patient outcome is:

- Death
- Life-threatening
- Hospitalization - initial or prolonged
- Disability or permanent damage
- Congenital anomaly/birth defect
- Required intervention to prevent permanent impairment or damage (devices)
- Other serious (important medical events)

Report even if:

- You're not certain the product caused the event
- You don't have all the details

How to report:

- Just fill in the sections that apply to your report
- Use section D for all products except medical devices
- Attach additional pages if needed
- Use a separate form for each patient
- Report either to FDA or the manufacturer *(or both)*

Other methods of reporting:

- 1-800-FDA-0178 - To FAX report
- 1-800-FDA-1088 - To report by phone
- www.fda.gov/medwatch/report.htm - To report online

If your report involves a serious adverse event with a device and it occurred in a facility outside a doctor's office, that facility may be legally required to report to FDA and/or the manufacturer. Please notify the person in that facility who would handle such reporting.

If your report involves a serious adverse event with a vaccine, call 1-800-822-7967 to report.

Confidentiality: The patient's identity is held in strict confidence by FDA and protected to the fullest extent of the law. FDA will not disclose the reporter's identity in response to a request from the public, pursuant to the Freedom of Information Act. The reporter's identity, including the identity of a self-reporter, may be shared with the manufacturer unless requested otherwise.

-Fold Here-

The public reporting burden for this collection of information has been estimated to average 36 minutes per response, including the time for reviewing instructions, searching existing data sources, gathering and maintaining the data needed, and completing and reviewing the collection of information. Send comments regarding this burden estimate or any other aspect of this collection of information, including suggestions for reducing this burden to:

Department of Health and Human Services
Food and Drug Administration
Office of Chief Information Officer (HFA-710)
5600 Fishers Lane
Rockville, MD 20857

Please DO NOT
RETURN this form
to this address.

OMB statement:
"An agency may not conduct or sponsor, and a person is not required to respond to, a collection of information unless it displays a currently valid OMB control number."

U.S. DEPARTMENT OF HEALTH AND HUMAN SERVICES
Food and Drug Administration

FORM FDA 3500 (1/09) (Back)   Please Use Address Provided Below -- Fold in Thirds, Tape and Mail

---

DEPARTMENT OF
HEALTH & HUMAN SERVICES

Public Health Service
Food and Drug Administration
Rockville, MD 20857

Official Business
Penalty for Private Use $300

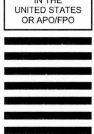

BUSINESS REPLY MAIL
FIRST CLASS MAIL PERMIT NO. 946 ROCKVILLE MD

POSTAGE WILL BE PAID BY FOOD AND DRUG ADMINISTRATION

MEDWATCH
The FDA Safety Information and Adverse Event Reporting Program
Food and Drug Administration
5600 Fishers Lane
Rockville, MD 20852-9787

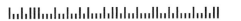

U.S. Department of Health and Human Services

(CONTINUATION PAGE)

**For VOLUNTARY reporting of
adverse events and product problems**

MEDWATCH

**The FDA Safety Information and
Adverse Event Reporting Program**

B.5. **Describe Event or Problem** *(continued)*

B.6. **Relevant Tests/Laboratory Data, Including Dates** *(continued)*

B.7. **Other Relevant History, Including Preexisting Medical Conditions** *(e.g., allergies, race, pregnancy, smoking and alcohol use, hepatic/renal dysfunction, etc.) (continued)*

F. **Concomitant Medical Products and Therapy Dates** *(Exclude treatment of event) (continued)*

General Instructions for Completing the MedWatch Form FDA 3500

For use by health professionals and consumers for **VOLUNTARY** reporting of adverse events, product use errors and product quality problems with:

- Drugs

- Biologics (including blood components, blood derivatives, allergenics, human cells, tissues, and cellular and tissue-based products (HCT/Ps)

- Medical devices (including *in-vitro* diagnostics)

- Combination products (e.g. drug-device, biologic-device)

- Special nutritional products (dietary supplements, infant formulas, medical foods)

- Cosmetics

Adverse events involving **vaccines** should be reported to the Vaccine Adverse Event Reporting System (VAERS), http://vaers.hhs.gov/pdf/vaers_form.pdf Adverse events involving **investigational (study) drugs, such as those relating to Investigational New Drug (IND) applications**, should be reported as required in the study protocol and sent to the address and contact person listed in the study protocol. They should generally not be submitted to FDA MedWatch as voluntary reports.

Note for consumers: If possible, please take the 3500 form to your health professional (e.g., doctor or pharmacist) so that information based on your medical record that can help in the evaluation of your report will be provided. If, for whatever reason, you do not wish to have your health professional fill out the form, you are welcome to do so yourself.

GENERAL INSTRUCTIONS

- Please make sure that all entries are either typed, printed in a font no smaller than 8 point, or written using black ink.

- Please complete all sections that apply to your report.

- Dates should be entered as mm/dd/yyyy (e.g., June 3, 2005 = 06/03/2005). If exact dates are unknown, please provide the best estimate (see block **B3**).

- For narrative entries, if the fields do not provide adequate space, attach additional pages as needed.

- If attaching additional pages, please do the following:

  - Identify all attached pages as Page __ of __

  - Indicate the appropriate section and block number next to the narrative continuation.

- Include the phrase continued at the end of each field that has additional information continued on to another page.

- **Section D,** Suspect product(s), should be used to report on special nutritional products and cosmetics as well as drugs or biologics, including human cells, tissues, and cellular and tissue-based products (HCT/Ps).

- If your report involves a serious adverse event with a device and it occurred in a facility other than a doctor's office, that facility may be legally required to report to FDA and/or the manufacturer. Please notify the person in that facility who would handle such reporting.

SECTION A: PATIENT INFORMATION

Complete a separate form for each patient, unless the report involves a medical device where multiple patients were adversely affected through the use of the same device. In that case, please indicate the number of patients in block **B5** (Describe event or problem) and complete Section A and blocks **B2**, **B5**, **B6**, **B7**, and **F** for each patient. Enter the corresponding patient identifier in block **A1** for each patient involved in the event.

Parent-child/fetus report(s) are those cases in which either a fetus/breast-feeding infant or the mother, or both have an adverse event that is possibly associated with a product administered to the mother during pregnancy. Several general principles are used for filing these reports:

- If there has been no event affecting the child/fetus, report only on the parent.
- For those cases describing fetal death, miscarriage or abortion, report the parent as the patient in the report.
- When only the child/fetus has an adverse reaction/event (other than fetal death, miscarriage or abortion), the information provided in **Section A** applies to the child/fetus. However, the information in **Section D** would apply to the parent who was the source of exposure to the product.
- When a newborn baby is found to have a birth defect/congenital anomaly that the initial reporter considers possibly associated with a product administered to the mother during pregnancy, the patient is the newborn baby.
- If both the parent and the child/fetus have adverse events, separate reports should be submitted for each patient.

A1:   Patient Identifier

Please provide the patient's initials or some other type of identifier that will allow you, the reporter, to readily locate the case if you are contacted for more information. Do not use the patient's name or social security number.

The patient's identity is held in strict confidence by FDA and protected to the fullest extent of the law. FDA will not disclose the reporter's identity in response to a request from the public, pursuant to the Freedom of Information Act.

If no patient was involved (such as may be the case with a product problem), enter none.

A2:   Age at Time of Event or Date of Birth

Provide the most precise information available. Enter the patient's birth date, if known, or the patient's age at the time of event onset. For age, indicate time units used (e.g., years, months, days):

- If the patient is 3 years or older, use years (e.g., 4 years).
- If the patient is less than 3 years old, use month (e.g., 24 months).
- If the patient is less than 1 month old, use days (e.g., 5 days).
- Provide the best estimate if exact age is unknown.

A3:   Sex

Enter the patient's gender. If the adverse event is a congenital anomaly/birth defect, report the sex of the child.

A4:   Weight

Indicate whether the weight is in pounds (lb) or kilograms (kg). Make a best estimate if exact weight is unknown.

SECTION B: ADVERSE EVENT, PRODUCT PROBLEM, PRODUCT USE ERROR

B1: Adverse Event, Product Problem, Product Use Error, or Problem with Different Manufacturer of Same Medicine.

Choose the appropriate box(es). If a product problem may have caused or contributed to the adverse event, check both boxes.

Adverse event: Any incident where the use of a medication (drug or biologic, including HCT/P), at any dose, a medical device (including *in-vitro* diagnostics) or a special nutritional product (e.g., dietary supplement, infant formula or medical food) is suspected to have resulted in an adverse outcome in a patient.

To report, it is not necessary to be certain of a cause/effect relationship between the adverse event and the use of the medical product(s) in question. Suspicion of an association is sufficient reason to report. Submission of a report does not constitute an admission that medical personnel or the product caused or contributed to the event.

Please limit your submissions to those events that are serious. An event is classified as serious when the patient outcome is:

- Death
- Life-threatening
- Hospitalization (initial or prolonged)
- Disability or Permanent Damage
- Congenital Anomaly/Birth Defect
- Required Medical or Surgical Intervention to Prevent Permanent Impairment or Damage (Devices)
- Other Serious (Important Medical Events)

Please see instructions for block **B2** for further information on each of these criteria.

Product problem (e.g., defects/malfunctions): Any report regarding the quality, performance, or safety of any medication, medical device or special nutritional product. In addition, please select this category when reporting device malfunctions that could lead to a death or serious injury if the malfunction were to recur. Product problems include, but are not limited to, such concerns as:

- Suspected counterfeit product
- Suspected contamination
- Questionable stability
- Defective components
- Therapeutic failures (product didn't work)
- Product confusion (caused by name, labeling, design or packaging)
- Suspected superpotent or subpotent medication
- Labeling problems caused by printing errors/omissions

Product Use Error:

Medication Use Error: Any report of a medication error regardless of patient involvement or outcome. Also report circumstances or events that have the capacity to cause error (e.g., similar product appearance, similar packaging and labeling, sound-alike/look-alike names, etc.).

Medication errors can and do originate in all stages of the medication use system, which includes selecting and procuring drugs, prescribing, preparing and dispensing, administering and monitoring. A medication error is defined as "any preventable event that may cause or lead to inappropriate medication use or patient harm while the medication is in the control of the health care professional, patient, or consumer. Such events may be related to professional practice, health care products, procedures, and systems, including prescribing, order communication, product labeling, packaging, nomenclature, compounding, dispensing, distribution, administration, education, monitoring and use."

Medical Device Use Error: Health care professionals, patients, and consumers can unintentionally cause harm to patients or to themselves when using medical devices. These problems can often arise due to problems with the design of the medical device or the manner in which the device is used. Often, use errors are caught and prevented before they can do harm (close call). Report use errors regardless of patient involvement or outcome. Also report circumstances or events that could cause use errors. Medical device use errors usually occur for one or more of the following reasons:

- Users expect devices to operate differently than they do.
- Product use is inconsistent with use's expectations or intuition.
- Product use requires physical, perceptual, or cognitive abilities that exceed those of the user.
- Devices are used in ways not anticipated by the manufacturer.
- Product labeling or packaging is confusing or inadequate.
- The environment adversely affects or influences device use.

Problem with Different Manufacturer of Same Medicine: Any incident, to include, but not be limited to, differences in noted therapeutic response, suspected to have resulted from a switch, or change, from one manufacturer to another manufacturer of the **same** medicine or drug product. This could be changes from a brand name drug product to a generic manufacturer's same product, or from a generic manufacturer's product to the same

(continued on next page)

product as supplied by a different generic manufacturer, or from a generic manufacturer's product to a brand name manufacturer of the same product. In order to fully evaluate the incident, please include in **Section B5**, if available, specific information relative to the switch between different manufacturers of the same medicine, to include, but not be limited to, the names of the manufacturers, length of treatment on each manufacturer's product, product strength, and any relevant clinical data.

B2: Outcomes Attributed to Adverse Event: Indicate all that apply to the reported event:

Death: Check ony if you suspect that the death was an outcome of the adverse event, and include the date if known.

Do not check if:

- The patient died while using a medical product, but there was no suspected association between the death and the use of the product
- A fetus is aborted because of a congenital anomaly (birth defect), or is miscarried

Life-threatening: Check if suspected that:

- The patient was at substantial risk of dying at the time of the adverse event, or
- Use or continued use of the device or other medical product might have resulted in the death of the patient

Hospitalization (initial or prolonged): Check if admission to the hospital or prolongation of hospitalization was a result of the adverse event.

Do not check if:

- A patient in the hospital received a medical product and subsequently developed an otherwise nonserious adverse event, unless the adverse event prolonged the hospital stay

Do check if:

- A patient is admitted to the hospital for one or more days, even if released on the same day
- An emergency room visit results in admission to the hospital. Emergency room visits that do not result in admission to the hospital should be evaluated for one of the other serious outcomes (e.g., life-threatening; required intervention to prevent permanent impairment or damage; other serious (medically important event)

Disability or Permanent Damage: Check if the adverse event resulted in a substantial disruption of a person's ability to conduct normal life functions. Such would be the case if the adverse event resulted in a significant, persistent or permanent change, impairment, damage or disruption in the patient's body function/structure, physical activities and/or quality of life.

Congenital Anomaly/Birth Defect: Check if you suspect that exposure to a medical product prior to conception or during pregnancy may have resulted in an adverse outcome in the child.

Required Intervention to Prevent Permanent Impairment or Damage (Devices): Check if you believe that medical or surgical intervention was necessary to preclude permanent impairment of a body function, or prevent permanent damage to a body structure, either situation suspected to be due to the use of a medical product.

Other Serious (Important Medical Events): Check when the event does not fit the other outcomes, but the event may jeopardize the patient and may require medical or surgical intervention (treatment) to prevent one of the other outcomes. Examples include allergic brochospasm (a serious problem with breathing) requiring treatment in an emergency room, serious blood dyscrasias (blood disorders) or seizures/convulsions that do not result in hospitalization. The development of drug dependence or drug abuse would also be examples of important medical events.

B3: Date of Event

Provide the actual or best estimate of the date of first onset of the adverse event. If day is unknown, month and year are acceptable. If day and month are unknown, year is acceptable.

- When a newborn baby is found to have a congenital anomaly, the event onset date is the date of birth of the child.
- When a fetus is aborted because of a congenital anomaly, or is miscarried, the event onset date is the date pregnancy is terminated.
- If information is available as to time during pregnancy when exposure occurred, indicate that information in narrative block **B5**.

B4: Date of this Report

The date the report is filled out.

B5: Describe Event, Problem or Product Use Error

For an **adverse event:**

Describe the event in detail, including a description of what happened and a summary of all relevant clinical information (medical status prior to the event; signs and/or symptoms; differential diagnosis for the event in question; clinical course; treatment; outcome, etc.). If available and if relevant, include synopses of any office visit notes or the hospital discharge summary. To save time and space (and if permitted by your institution), please attach copies of these records with any confidential information deleted. **Do not identify any patient, physician, or institution by name. The reporter's identity should be provided in full in Section G.**

(continued on next page)

SECTION B: ADVERSE EVENT, PRODUCT PROBLEM, PRODUCT USE ERROR *(continued)*

Information as to any environmental conditions that may have influenced the event should be included, particularly when (but not exclusive to) reporting about a device.

- Results of relevant tests and laboratory data should be entered in block **B6**. (See instructions for **B6**.)
- Preexisting medical conditions and other relevant history belong in block **B7**. Be as complete as possible, including time courses for preexisting diagnoses (see instructions for **B7**).

If it is determined that reuse of a medical device labeled for single use may have caused or contributed to an adverse patient outcome, please report in block **B5** the facts of the incident and the perceived contribution of reuse to the occurrence.

For a product problem: Describe the problem (quality, performance, or safety concern) in sufficient detail so that the circumstances surrounding the defect or malfunction of the medical product can be understood.

- If available, the results of any evaluation of a malfunctioning device and, if known, any relevant maintenance/service information should be included in this section.
- For a medication or special nutritional product problem, please indicate if you have retained a sample that would be available to FDA.

For a product use error: Describe the sequence of events leading up to the error in sufficient detail so that the circumstances surrounding the error can be understood.

- **For Medication Use Errors:** Include a description of the error, type of staff involved, work environment in which the error occurred, indicate causes or contributing factors to the error, location of the error, names of the products involved (including the trade (proprietary) and established (proper) name), manufacturer, dosage form, strength, concentration, and type and size of container.

- **For Medical Device Use Errors:** Report circumstances or events that could cause use errors. Medical device use errors usually occur for one or more of the following reasons:

  - Users expect devices to operate differently than they do.
  - Product use is inconsistent with user's expectations or intuition.
  - Product use requires physical, perceptual, or cognitive abilities that exceed those of the user.
  - Devices are used in ways not anticipated by the manufacturer.
  - Product labeling or packaging is confusing or inadequate.
  - The environment adversely affects or influences device use.

For a problem with a different manufacturer of the same medicine:

Please include specific information relative to the switch between different manufacturers of the same medicine, to include, but not be limited to, the names of the manufacturers, length of treatment on each manufacturer's product, product strength, and any relevant clinical data.

B6: Relevant Tests/Laboratory Data, Including Dates

Please provide all appropriate information, including relevant negative test and laboratory findings, in order to most completely convey how the medical work-up/assessment led to strong consideration of medical product-induced disease as etiology for clinical status, as other differential diagnostic considerations were being eliminated.

Please include:

- Any relevant baseline laboratory data prior to the administration or use of the medical product
- All laboratory data used in diagnosing the event
- Any available laboratory data/engineering analyses (for devices) that provide further information on the course of the event

If available, please include:

- Any pre- and post-event medication levels and dates (if applicable)
- Synopses of any relevant autopsy, pathology, engineering, or lab reports

If preferred, copies of any reports may be submitted as attachments, with all confidential information deleted. **Do not identify any patient, physician or institution by name.** The initial reporter's identity should be provided in full in **Section G.**

B7: Other Relevant History, Including Preexisting Medical Conditions

Knowledge of other risk factors can help in the evaluation of a reported adverse event. If available, provide information on:

- **Other known conditions in the patient, e.g.,**
  - Hypertension (high blood pressure)
  - Diabetes mellitus
  - Liver or kidney problems

- **Significant history**
  - Race
  - Allergies
  - Pregnancy history
  - Smoking and alcohol use, drug abuse
  - Setting

SECTION C: PRODUCT AVAILABILITY

Product available for evaluation? (Do not send the product to FDA.)
To evaluate a reported problem with a medical product, it is often critical to be able to examine the product. Please indicate whether the product is available for evaluation. Also indicate if the product was returned to the manufacturer and, if so, the date of the return.

SECTION D: SUSPECT PRODUCT(S)

For adverse event reporting:

A suspect product is one that you suspect is associated with the adverse event. In **Section F** enter other concomitant medical products (drugs, biologics including human cells, tissues, and cellular and tissue-based products (HCT/Ps), medical devices, etc.) that the patient was using at the time of the event but which you do not think were involved in the event.

Up to two (2) suspect products may be reported on one form (#1=first suspect product, #2=second suspect product). Attach an additional form if there were more than two suspect products associated with the reported adverse event.

For product quality problem reporting:

A suspect product is the product that is the subject of the report. A separate form should be submitted for each individual product problem report.

Identification of the labeler/distributor and pharmaceutical manufacturer and labeled strength of the product is important for prescription or non-prescription products.

This section may also be used to report on special nutritional products (e.g., dietary supplements, infant formula or medical foods), cosmetics, human cells, tissues, or cellular and tissue-based products (HCT/Ps) or other products regulated by FDA.

If reporting on a special nutritional or drug product quality problem, please attach labeling/packaging if available.

If reporting on a special nutritional product only, please provide directions for use as listed on the product labeling.

D1: Name, Strength, Manufacturer

Use the trade/brand name. If the trade/brand name is not known or if there is no trade/brand name, use the generic product name and the name of the manufacturer or labeler. These names are usually found on the product packaging or labeling. Strength is the amount in each tablet or capsule, the concentration of an injectable, etc. (such as "10mg", "100 units/cc", etc.).

For human cells, tissues, and cellular and tissue-based products (HCT/Ps), please provide the common name of the HCT/P. You can also indicate if the HCT/P has a proprietary or trade name. Examples: Achilles tendon, Iliac crest bone or Islet cells.

D2: Dose or Amount, Frequency, Route

Describe how the product was used by the patient (e.g., 500 mg QID orally or 10 mg every other day IV). For reports involving overdoses, the amount of product used in the overdose should be listed, not the prescribed amount. (See **APPENDIX** for list of **Routes of Administration** on the next page.)

D3: Dates of Use

Provide the date administration was started (or best estimate) and the date stopped (or best estimate). If no dates are known, an estimated duration is acceptable (e.g., 2 years) or if therapy was less than one day, then duration is appropriate (e.g., 1 dose or 1 hour for an IV).

For human cells, tissues, and cellular and tissue-based products, provide the date of transplant and if applicable, the date of explanation.

D4: Diagnosis or Reason for Use (Indication)

Provide the reason or indication for which the product was prescribed or used in this particular patient.

D5: Event Abated After Use Stopped or Dose Reduced

If available, this information is particularly useful in the evaluation of a suspected adverse event. In addition to checking the appropriate box, please provide supporting lab tests and dates, if available, in block **B6**.

D6: Lot #

If known, include the lot number(s) with all product quality problem reports, or any adverse event report with a biologic, or medication.

D7: Expiration Date

Please include if available.

(continued on next page)

SECTION D: SUSPECT PRODUCT(S) *(continued)*

D8: Event Reappeared After Reintroduction

This information is particularly useful in the evaluation of a suspected adverse event. In addition to checking the appropriate box, please provide a description of what happened when the drug was stopped and then restarted in block **B5**, and any supporting lab tests and dates in block **B6**.

D9: NDC # or Unique ID

The national drug code (NDC #) is requested only when reporting a drug product problem. Zeros and dashes should be included as they appear on the label. NDC # can be found on the original product label and/or packaging, but is usually not found on dispensed pharmacy prescriptions.

If the product has a unique or distinct identification code, please provide this here. This is applicable to human cells, tissues, and cellular and tissue-based products (HCT/Ps).

Appendix - Routes of Administration

Auricular (otic) 001	Intracerebral 018	Intrasynovial 035	Perineural 052
Buccal 002	Intracervical 019	Intratumor 036	Rectal 053
Cutaneous 003	Intracisternal 020	Intrathecal 037	Respiratory (inhalation) 054
Dental 004	Intracorneal 021	Intrathoracic 038	Retrobulbar 055
Endocervical 005	Intracoronary 022	Intratracheal 039	Subconjunctival 056
Endosinusial 006	Intradermal 023	Intravenous bolus 040	Subcutaneous 057
Endotracheal 007	Intradiscal (intraspinal) 024	Intravenous drip 041	Subdermal 058
Epidural 008	Intrahepatic 025	Intravenous (not otherwise specified) 042	Sublingual 059
Extra-amniotic 009	Intralesional 026	Intravesical 043	Topical 060
Hemodialysis 010	Intralymphatic 027	Iontophoresis 044	Transdermal 061
Intra corpus cavernosum 011	Intramedullar (bone marrow) 028	Occlusive dressing technique 045	Transmammary 062
Intra-amniotic 012	Intrameningeal 029	Ophthalmic 046	Transplacental 063
Intra-arterial 013	Intramuscular 030	Oral 047	Unknown 064
Intra-articular 014	Intraocular 031	Oropharingeal 048	Urethral 065
Intra-uterine 015	Intrapericardial 032	Other 049	Vaginal 066
Intracardiac 016	Intraperitoneal 033	Parenteral 050	
Intracavernous 017	Intrapleural 034	Periarticular 051	

SECTION E: SUSPECT MEDICAL DEVICE

The suspect medical device is 1) the device that may have caused or contributed to the adverse event or 2) the device that malfunctioned.

In **Section F**, report other concomitant medical products (drugs, biologics including HCT/Ps, medical devices, etc.) that the patient was using at the time of the event but which you do not think were involved in the event.

If more than one suspect medical device was involved in the event, complete all of **Section E** for the first device and attach a separate completed **Section E** for each additional device.

If the suspect medical device is a single-use device that has been reprocessed, then the reprocessor is now the device manufacturer.

E1: Brand Name

The trade or proprietary name of the suspect medical device as used in product labeling or in the catalog (e.g., Flo-Easy Catheter, Reliable Heart Pacemaker, etc.). This information may 1) be on a label attached to a durable device, 2) be on a package of a disposable device, or 3) appear in labeling materials of an implantable device. Reprocessed single-use devices may bear the Original Equipment Manufacturer (OEM) brand name. If the suspect device is a reprocessed single-use device, enter "NA".

E2: Common Device Name

The generic or common name of the suspect medical device or a generally descriptive name (e.g., urological catheter, heart pacemaker, patient restraint, etc.). Please do not use broad generic terms such as "catheter", "valve", "screw", etc.

E3: Manufacturer Name, City and State

If available, list the full name, city and state of the manufacturer of the suspected medical device. If the answer of block **E8** is "yes", then enter the name, city and state of the reprocessor.

E4: Model #, Catalog #, Serial #, Lot #, Expiration Date, Other

If available, provide any or all identification numbers associated with the suspect medical device exactly as they appear on the device or device labeling. This includes spaces, hyphens, etc.

Model #:

The exact model number found on the device label or accompanying packaging.

Catalog #:

The exact number as it appears in the manufacturer's catalog, device labeling, or accompanying packaging.

Serial #:

This number can be found on the device label or accompanying packaging; it is assigned by the manufacturer, and should be specific to each device.

Lot #:

This number can be found on the label or packaging material.

Expiration Date (mm/dd/yyyy):

If available, this date can often be found on the device itself or printed on the accompanying packaging.

Other #:

Any other applicable identification number (e.g., component number, product number, part bar-coded product ID, etc.)

E5: Operator of Device

Indicate the type (not the name) of person operating or using the suspect medical device on the patient at the time of the event as follows:

- Health professional = physician, nurse, respiratory therapist, etc.
- Lay user/patient = person being treated, parent/ spouse/friend of the patient
- Other = nurses aide, orderly, etc.

E6: If Implanted, Give Gate (mm/dd/yyyy)

For medical devices that are implanted in the patient, provide the implant date or your best estimate. If day is unknown, month and year are acceptable. If month and day are unknown, year is acceptable.

E7: If Explanted, Give Date (mm/dd/yyyy)

If an implanted device was removed from the patient, provide the explantation date or your best estimate. If day is unknown, month and year are acceptable. If month and day are unknown, year is acceptable.

E8: Is this a Single-use Device that was returned before Reprocessed and Reused on a Patient?

Indicate "Yes" or "No".

E9: If Yes to Item No. 8, Enter Name and Address of Reprocessor

Enter the name and address of the reprocessor of the single-use device. Anyone who reprocesses single-use devices for reuse in humans is the manufacturer of the reprocessed device.

SECTION F: OTHER (CONCOMITANT) MEDICAL PRODUCTS

Product names and therapy dates (exclude treatment of event)

Information on the use of concomitant medical products can frequently provide insight into previously unknown interactions between products, or provide an alternative explanation for the observed adverse event. Please list and provide product names and therapy dates for any other medical products (drugs, biologics including HCT/Ps, medical devices, etc.) that the patient was using at the time of the event. Do not include products used to treat the event.

SECTION G: REPORTER

FDA recognizes that confidentiality is an important concern in the context of adverse event reporting. The patient's identity is held in strict confidence by FDA and protected to the fullest extent of the law. However, to allow for timely follow-up in serious cases, the reporter's identity may be shared with the manufacturer unless specifically requested otherwise in block G5. FDA will not disclose the reporter's identity in response to a request from the public, pursuant to the Freedom of Information Act.

G1: Name, Address, Phone #, E-mail

Please provide the name, mailing address, phone number and E-mail address of the person who can be contacted to provide information on the event if follow-up is necessary. While optional, providing the fax number would be most helpful, if available. This person will also receive an acknowledgment letter from FDA on receipt of the report.

G2: Health Professional?

Please indicate whether you are a health professional (e.g., physician, pharmacist, nurse, etc.) or not.

G3: Occupation:

Please indicate your occupation (particularly type of health professional), and include specialty, if appropriate.

G4: Also Reported to:

Please indicate whether you have also notified or submitted a copy of this report to the manufacturer and/ or distributor of the product, or, in the case of medical device reports only, to the user facility (institution) in which the event occurred. This information helps to track duplicate reports in the FDA database.

G5: Release of reporter's Identity to the manufacturer

In the case of a serious adverse event, FDA may provide name, address and phone number of the reporter denoted in block **G1** to the manufacturer of the suspect product. If you do not want your identity released to the manufacturer, please put an X in this box.

Answer Key

Chapter 1 Answer Key

Multiple Choice

1. D	2. C	3. B	4. B	5. C	6. C
7. C	8. A	9. B	10. A	11. C	12. D
13. B	14. C	15. D			

Case Study

A tracheostomy would have provided an airway for the patient to be able to breathe through. His condition was most likely caused by epiglottitis, which swells the epiglottis to 10 times its normal size. Therefore, the tracheostomy would have saved his life.

Chapter 2 Answer Key

Multiple Choice

1. C	2. C	3. B	4. D	5. B	6. A
7. A	8. C	9. B	10. A	11. C	12. D
13. A	14. D	15. D			

Case Study

1. Most likely, this patient has berylliosis.
2. Steroid drugs, such as prednisone, would be the drugs of choice to control his symptoms.

Chapter 3 Answer Key

Multiple Choice

1. C	2. B	3. A	4. B	5. D	6. A
7. B	8. C	9. D	10. B	11. A	12. D
13. B	14. D	15. B			

Case Study

1. Generic drugs may save the patient money as compared to the cost of trade name drugs because they are not as expensive.
2. A trade name drug may contain slightly different ingredients than a generic version of the same drug. Sometimes these different ingredients may have preferred effects to those of the generic formulation.

Chapter 4 Answer Key

Multiple Choice

1. D	2. B	3. D	4. B	5. D	6. C
7. D	8. B	9. B	10. D	11. C	12. A
13. D	14. A	15. C			

Case Study

1. Because this patient had liver impairment, the phenobarbital and warfarin could not be metabolized quickly enough, and a drug toxicity occurred. As a result, there is a possibility that he developed a thrombosis, which caused a stroke.
2. Elderly patients should have much lower doses of many medications because their livers cannot process drugs as efficiently as the livers of younger adults. His cirrhosis further reduced his liver's ability to function normally.

Chapter 5 Answer Key

Multiple Choice

1. B	2. B	3. C	4. B	5. A	6. B
7. D	8. A	9. B	10. A	11. C	12. B
13. A	14. D	15. B			

Case Study

1. The physician or nurse should have explained to the patient that the suppositories were to be inserted vaginally; they should not have assumed that she understood how a suppository should be used. The pharmacist also should have consulted with the patient to make sure she understood.
2. If the labeling did not clearly explain the correct usage of the suppositories, the pharmacy technician who prepared the package, as well as the

pharmacist who is responsible for the pharmacy technician's actions, are both responsible.

Chapter 6 Answer Key
Multiple Choice

1. B 2. C 3. B 4. D 5. B 6. B
7. B 8. C 9. D 10. C 11. B 12. A
13. C 14. B 15. D

Case Study

1. The physician should discuss the situation with the nurse. He should explain to the patient's parents that the injection was into a deeper area than the surface of the skin. He should also report this incorrect route of administration to the nurse's supervisor at the clinic.
2. The physician should refer the patient and her parents to a pediatric surgeon so that the abscess may be removed and appropriate antibiotics can be started.

Chapter 7 Answer Key
Fill in the Blank

1. 1000
2. 1000
3. 0.01
4. 1000
5. 0.001
6. 0.001
7. 0.001
8. 0.001
9. 0.000001
10. 2
11. 480
12. 12
13. 4
14. 2
15. $\frac{1}{15}$
16. 5
17. 8
18. 2
19. 3
20. 240
21. 960
22. 15
23. 2.2
24. 2
25. 60

Calculate the Amount to Administer

1. 2
2. 20
3. 2
4. 1
5. 7.5

Calculate the Amount for a Single Dose

1. 1
2. 0.8
3. 0.4
4. 2
5. 0.75

Case Study

1. Using Clark's rule,

$$\frac{28 \text{ (pounds)}}{150 \text{ (pounds)}} \times 400 \text{ (mg)} = 75 \text{ mg (rounded)}$$

Therefore, Amanda should receive 75 mg every 6 hours by mouth.
2. Using Fried's rule,

$$\frac{11 \text{ months of age}}{150 \text{ (pounds)}} \times 400 \text{ (mg)} = 29 \text{ mg (rounded)}$$

Chapter 8 Answer Key
Multiple Choice

1. D 2. C 3. D 4. B 5. A 6. B
7. B 8. D 9. A 10. B 11. C 12. B
13. C 14. D 15. A

Case Study

1. Protamine sulfate is used to counteract heparin overdosage.
2. Other signs and symptoms of heparin overdosage include fever, chills, skin rashes, elevated blood pressure, cyanosis, and many others.

Chapter 9 Answer Key
Multiple Choice

1. D 2. B 3. B 4. A 5. D 6. B
7. C 8. D 9. D 10. C 11. B 12. A
13. C 14. A 15. C

Case Study

1. The respiratory therapist should take the patient's history and conduct a physical examination. To diagnose the condition, an EKG can be used along with a stress test. The patient's blood must also be tested to rule out myocardial infarction.
2. The respiratory therapist should advise the patient to use nitroglycerin if another angina attack occurs, then call the physician and wait until the physician gives other instructions. If

there are other signs and symptoms, the condition may be more serious.

Chapter 10 Answer Key

Multiple Choice

1. B 2. D 3. B 4. A 5. C 6. B
7. B 8. A 9. C 10. B 11. D 12. A
13. C 14. B 15. A

Case Study

The respiratory therapist must start CPR and remember the ABCs of life support.

Chapter 11 Answer Key

Multiple Choice

1. D 2. B 3. A 4. B 5. A 6. C
7. B 8. D 9. B 10. A 11. D 12. A
13. C 14. B 15. A

Case Study

1. It is most likely pheochromocytoma.
2. Treatment should begin with injection of phentolamine, followed by surgery to remove the tumor.

Chapter 12 Answer Key

Multiple Choice

1. C 2. B 3. A 4. B 5. D 6. B
7. B 8. A 9. C 10. B 11. A 12. B
13. D 14. A 15. C

Case Study

1. In elderly people, the doses of ACE inhibitors should be reduced because of impaired renal clearance, which can result in a toxic effect (causing severe hypotension). Average adult dosages should not be given to elderly patients.
2. The patient should be given reduced doses of the ACE inhibitor based on his age, or other medications can be given for treatment of left-sided heart failure.

Chapter 13 Answer Key

Multiple Choice

1. C 2. D 3. B 4. B 5. B 6. A
7. B 8. D 9. B 10. A 11. C 12. B
13. D 14. A 15. C

Case Study

1. Yes, hypokalemia is an adverse effect of loop diuretics.
2. Both loop diuretics and thiazide diuretics can cause hypokalemia.
3. Hypokalemia can be prevented by supplying additional potassium ions through diet, drug treatment, or both.

Chapter 14 Answer Key

Multiple Choice

1. A 2. C 3. D 4. C 5. B 6. C
7. D 8. A 9. C 10. D 11. C 12. C
13. A 14. D 15. B

Case Study

1. Heparin is effective immediately because it is administered by injection. Warfarin must be taken orally and takes at least 1 week to become effective.
2. Prothrombin time (PT) is a laboratory test often used during therapy with the anticoagulant warfarin, so she will be given this blood test.

Chapter 15 Answer Key

Multiple Choice

1. D 2. D 3. B 4. C 5. B 6. C
7. A 8. D 9. A 10. B 11. D 12. B
13. C 14. B 15. C

Case Study

1. The girl would be given oxygen and a beta-blocker because it is the drug class of choice.
2. For home use, the patient would most likely be prescribed a long-acting bronchodilator with an inhaled corticosteroid.

Chapter 16 Answer Key

Multiple Choice

1. B 2. A 3. C 4. D 5. B 6. A
7. B 8. B 9. A 10. A 11. C 12. B
13. B 14. C 15. D

Case Study

1. The primary diagnosis most likely will be lung cancer.
2. The first treatment should be for the bacterial pneumonia because surgery or chemotherapy for the cancer is not safe while the patient has this type of pneumonia.

Chapter 17 Answer Key
Multiple Choice

1. C   2. A   3. D   4. B   5. D   6. B
7. A   8. A   9. C   10. C   11. B   12. B
13. A   14. D   15. C

Case Study

1. The patient probably was taking an antihistamine, in which case she shouldn't have been driving.
2. The adverse effects of the most commonly used antiallergy drugs, such as antihistamines, include drowsiness, dizziness, disturbed coordination, weakness, and confusion, among many others.

Chapter 18 Answer Key
Multiple Choice

1. C   2. D   3. C   4. A   5. B   6. D
7. B   8. C   9. C   10. A   11. C   12. A
13. B   14. D   15. B

Case Study

1. The possible cause of Samantha's condition is an allergy to penicillin. Even though she had six previous shots of penicillin with no reaction, penicillin can cause anaphylactic shock, which is life threatening.
2. Because her situation is life threatening, she should immediately receive oxygen, norepinephrine, cortisone, antihistamine, and, if required, cardiopulmonary resuscitation (CPR).

Chapter 19 Answer Key
Multiple Choice

1. D   2. A   3. D   4. B   5. C   6. B
7. D   8. A   9. C   10. A   11. B   12. C
13. B   14. A   15. D

Case Study

1. The probable cause of death is sudden infant death syndrome (SIDS), which is also known as crib death. It is more common in the fall or winter and affects infants between 2 and 4 months of age while they are sleeping. While asleep, they may suddenly stop breathing, become cyanotic, and die as a result of oxygen deficiency.
2. Unfortunately, there is no prevention for SIDS. However, there are some devices that alert parents when an infant changes position. They work by sensing pressure changes that indicate the baby is rolling over. It is preferred that infants sleep on their backs, not on their stomachs, because more cases of SIDS have occurred when they sleep face down.

Chapter 20 Answer Key
Multiple Choice

1. D   2. D   3. A   4. C   5. D   6. A
7. C   8. C   9. B   10. C   11. B   12. B
13. C   14. B   15. D

Case Study

1. Most likely, this man has shingles, which is more common after age 60 years.
2. The herpes zoster vaccine is used to prevent the development of shingles and is recommended for adults after age 60 years.

Chapter 21 Answer Key
Multiple Choice

1. C   2. D   3. C   4. A   5. B   6. C
7. B   8. A   9. B   10. C   11. C   12. A
13. C   14. C   15. B

Case Study

1. Sleep disturbances may indicate chronic illnesses and changes in the central nervous system due to aging. She may have sleep apnea, which causes her to stop breathing many times during the night for short intervals until her respiratory system awakens her as she gasps for air.
2. A person's quality of sleep does deteriorate as a result of aging. The time spent in REM sleep and the deeper stages of non-REM sleep shortens, causing older adults to awaken more often during the night.

Chapter 22 Answer Key
Multiple Choice

1. C   2. C   3. A   4. D   5. B   6. D
7. A   8. B   9. A   10. C   11. C   12. B
13. A   14. C   15. B

Case Study

1. As an anticholinergic, benztropine blocks the parasympathetic nerves to allow the sympathetic nervous system to dominate. It is given as an adjunct in Parkinson disease to reduce muscular tremor and rigidity.
2. Anticholinergics may produce a wide variety of adverse effects. These include decreased heart rate, dilated pupils, decreased peristalsis, and decreased salivation.

Glossary

A

Abbreviations Shortened forms of words or phrases; for example, the abbreviation for chronic obstructive pulmonary disease is COPD.

Abruptio placentae Separation of the placenta from the uterus before delivery of the fetus.

Absorption The movement of a drug from the site of administration into the bloodstream.

Acetylcholine (ACh) The neurotransmitter that is released by preganglionic sympathetic neurons and preganglionic and postganglionic fibers of the parasympathetic nervous system.

Acidosis A chemical state where the pH of the blood drops significantly below 7.35.

Acne rosacea A chronic skin condition involving redness and occasionally pimples; it primarily affects women between 30 and 60 years of age and can lead to more serious skin damage.

Action potential The sequence of electrical changes that occurs in a portion of a nerve cell membrane that is exposed to a stimulus.

Active immunity The production of antibodies against a specific agent by the immune system.

Administration errors Errors made during the administration of medications to a patient, including giving a drug to the wrong patient, administering the incorrect drug strength, administrating medications too frequently or not frequently enough, and administering incorrect dosage forms.

Adrenal medulla The center portion of the adrenal gland; it releases adrenaline (epinephrine) and norepinephrine as part of the fight-or-flight response.

Adrenergic fibers Nerve fibers that secrete norepinephrine.

Adrenergic receptors Those that bind to norepinephrine.

Adverse effects Those that are harmful and undesired.

Aerobic Requiring oxygen and producing carbon dioxide.

Aerobic metabolism The process that generates carbon dioxide in peripheral tissues.

Affinity The ability to bind or combine.

Agonist A drug that binds to a receptor to alter its activity.

Agranulocytosis A marked increase in granulocytes, potentially leading to frequent, chronic bacterial infections.

Albumin Any water-soluble protein that coagulates when heated.

Aldosterone A hormone produced in the adrenal glands that increases the reabsorption of sodium and water and releases potassium in the kidneys, thereby increasing blood volume and pressure.

Allergens Foreign substances that can cause allergic reactions.

Angina pectoris A sudden outburst of chest pain frequently caused by myocardial anoxia, atherosclerosis, or coronary artery spasm.

Anoxia Lack of oxygen.

Antagonist A drug that blocks a receptor's response to an agonist.

Anthracosis A form of pneumoconiosis that develops from the inhalation of carbon, such as found in coal. Anthracosis may further develop into black lung disease.

Antibiotic An antibacterial drug derived from a natural rather than synthetic source.

Anticholinergics Agents that block the effects of acetylcholine in the nervous system.

Antidiuretic hormone (ADH) Vasopressin; it prevents the production of dilute urine.

Antidote   An agent that counteracts the effects of another agent.

Anti-infective   An agent used to treat an infection due to a microorganism; anti-infectives include antibacterials, antivirals, antiprotozoals, and antifungals.

Antitussives   Cough suppressants; agents that reduce coughing.

Antivirals   Drugs that kill or inhibit the reproduction of viruses.

Aorta   The largest arterial blood trunk in the entire body; it brings oxygenated blood to all parts of the body via the systemic circulation.

Aortic valve   Located at the base of the aorta, this valve opens to allow blood to leave the left ventricle when it contracts.

Arrhythmia   A disturbance of heart rhythm. Also see *dysrhythmia*.

Asbestosis   A form of pneumoconiosis that develops from the inhalation of asbestos. Asbestosis causes an increased risk of various lung cancers.

Aseptic technique   A set of specific procedures and practices designed to reduce potential contamination by pathogens.

Asphyxia   Deficient oxygen supply due to abnormal breathing.

Asthma   A disease characterized by increasing irritability of the tracheobronchial tree, either from allergic or nonallergic stimuli.

Asymptomatic   Without symptoms; a condition that does not exhibit its normal symptoms, but the symptoms may develop at a later time.

Ataxia   Inability to coordinate muscle activity.

Atelectasis   Incomplete expansion or collapse of part or all of a lung.

Atherosclerosis   Hardening or thickening of the arterial walls.

Atria   The upper two chambers of the heart.

Attenuated vaccine   One that has been made less harmful but has not been killed.

Automaticity   A property of specialized, excitable tissue that allows self-activation through spontaneous development of an action potential, as in the pacemaker cells of the heart.

Autosomal   Existing in equivalent amounts in males and females; autosomes are chromosomes that are identical in both sexes, and the sex chromosomes (X and Y) are different between the two sexes.

Axons   Nerve cell structures that carry impulses away from cell bodies to dendrites.

B

B lymphocytes   White blood cells that play a large role in the humoral immune response; they primarily make antibodies against antigens.

Bacteremia   The presence of bacteria in the blood.

Bactericidal   An agent capable of killing bacteria.

Bacteriostatic   An agent capable of stopping the growth and reproduction of bacteria.

Beta-lactam antibiotics   The type of antibiotics that includes penicillins, which work by inhibiting the synthesis of bacterial cell walls.

Bevel   The sloped surface of a needle that creates its sharpened edge.

Bioavailability   Measurement of the rate of absorption and total amount of a drug that reaches the systemic circulation.

Biopharmaceutical   A medical drug produced by methods other than direct extraction from a native biological source. An example of a biopharmaceutical is human insulin.

Biotransformation   The modification of a chemical compound by the body.

Blepharitis   Inflammation of the eyelid margins.

Blood–brain barrier   A separation of circulating blood and cerebrospinal fluid (CSF) in the central nervous system.

Bone marrow   The flexible tissue inside the hollow interior of bones; it is one of the two primary lymphoid tissues.

Booster   An additional dose or injection that reexposes a patient to a particular antigen; it is intended to increase immunity against a certain disease.

Bradyarrhythmias   Heart rhythm disturbances that result in a heartbeat of less than 60 beats per minute.

Bradycardia   Abnormally slow heartbeat.

Bradykinin   A protein that is a potent vasodilator.

Brain   The center of the nervous system. It is divided into four major portions: cerebrum, diencephalon, brainstem, and cerebellum.

Brainstem   The extension of the spinal cord into the brain; it consists of the midbrain, pons, and medulla oblongata.

Broad spectrum   An antibiotic that is effective against a wide range of bacterial species.

Bronchial tree   The branched parts of the primary bronchi in the lungs.

Bronchiectasis   A condition of permanent dilation of the bronchi and bronchioles.

Bronchiolectasis   Chronic dilation of the bronchioles.

Bronchiolitis   Respiratory syncytial viral infection that usually causes inflammation in the lower respiratory tract.

Bronchitis   Inflammation of the mucous membranes of the lung bronchi.

Bronchodilators   Agents that widen the diameter of the bronchioles.

Bronchogenic carcinoma   The most common fatal cancer in the United States; it is seen in nearly 95% of primary lung tumors.

C

Candidemia   A genus of yeastlike fungi that appears in the bloodstream.

Capillaries   The smallest blood vessels in the body; they enable the transfer of substances between the blood and tissues.

Caplets   Tablets that are shaped like capsules and have special film coatings.

Capsules   Drugs usually encased in soft or hard gelatin shells.

Carbaminohemoglobin   A compound of carbon dioxide and hemoglobin; it is bluish in color and makes the veins appear blue.

Carbonic anhydrase   The enzyme in red blood cells that converts carbon dioxide to carbonic acid.

Carcinogens   Substances that may cause cancer, including silica, asbestos, carbon, vinyl chloride, tobacco products, and others.

Cardiac cycle   The period between the start of one heartbeat and the start of the next heartbeat.

Cardiac veins   Those that branch out to drain blood from the myocardial capillaries.

Cardiotonic   Having a favorable effect upon the heart.

Catecholamine   Any one of a group of sympathomimetic compounds; some catecholamines are produced naturally by the body and function as key neurologic chemicals.

Cell-mediated immunity   An immune response that involves the activation of macrophages, NK cells, T lymphocytes, and substances that respond to antigens.

Central nervous system (CNS)   One of the two major divisions of the nervous system; it consists of the brain and spinal cord.

Cerebellum   The brain's center for coordination of skeletal muscle movements and maintenance of posture.

Cesarean section   A surgical procedure wherein an opening is made through the mother's abdomen and uterus to deliver the baby.

Cholinergic fiber   A nerve fiber that secretes acetylcholine.

Cholinergic receptor   One that binds to acetylcholine; it may be either a muscarinic or nicotinic receptor.

Clearance   The rate at which drug molecules disappear from the circulation.

Coagulation   Blood clotting; the third event in the process of hemostasis.

Collecting ducts   A system of vessels that connect the nephrons in a kidney to its ureter; they collect tubular fluid from the collecting tubules.

Collecting tubules   A system of vessels that collect tubular fluid from the distal convoluted tubules.

Commission errors   Errors that occur when a drug that has been discontinued for a patient is accidentally restarted or when a drug is added to a patient's medication history in error.

Conduction velocity   The speed with which an electrical impulse can be transmitted through excitable tissue.

Conjunctivitis   Inflammation of the outermost layer of the eye and innermost layer of the eyelids; commonly known as pink eye.

Consolidation   The increasing or strengthening of a condition.

Cor pulmonale   A change in structure and function of the right ventricle caused by a respiratory disorder.

Coronary arteries   The first two branches of the aorta that supply blood to the heart's tissues.

Coronary sinus   A collection of veins that forms a large vessel that collects blood from the myocardium and empties it into the right atrium.

Cotinine   A metabolite of nicotine; the level of cotinine in the blood is proportionate to the amount of tobacco smoke the patient has been exposed to.

Creams   Usually, topical medications in a water–oil base that are thicker than lotions and often white in color.

Cricoid cartilage   Laryngeal cartilage that helps to protect the glottis and entrance to the trachea.

Cytotoxic T cells   Lymphocytes that can cause the death of infected somatic or tumor cells.

D

Decongestants   Drugs that decrease nasal congestion related to the common cold, allergic rhinitis, and sinusitis.

Defibrillation   Electrically shocking the heart to restore a normal sinus rhythm.

Dendrites   Nerve cell processes that carry nervous impulses toward cell bodies.

Depolarization   A change in a cell's membrane potential that makes it more positive or less negative; it may result in an action potential.

Desired dose   The amount of medication to be administered to a patient.

Diaphragm   The thoracic muscle across the bottom of the rib cage that is very important for respiration.

Diastole   Relaxation of a heart chamber.

Diastolic heart failure   Heart failure due to a defect in ventricular filling caused by an abnormality in diastolic function.

Diluent   A liquid substance used to dilute another substance.

Dispensing errors   Errors made when a medication is dispensed by a pharmacist, pharmacy technician, or another pharmacy assistant.

Distribution   The movement of a drug through the bloodstream into the tissues and cells.

Diuresis   The process of removing fluids from the body by producing urine and excreting water and electrolytes.

Diuretic   Any substance that causes diuresis.

Dosage ordered   The exact amount of medication ordered, along with the frequency with which it should be given.

Dose   The strength of a drug in one dosage unit.

Dose–effect relationship   The effect of differing levels of a drug on the body over time.

Dyspnea   Shortness of breath.

Dysrhythmia   A disturbance of heart rhythm. Also see *arrhythmia*.

Dysthymia   A chronic form of depression that causes the patient to function less than normally and to feel as if he or she is ill.

E

ECG   Abbreviation for an electrocardiogram. Also see *EKG*.

Efficacy   How well a drug produces its desired effect.

EKG   Abbreviation for an electrocardiogram. Also see *ECG*.

Electrocardiogram   A graphic depiction of the heart's electrical impulses.

Elixirs   Liquid mixtures of alcohol, sugar, water, and a flavoring agent that may or may not contain a medication.

Emphysema   A form of chronic obstructive pulmonary disease (COPD) that is usually caused by smoking tobacco products.

Emulsion   A mixture of two agents that cannot ordinarily be mixed, usually oil in water or water in oil.

Endocardium   The innermost layer of tissue that lines the heart's inner surfaces.

Endogenous   Anything that comes from within the body.

Endothelial   The layer of cells lining the inside of the blood vessels and other related structures.

Epicardium   The outermost layer of tissue that lines the heart's outer surface.

Epiglottis   Laryngeal cartilage that forms a lid over the glottis.

Epiglottitis   Inflammation of the epiglottis (the flap at the base of the tongue that keeps food out of the trachea); may become a medical emergency.

Epithelial   Lining the cavities and surfaces of body structures.

Erythropoietin   A hormone that controls red blood cell production.

Esophagus   The muscular tube through which food passes from the pharynx to the stomach.

Eustachian tubes   The auditory tubes; they link the pharynx to the middle ear.

Excretion   The removal of a drug, or what the drug became after metabolism, from the body.

Exfoliative dermatitis   Erythroderma; a rare yet serious skin disorder that may lead to T-cell lymphoma.

Exogenous   Anything that comes from outside a system, such as a pathogen that enters the body from the external environment.

Expectorants   Drugs that help to bring up mucus and other material from the respiratory system.

Expiration   Exhalation; the opposite of inspiration (or inhalation).

External respiration   The exchange of oxygen and carbon dioxide between the alveoli of the lungs and the pulmonary capillaries.

F

Fibrillation   Very rapid, irregular contractions or twitching of muscle fibers.

Filtrate   The combined substance of water and dissolved solutes involved in urine formation.

Filtration   A process that contributes to urine formation; it involves filtrate moving out of each glomerulus into the renal corpuscle because of pressure differences across the filtration membrane.

First-pass effect   The immediate exposure of orally administered medications to metabolism by the liver enzymes before they reach the systemic circulation.

Flutter   Rapid, regular atrial contractions or rapid ventricular tachycardia.

Foramen magnum   The large hole in the occipital bone of the skull through which the medulla oblongata passes.

Foxglove plant   An herb with tubular pinkish purple flowers that is the source of the drug digitalis.

Fungi   The plural form of *fungus*.

G

Gag reflex   One that occurs in the back of the throat to prevent choking.

Gamma globulins   Blood proteins, which include the immunoglobulins; injections of gamma globulins are commonly given to boost a patient's immunity.

Gastric reflux   A condition wherein the relaxation of the gastroesophageal sphincter allows acidic stomach contents to enter the esophagus.

Gastritis   Inflammation of the lining of the stomach due to a variety of causes.

Gauge   The outside diameter of a needle; the gauge is a higher number for a smaller size needle; for example, a 20 gauge is smaller than a 14 gauge.

Gelcaps   Oil-based medications contained in soft gelatin capsules.

Genes   Units in a living organism that hold information to build and maintain cells and pass genetic traits to offspring.

Glial cells   Supporting cells in the CNS; also called neuroglia.

Gram-negative bacteria   Retaining a pink color from the Gram method of staining microorganisms.

Gram-positive bacteria   Retaining a violet color from the Gram method of staining microorganisms.

Granuloma   A ball-like formation of immune cells that occurs when the immune system is fighting off foreign substances that it cannot eliminate.

Gynecomastia   The development of enlarged mammary glands and breasts in a male patient.

H

Half-life   The time needed for a drug's effectiveness to decrease by 50%.

Helper T cells   Lymphocytes that direct or activate other immune cells; they have no cytotoxic or phagocytic ability of their own.

Hemagglutinin   A substance that causes red blood cells to agglutinate.

Hematomas   Collections of blood outside of the blood vessels; usually as a result of internal bleeding.

Hemoglobin (Hb)   The protein in red blood cells that contains iron and transports oxygen.

Hemophilia   A rare bleeding disorder that prevents the blood from clotting normally.

Hemoptysis   Coughing up blood or bloody sputum.

Hemostasis   A physiologic progression of three events that stops all but the most catastrophic bleeding in the body.

Heparin   A mucopolysaccharide found in many tissues but is most abundant in the lungs and liver; it is used medically as an anticoagulant.

Hepatic encephalopathy   A brain disorder caused by toxic substances that the liver cannot remove from the blood.

Hepatosplenomegaly   Enlargement of the liver and spleen.

Heredity   The passing of traits from a parent or ancestor to their offspring.

Hilt   The connection point of a needle's hub and syringe.

Hilum   The concave, medial border of each kidney where vessels, nerves, and the ureter connect to the kidney.

Histamine   A substance involved in allergic reactions that dilates blood vessels and makes the walls of the vessels excessively permeable.

Histoplasmosis   A fungal lung disease that commonly arises because of an inadequate immune system, caused by inhalation of a specific dust.

Homeostasis   The ability to maintain balance in the body by adjusting physiological processes.

Hub   The piece, usually plastic, that fits onto the syringe.

Hypercapnia   Excessive carbon dioxide in the blood.

Hyponatremia   An electrolyte disturbance in which plasma sodium is lower than normal.

Hypovolemia   A decrease in volume of blood plasma; it is commonly caused by dehydration, bleeding, vomiting, burns, and certain drugs.

Hypoxemia   A general decrease in blood oxygen pressure.

I

Immunoglobulin E (IgE) antibodies   Types of antibodies elicited by an allergic response; the *E* stands for erythema (redness).

Immunoglobulins   Antibodies found in the blood and body fluids that help to identify and neutralize foreign objects and substances.

Inactivated vaccine   One that contains virus particles killed by heat or chemicals.

Incubator   A device that maintains a constant, preset temperature.

Infants   Babies between age 29 days and approximately 1 year.

Inotropic   Affecting the force of muscle contraction.

Inspiration   Inhalation; the opposite of expiration (exhalation).

Internal respiration   The exchange of oxygen and carbon dioxide between the systemic capillaries and body tissues and cells.

Interstitial fluid   A solution that surrounds the cells in the interstitial (tissue) spaces of the body; it is the main component of extracellular fluid, including the plasma.

Ischemia   A restriction in blood supply that causes tissue damage.

J

Juxtaglomerular apparatus   A group of cells near each renal glomerulus that work together to regulate blood pressure.

Juxtaglomerular cells   Modified smooth muscle cells of the afferent arteriole.

K

Kernicterus   Brain damage in infants caused by increased levels of bilirubin.

L

Lancet   A double-edged, bladed medical instrument that is similar to a scalpel.

Lethargic   Fatigued, sluggish, or inactive.

Leukocytes   White blood cells; they defend the body against both infectious disease and foreign materials.

Leukotriene   A lipid compound related to the prostaglandins that mediates the body's inflammatory response.

Lipophilic   The ability of a chemical compound to dissolve in lipids, fats, or oils.

Loading dose   A first dose of a drug administered in excess of the maintenance dose to rapidly achieve therapeutic drug levels.

Lotion   A liquid suspension containing water and an oil that is intended to be patted onto the skin; must be shaken before use.

Lumen   The interior diameter of a needle.

M

Macrophages   White blood cells that ingest foreign material and are important for the body's immune response.

Major calyces   Kidney structures that collect urine from the minor calyces.

Manufacturing errors   Errors made during the creation or packaging of a drug product, including contamination, mislabeling, incorrect drug, incorrect concentration, or incorrect dose.

Mast cell stabilizers   Medications used for allergic conditions that stabilize mast calls and prevent the release of histamine and other substances.

Mast cells   Basophils that secrete histamine and heparin in response to allergies, inflammation, and to defend against pathogens.

Mediastinum   The central compartment of the thoracic cavity; it separates the right and left lungs and contains the heart.

Medication error   Anything that has the potential to cause harm to a patient or lead to incorrect use of a medication; these errors can be made by anyone in the healthcare profession, as well as by patients.

Medulla oblongata   The lower part of the brainstem, which controls vital visceral activities including respiration, heart rate, and blood pressure.

Metabolism   The conversion of a drug into another substance or substances.

Metabolites   Chemical products that result from metabolism.

Metric system   Internationally used system of measurement based on the decimal system; uses the number 10 as its basic unit.

Microfibrillar collagen   A substance that causes the aggregation of platelets and formation of clots during surgical procedures.

Midbrain   The mesencephalon; the portion of the brainstem that contains the centers for visual and auditory reflexes.

Milliliter   One one-thousandth of a liter; used to measure liquid volumes.

Minor calyces   Kidney structures that collect urine from the renal pyramids.

Mitral valve   The left atrioventricular valve, located between the left atrium and left ventricle.

Mucolytics   Drugs that dissolve thick mucus.

Muscarinic receptor   A cholinergic receptor that is more sensitive to muscarine than nicotine; muscarine is a parasympathomimetic substance that mimics the effects of acetylcholine.

Muscle cells   Those that comprise a muscle or muscular structure in the body.

Mycoplasma pneumonia   A type of bacterial pneumonia that has a long duration, lack of sputum production, and many extrapulmonary symptoms.

Myocardial infarction   A heart attack that is caused when the blood supply to the heart is reduced, resulting in the death of some heart cells.

Myocardium The muscular heart wall that forms the atria and ventricles.

N

Nasal flaring Widening of the nostrils on inspiration; a sign of respiratory distress.

Nasal septum The wall that divides the nasal cavity into right and left portions.

National Drug Code The American coding system for prescription drugs whereby each drug is individually identified down to its package size.

Natural killer (NK) cells Cytotoxic leukocytes that kill viruses and tumors; they release small protein granules that infiltrate target cells and kill them by causing various cell components to fragment.

Necrosis Premature death of living cells and tissue.

Needlesticks Injuries to the body by needle points or other sharp objects.

Neonates Babies who are 28 days of age or younger.

Nephron The functional filtration unit of a kidney; there are about 2.5 million nephrons in both kidneys combined.

Nephrotic syndrome A disorder in which the kidneys leak large amounts of protein from the blood into the urine.

Neuraminidase An enzyme found in the respiratory and intestinal tracts that removes sialic acid from mucoproteins.

Neurons Nerve cells capable of sending and receiving electrical impulses throughout the body; they are the basic structural and functional units of the nervous system.

Neurotransmitters Chemicals located and released in the brain that allow impulses to pass between nerve cells.

Nicotine The agent in tobacco that acts as a stimulant; nicotine is highly addictive.

Nicotinic receptor A cholinergic receptor that is more sensitive to nicotine than muscarine; nicotine is an alkaloid that has stimulating effects throughout the body.

Nomogram A numerical relationship chart used to calculate a child's body surface area by using his or her weight and height.

Norepinephrine (NE) The neurotransmitter secreted by most sympathetic postganglionic neurons.

O

Ointment Topical medications in either a water or oil base, with a greasy consistency.

Omission errors Errors involving the failure to administer a prescribed medication.

Ounces Units of mass that may be used to measure weight or volume. Ounces are used in both the apothecary and household systems, with slightly different equivalencies—a liquid ounce is equivalent to 2 tablespoons.

Oxygen sensor A device that measures the proportion of oxygen in a gas or liquid.

P

Parenteral A route of administration that involves the piercing of the skin or a mucous membrane.

Parietal pleura The serous membrane that forms part of the mediastinum and lines the inner thoracic cavity walls.

Passive immunity The transfer of active humoral immunity from one individual to another; it can occur naturally or artificially.

Pathogens Infectious agents that can cause disease or illness in a host.

Patient error Any error involving self-administration of medications; patient errors may occur because of lack of knowledge, confusion, similar drugs prescribed by different physicians, lack of instruction, and lack of drug regimen review.

Peptic ulcer An erosion of a part of the gastrointestinal tract, usually due to acidic conditions, which makes it extremely painful; most peptic ulcers are caused by the bacterium *Helicobacter pylori*.

Peripheral Located away from the center of the body.

Peripheral nervous system (PNS) The second of the two major divisions of the nervous system; it includes the cranial and spinal nerves.

Peristalsis The rhythmic movements of the intestines.

Phagocytic cells Those that engulf targeted cells to remove bacteria, cell debris, and other microorganisms.

Pharmacodynamics The study of drug effects on the body.

Pharmacokinetics The study of the body's effects upon a drug.

Pheochromocytoma A malignant tumor of the adrenal medulla characterized by hypersecretion of epinephrine and norepinephrine that causes persistent or intermittent hypertension.

Phosphodiesterase One of a group of enzymes that break phosphodiester (phosphorus and ester) bonds to increase amounts of calcium available for myocardial contraction.

Pill A round or oval single-dose medication made by mixing a powdered drug with a liquid (usually a syrup).

Placenta previa   An obstetric complication wherein the placenta attaches to the uterine wall and may partially or totally cover the cervix.

Plasma cells   White blood cells that produce large volumes of antibodies; they are transported by the blood plasma and the lymphatic system.

Platelet plug   A sticky mass of platelets that help to plug a torn blood vessel; platelet plug formation is the second event in the process of hemostasis.

Pleural effusion   Excess fluid that accumulates in the pleural cavity.

Pleurisy   Inflammation of the pleura, also called pleuritis, which is usually caused by other conditions, injuries, or a tumor.

Pneumoconiosis   An occupational lung disease caused by dust inhalation; types of pneumoconiosis include silicosis, anthracosis, asbestosis, and others.

Pneumonia   Lung inflammation with fluid accumulation in the alveoli and bronchioles.

Pneumothorax   A potential medical emergency wherein air or gas accumulates in the pleural cavity.

Pons   The part of the brainstem situated above the medulla oblongata, which also aids in control of the respiratory centers.

Postural hypotension   Also known as orthostatic hypotension; it is defined as a decrease in blood pressure when a person stands up.

Potency   An amount of a drug required to produce a particular response.

Prescribing errors   Errors made when medications are prescribed by physicians and other licensed healthcare practitioners.

Primary hyperaldosteronism   A condition wherein the adrenal gland releases too much aldosterone; most commonly caused by a benign adrenal tumor.

Prolapse   To flop backwards, as in mitral valve prolapse. In this condition, the thin mitral valve structures flop backwards into the left atrium, sometimes allowing blood leakage.

Prophylaxis   Prevention; commonly referred to as preventing disease.

Prototype   The first, or primitive, form of a drug to which subsequent versions of the drug conform.

Protozoa   Unicellular parasites that ingest food.

Pulmonary edema   Fluid accumulation in the lungs.

Pulmonary emboli   Obstructions of blood vessels in the lungs, usually due to blood clots.

Pulmonary embolism   A condition wherein an object causes a blockage (or occlusion) of a pulmonary vessel.

Pulmonary fibrosis   An interstitial lung disease wherein excess fibrous tissue forms in the lungs and surrounding structures.

Pulmonary hypertension   Increase in blood pressure in the pulmonary vessels.

Pulmonary valve   The heart valve that allows blood to flow from the right ventricle while preventing backflow into the ventricle.

R

Radiant warmer   A warming device that resembles a baby cradle; provides consistent heat to the body of a pediatric patient.

Rebound congestion   A condition caused by use of decongestants for more than 3 consecutive days wherein the nasal mucosa swells and blocks the nasal passageways; if additional decongestant is administered, the mucosa starts to become addicted and needs the decongestant to temporarily remain open.

Receptor   The site (either on a cell surface or inside a cell) that binds with a specific substance or drug.

Reconstitute   To restore a powdered or concentrated liquid medication to its proper strength by adding water or another liquid.

Reflex tachycardia   Accelerated heart rate in response to a stimulus conveyed through the cardiac nerves.

Renal columns   Extensions of the renal cortex that allow it to be anchored with more strength.

Renal cortex   The outer portion of each kidney; between the renal capsule and renal medulla.

Renal medulla   The innermost portion of each kidney; it is divided into sections known as renal pyramids.

Renal papilla   The part of the kidney where the pyramids empty urine into the renal pelvis.

Renal pelvis   The funnel-shaped, dilated kidney structure that transports urine into the ureter.

Renal pyramids   Cone-shaped kidney tissues; between 8 and 18 of these pyramids make up each kidney.

Renal sinus   An internal space within each kidney that contains the renal pelvis, calyces, blood vessels, nerves, and fat.

Renin   An enzyme produced in the kidneys that facilitates the conversion of angiotensinogen to angiotensin I. Because angiotensin I and its metabolite, angiotensin II, cause blood vessels to constrict, renin plays a major role in controlling blood pressure.

Respiration   The processes of breathing in the respiratory system.

Respiratory acidosis   Increased concentration of acid in the blood caused by the retention of carbon dioxide due to inadequate pulmonary ventilation.

Respiratory failure   The inability to maintain an adequate exchange of oxygen and carbon dioxide in the lungs.

S

Sepsis   An inflammatory state that affects the entire body.

Septicemia   The presence of bacteria in the blood (bacteremia), often associated with severe infections.

Septum   One of the heart's wall-like structures that separates the right and left atrium, as well as the right and left ventricle.

Serotonin   A neurotransmitter that causes vascular spasms, the first step in hemostasis.

Shaft   The main body of a needle, usually made of stainless steel.

Sickle cell anemia   A red blood cell disorder that causes the cells to assume an elongated sickle shape; it shortens life expectancy, primarily in African Americans.

Side effects   Unintended effects of a drug.

Silicosis   A form of pneumoconiosis caused by the inhalation of silica dust.

Sinus node   The sinoatrial node; it generates the regular electric impulses of the heartbeat.

Solution   A liquid mixture of one or more drugs in an appropriate solvent.

Spores   Forms that some bacteria assume to increase their chances of surviving heat, dehydration, antiseptics, or antibiotics; when the bacteria are no longer threatened, they revert to their normal state and continue to live and reproduce.

Stable angina   Also called classic angina; this type may be caused by atherosclerosis or increased physical exertion and is the most common form.

Standing orders   Ongoing prescription orders used in certain care settings.

Stenosis   Abnormal narrowing of a blood vessel or other structure.

Sterility   Free of living bacteria or other microorganisms.

Stevens-Johnson syndrome   A serious, sometimes fatal inflammatory disease that affects children and young adults.

Stillbirth   The death of a baby in the womb after the 20th week of pregnancy.

Stridor   A high-pitched sound caused by turbulent airflow in the upper parts of the respiratory system.

Stroke volume   The volume of blood pumped from one ventricle of the heart with each heartbeat.

Surfactant   A combination of lipids and proteins that lines the alveoli and smallest bronchioles; it reduces surface tension throughout the lung.

Sustained release   Designed to be released into the body over an extended period of time.

Sympathetic   Increasing heart rate, force, and oxygen use; related to the actions of the sympathetic nervous system.

Sympathetic division   The part of the nervous system that adapts the body for many types of physical activity; also known as the thoracolumbar division.

Sympathetic nerves   Those that are part of the sympathetic nervous system; they oppose the effects of nerves in the parasympathetic nervous system.

Sympathomimetic   An agent that produces effects similar to those of impulses of the sympathetic nervous system.

Synapses   Functional connections between neurons or between neurons and other types of cells; most synapses connect axons to dendrites.

Systole   Contraction of a heart chamber.

Systolic heart failure   Heart failure due to a defect in the expulsion of blood, caused by abnormal systolic function.

T

T lymphocytes   White blood cells that play a central role in cell-mediated immunity; they have special T-cell receptors on their surfaces.

Tablets   Compressed powdered drugs, which are usually formed into cylindrical shapes that may or may not be specially coated.

Tachyarrhythmias   Heart rhythm disturbances that result in a heartbeat of more than 100 beats per minute.

Tachycardia   Abnormally fast heartbeat.

Thalamus   Part of the diencephalon that relays sensory impulses from parts of the nervous system to the cerebral cortex.

Therapeutic duplication   A situation wherein a medication is prescribed that the patient is already receiving, even if it is not exactly the same medication, increasing the chance for a medication error to occur.

Therapeutic effects   Those with the ability to heal or to improve a patient's health condition.

Therapeutic index   The relationship of the effective dose 50% to the lethal dose 50%.

Thrombocytopenia   A persistent decrease in the amount of platelets in the blood.

Thromboembolism   Formation of a clot (thrombus) in a blood vessel that breaks off and is carried to another blood vessel.

Thrombus   A blood clot that forms in the cardiovascular system.

Thymus gland   An organ located in the upper chest cavity just under the sternum; it is one of the two primary lymphoid tissues in the body.

Thyroid cartilage   The type that forms most of the anterior and lateral laryngeal walls.

Toddlers   Babies between 1 and 3 years of age.

Tourniquets   Devices that constrict or compress body parts to slow blood circulation to a specific area of the body.

Toxoid vaccine   One that contains inactivated toxic compounds that otherwise are able to cause disease.

Tracheostomy   A surgical operation to make a semipermanent or permanent opening in the trachea, allowing the patient to breathe.

Tracheotomy   The emergency procedure of cutting into the trachea to create an alternate airway for breathing.

Trichomoniasis   Any infection via a species of *Trichomonas*; certain species may infect the intestines or mouth, but this term is most commonly used in reference to genitourinary infections.

Tricuspid valve   The right atrioventricular valve, located between the right atrium and right ventricle.

Tuberculosis   An infectious bacteriological disease that initially affects the respiratory system but may attack other body systems and potentially cause death.

Tubular fluid   The fluid in the kidney tubules; it begins as renal ultrafiltrate and ends up as urine.

Tubular reabsorption   The flow of glomerular filtrate from the proximal tubule of each nephron into the peritubular capillaries.

Tubular secretion   The transfer of materials from the peritubular capillaries to the renal tubular lumen, mainly by active transport.

U

Unit   A quantity expressed in terms of similar quantities. In medicine, units are commonly used to measure quantities of vitamins, aspirin, and other substances.

Unit–dose   The amount of medication to be administered to a patient in a single dose.

Universal precautions   The actions taken to avoid contact with a patient's bodily fluids by wearing personal protective clothing and equipment.

Unstable angina   A form of angina that occurs during resting or sleeping that is caused by severely decreased coronary blood flow.

Ureters   Tubes that conduct urine from the kidneys to the urinary bladder.

Urethra   The tube that conducts urine from the urinary bladder to the outside of the body.

Urinary bladder   The sac that expands to contain urine prior to urination.

Urine   Liquid waste; normally clear with an amber color.

Urticaria   Hives; raised, red, and sometimes itchy welts on the skin.

V

Vagal   Related to the actions of the vagus nerve, which is primarily responsible for the nerve supply of the viscera.

Vaporize   The conversion of a substance from a liquid to a gaseous state.

Variant angina   A rare form of angina caused by sudden coronary artery spasms that can induce ischemia and lead to sudden death.

Vasodilation   Dilation of blood vessels.

Vasospasms   Spasms of the blood vessels.

Ventricular asystole   No electrical activity in the heart's ventricles. Asystole is also known as flatline or flatlining, meaning that the patient may be considered dead due to no electrical activity in the heart.

Ventricular fibrillation   Uncontrolled contraction of the ventricles of the heart.

Viruses   The smallest microorganisms; they are not visible with ordinary microscopes. Viruses do not exist as cells; they are composed only of a single strand of nucleic acid with an enveloping protein sheath.

Visceral pleura   A layer of serous membrane that covers the surface of each lung; also known as the pulmonary pleura.

Index

Barbiturates, 222, 227
Beclomethasone, 154
Benazepril, 115
Benzodiazepines, 220–223, 227
Benzonatate, 167
Berylliosis, 30
Beta-adrenergic agonists, for asthma, 151–152, 190
Beta-adrenergic blockers
    for angina pectoris, 98–100
    for arrhythmias, 105–108
    for heart failure, 124, 125
    for hypertension, 116–117
Beta-blockers, list of generic/trade, 244
Beta-lactam antibiotics, 174
Beta$_1$ and beta$_2$ agonists, 235, 236–237
Beta receptor antagonists, 237–238
Betaxolol, 117
Bethanechol, 238
Bevel, 69
Bioavailability, 55, 106
Biopharmaceutical agents, 38
Biotransformation, 57
Bipolar depression, 223–225
Bisoprolol, 117, 125
Blepharitis, 177
Blood-brain barrier, 56
Blood clotting, 140, 141
Blood pressure, 8
    classification and regulation of, 114
Blood supply to the heart, 6–7
Blood vessels, 7–8
Body surface area, calculating dosage based on, 85–86
Bone marrow, 196
Boosters, 203
Bradyarrhythmias, 104
Bradycardia, 100
Bradykinin, 115
Brain, cross-section and parts of, 12, 14–15, 218–219
Brainstem, 14, 219
Breathing mechanism and control, 10, 12
Bretylium, 105
Broad-spectrum antibacterial drugs, 177
Bronchial tree, 9–10
Bronchiectasis, 27, 28
Bronchiolectasis, 28
Bronchiolitis, 27
    acute, in infants, 189
Bronchitis, 26–27
Bronchodilators, 150–153, 244
Bronchogenic carcinoma, 31
Budesonide, 154, 155
Bumetanide, 133
Bupropion, 162, 163, 224, 225
Buspirone, 220, 221

C

Calcium channel blockers
    for angina pectoris, 98, 100
    for arrhythmias, 105, 106, 109–110
    for hypertension, 118
    list of generic/trade, 244
Cancer, lung, 31
Candesartan, 115, 124

Candidemia, 181
Capillaries, 8, 68
Caplets, 62
Capreomycin, 184
Capsules, 61
Captopril, 115
Carbachol, 238
Carbaminohemoglobin, 13
Carbenicillin, 175
Carbonic anhydrase, 13
Carbonic anhydrase inhibitors, 135–136
Carcinogens, 31
Cardiac arrest, 25
Cardiac cycle, 8
Cardiac glycosides, 124
Cardiac veins, 6
Cardiomyopathy, 24–25
Cardiotonic action, 124
Cardiovascular disorders
    angina pectoris, 23
    cardiac arrest, 25
    cardiomyopathy, 24–25
    carditis, 25
    coronary artery disease, 23
    dysrhythmias, 24
    heart failure, 25
    hypertension, 24
    myocardial infarction, 23–24
Cardiovascular system
    effects of smoking on, 159
    organs and role of, 4–8
Cardioversion, 110
Carditis, 25
Carvedilol, 117, 124, 125
Caspofungin, 181
Catecholamines, 108, 235
Cefazolin, 176
Cell-mediated immunity, 197, 198
Cells, 196
Central alpha$_2$-adrenergic agonists, 117–118
Central nervous system (CNS)
    brain, 14–15, 218–219
    effects of drugs on, 217–229
    spinal cord, 15, 219
Cephalosporins, 175–176
Cerebellum, 14–15, 219
Cerebrospinal fluid (CSF), 15
Cerebrum, 14, 218–219
Cesarean section, 189
Cetirizine, 169
Cevimeline, 238
Cherry bark, wild, 168
Chickenpox, 201
Children. See Immunization; Pediatrics; Vaccines
Chloramphenicol, 179–180
Chloroquine, 182
Chlorothiazide, 133, 134
Chlorpheniramine-hydrocodone, 167
Chlorthalidone, 133, 134
Cholinergic agonists, 238
Cholinergic antagonists, 238–239
Cholinergic fiber, 234
Cholinergic receptor, 234

Photo Credits

Chapter 5

5–1 © Mitar/ShutterStock, Inc.; **5–2** © Kesu/Shutter-Stock, Inc.; **5–4** © Juriah Mosin/Dreamstime.com

Chapter 6

6–4 © spfotocz/ShutterStock, Inc.; **6–5** © Bomshtein/ShutterStock, Inc.; **6–6 (top)** © Attila Németh/Dreamstime.com; **6–6 (bottom)** © Etiamos/Dreamstime.com; **6–10** © Tomasz Trojanowski/ShutterStock, Inc.; **6–14 (left)** © Jones and Bartlett Publishers. Courtesy of MIEMSS.; **6–14 (middle)** © Olga D. Van De Veer/Dreamstime.com; **6–14 (right)** © M. Dykstra/ShutterStock, Inc.

Chapter 7

7–2 (left) © Kimberly Hall/ShutterStock, Inc.; **7–2 (middle)** © Vladir09/Dreamstime.com; **7–2 (right)** © Keki/Dreamstime.com; **7–3** Reproduced from W. M. Boothby and R. B. Sandiford, Nomographic charts for the calculation of the metabolic rate by the gasomer method, *Boston Medical and Surgical Journal* 185 (1921): p. 337.

Chapter 15

15–1 (left) © Ann Baldwin/ShutterStock, Inc.; **15–1 (middle)** © David Davis/Dreamstime.com; **15–1 (right)** © Jones and Bartlett Publishers. Courtesy of MIEMSS

Chapter 18

18–1 (top left) Courtesy of Janice Haney Carr/CDC; **18–1 (top right)** Courtesy of Janice Haney Carr/CDC; **18–1 (middle left)** Courtesy of Janice Haney Carr/CDC; **18–1 (middle right)** Courtesy of Janice Haney Carr/CDC; **18–1 (bottom)** Courtesy of Bill Schwartz/CDC